T0291596

Female Circumcision and
Clitoridectomy in the United States

Rochester Studies in Medical History

Senior Editor: Theodore M. Brown
Professor of History and Preventive Medicine
University of Rochester

Additional Titles of Interest

Communities and Health Care: The Rochester, New York, Experiment
Sarah F. Liebschutz

The Neurological Patient in History
Edited by L. Stephen Jacyna and Stephen T. Casper

The Birth Control Clinic in a Marketplace World
Rose Holz

Bacteriology in British India: Laboratory Medicine and the Tropics
Pratik Chakrabarti

Barefoot Doctors and Western Medicine in China
Xiaoping Fang

Beriberi in Modern Japan: The Making of a National Disease
Alexander R. Bay

The Lobotomy Letters
Mical Raz

Plague and Public Health in Early Modern Seville
Kristy Wilson Bowers

Medicine and the Workhouse
Edited by Jonathan Reinarz and Leonard Schwarz

Stress, Shock, and Adaptation in the Twentieth Century
Edited by David Cantor and Edmund Ramsden

A complete list of titles in the Rochester Studies in Medical History series
may be found on our website, www.urpress.com.

Female Circumcision and Clitoridectomy in the United States

A History of a Medical Treatment

SARAH B. RODRIGUEZ

UNIVERSITY OF ROCHESTER PRESS

ed 2014
n paperback 2024

f Rochester Press
e Avenue, Rochester, NY 14620, USA
.com
& Brewer Limited
Voodbridge, Suffolk IP12 3DF, UK
andbrewer.com

3-1-58046-498-7 (hardcover)
3-1-64825-095-8 (paperback)
2715

ongress Cataloging-in-Publication Data

Sarah B., author.
rcumcision and clitoridectomy in the United States : a history of a
tment / Sarah B. Rodriguez.
— (Rochester studies in medical history, ISSN 1526-2715 ; v. 29)
bibliographical references and index.
1-58046-498-7 (hardcover : alk. paper)
 Series: Rochester studies in medical history. 1526–2715
1. Circumcision, Female—history—United States. 2. Clitoris—
ited States. 3. History, 19th Century—United States. 4. History, 20th
nited States. 5. Sexual Behavior—United States. 6. Sexuality—history—
s. WP 11 AA1]

9–dc23

                                                    2014016212

record for this title is available from the British Library.

to Javier & Pilar

Contents

Acknowledgments

As with any project years in the making, I have many people to thank, and my sincerest apologies if time has clouded my memory and I neglect someone. My on-again, off-again interest in the history of female circumcision and clitoridectomy in the United States began when I was an undergraduate at the University of Iowa, so I first want to thank Susan Lawrence. I am grateful for what I learned while in the history of science and medicine program at the University of Wisconsin–Madison, in particular from Judith Walzer Leavitt, and for the support I received from Toby Schonfeld, Patricia Leuschen, and Andrew Jameton at the University of Nebraska Medical Center, and from JoAnn Carrigan and Sharon Wood at the University of Nebraska at Omaha.

I thank Rose Holz for listening to me over lunches as I sorted out my ideas for an article that eventually appeared in the *Journal of the History of Medicine and Allied Sciences*. Though for a time after writing that article I thought I was finished with the history of female circumcision and clitoridectomy in the United States as medical therapy, I thank Lisa Campo-Engelstein for listening to me and reading various book proposals. During the process of researching and writing this book, I have had support and encouragement from many colleagues, in particular in the Medical Humanities and Bioethics Program at Northwestern University, especially from Tod Chambers and Alice Dreger. Alice has been a model and generous mentor who, in addition to listening to me work out my framing of this history, also read and edited a (nearly) final draft of this book. Thank you to Elizabeth Reis for suggesting I look more into gynecology books for information about clitoral surgeries and to Joseph Pincus for his thoughts on the use of medical textbooks as sources of clinical knowledge and acceptance. I further want to thank those who gave me feedback on various aspects of what became this book following talks at meetings of the American Association for the History of Medicine and at the American Society for Bioethics and Humanities and for comments following talks I gave at the University of Michigan at Dearborn, Grinnell College, the Wisconsin Medical College, and the University of Wisconsin–Madison. I am grateful for the comments I received from my students in the class I taught at Northwestern in the fall of 2011 regarding female circumcision and clitoridectomy globally. I thank Judy Leavitt for handing Ted Brown my proposal for this book. I thank the University of Rochester Press, in particular Ted for his encouragement and sympathetic understanding of deadlines, Sonia Kane and Julia Cook for helping me navigate the process, Ryan Peterson and Carrie Watterson for their precise editing work, Tracey Engel for her help with production, and Dave Prout for indexing this book. I also wish to thank the anonymous reviewers of the manuscript; I found their comments and suggestions quite useful and I appreciate the time and care they took in making them.

The Northwestern University Research Grants Committee has provided partial support for the publication of this book. I gratefully acknowledge this assistance. My research at the Kinsey Institute at Indiana University, my examination of the clitoris in anatomy texts, and some of the work I did concerning James Burt was supported by a generous grant from the Sexualities Project at Northwestern University. In addition to this grant, I am also appreciative of the comments I received from the anonymous reviewers who read my grant proposal. The findings and conclusions within this book are mine and do not necessarily reflect those of the Sexualities Project at Northwestern University.

I also want to acknowledge all of the librarians who assisted me in locating documents over the years. I could not have written this book without the help of the interlibrary loan departments at the University of Iowa, the University of Nebraska–Lincoln, the University of Nebraska Medical Center, and Northwestern University. I especially want to thank two librarians at Northwestern University's Galter Health Sciences Library, LaShanda Howard Curry in interlibrary loan (whose ability to retrieve everything I requested was amazing) and Ron Sims. I am grateful for the help of the librarians in Charles Deering McCormick Library of Special Collections for helping me discover the feminist health publications in their collection and for the help I received from the Pritzker Law Library reference librarians. Thank you to Shawn Wilson at the Kinsey Institute for his help with information about Kinsey and for help finding information about James Burt in that collection. In addition, I want to thank the librarians at the American Academy of Pediatrics, the University of Chicago Libraries, and the University of California, San Francisco, Archives and Special Collections. I am also appreciative of the help I received from the clerk of court of the Supreme Court of Ohio as well as from the librarians at the Dayton Metro Library and for the responses I received from several Ohio librarians (including those from Wright State University and the Ohio Historical Library) following a listserv query regarding collections that have information about James Burt.

Parts of chapters 1 and 4 originally appeared as "Rethinking the History of Female Circumcision and Clitoridectomy: American Medicine and Female Sexuality in the Late Nineteenth Century," *Journal of the History of Medicine and Allied Sciences* 63, no. 3 (2008): 323–47; and parts of chapter 7 appeared as "Female Sexuality and Consent in Public Discourse: James

Burt's 'Love Surgery,'" *Archives of Sexual Behavior* 42, no. 3 (2013): 343–51. I thank Oxford University Press and Springer Science+Business Media for permission to reproduce this material.

Finally, I am thankful to my nonacademic friends who have listened to me talk about my project over the years and to the caretakers who have tended to my children thus enabling me to work on this project. Thank you to my mother, Anne Webber, for reading a final draft of this book, and to both my mother and my father, Ivan Webber, for their unwavering support of their daughter's research into parts of the female body that often do not come up in typical conversation. And finally to my husband Pablo, who enjoyed bringing up his wife's research during typical conversation. I dedicate this book to our children, Javier and Pilar—though this project was my first child (and one that spent way too long in gestation), I love you both much more.

Introduction

Rethinking the History of Female Circumcision and Clitoridectomy in the United States

The history of the clitoris is part of the history of sexual difference generally and of the socialization of the body's pleasures . . . it is a story as much about socialization as about sex.

—Thomas Laqueur

In August 2012, Reuters carried a story entitled "Gynecologists Alarmed by Plastic Surgery Spread." The story concerned several surgeons across the United States performing gynecological surgery meant to enhance or enable women's sexual response. The surgeries, known collectively as female genital cosmetic surgery, include vaginal tightening, a reduction or removal of labia, and female circumcision. Women seeking to learn more about the surgeries, the article reported, run the gamut of ages, from teenagers to those in their late seventies. These women's interests in the surgeries, critics claim, are driven by impossible bodily ideals, ideals encouraged by the availability of pornography and marketing by physicians performing the surgeries.[1]

Though exact numbers of women who have undergone one or all of these surgeries are unavailable, their notoriety and increasing availability in certain parts of the United States has grown. Indeed, as I write this in the winter of 2014 from my office at Northwestern University's medical school in downtown Chicago, I know that if I went outside, walked west on Chicago Avenue, turned right on Michigan Avenue, and walked a few more blocks, I would be at the Watertower Building, where Otto J. Placik, a plastic surgeon, performs female circumcision (though he calls it "clitoral unhooding") for $1,000 plus operating room and anesthesia fees.[2] Placik is just one of many physicians who perform female genital cosmetic surgeries now in the United States and abroad; indeed, so many are now performing them that several international conferences have been established to, as the International Society of Cosmetogynecology says, "promote the advancement of knowledge, skill and excellence in female cosmetic medicine and surgery through education, training and fellowship."[3]

Both the popular media and academics have weighed in on what the rise in these surgeries means about the female body, female sexuality, and the role of medicine.[4] Activists have protested outside of clinics where physicians perform these surgeries, and though to a less dramatic extent, the American College of Obstetrics and Gynecology (ACOG) also protested them when in 2007 the college recommended practitioners not perform the surgeries since their safety and efficacy were unknown.[5] According to ACOG, the promotion of female genital cosmetic surgeries as sexually enhancing was not based on empirical evidence, nor were the surgeries considered clinically routine or medically indicated, all of which made them "untenable."[6]

Feminists and physicians are understandably concerned about these surgeries, and a look at a recent outcomes study illustrates more reason for concern. Despite (and in response to) ACOG's opposition, in late 2010 a dozen physicians published evidence of the sexual benefits of female genital cosmetic surgeries. A 2010 *Journal of Sexual Medicine* article claimed to provide evidence to support the surgeries' safety and efficacy in enhancing sexual experience. Of the 258 women who responded to a retrospective questionnaire, 91.6 percent indicated they were satisfied with the results of their surgery. The first question on the survey asked the women their initial reason for seeking surgery, with the first response option "to look better 'down there,'" a phrase the survey used to refer to women's genitalia. Moreover, satisfaction was measured not just by sexual enhancement for the women respondents but also by how the women perceived the satisfaction of their (presumably) male partners.[7] While the authors noted the existence of a natural diversity of how women look "down there," these physicians implicitly presented a very narrow range of what normal female genitals really look like, as well as a belief that the normality of female genitals includes a sexual function defined not solely (or even perhaps primarily) by the possessor of these genitals, but by her (assumed) male partner.

While medical practitioners and nonpractitioners have roundly criticized these surgeries, some physicians, even those who do not perform female genital cosmetic surgeries, see them as part of the future of plastic surgery.[8] Yet people tend to assume these surgeries are somehow new. In fact there is a long history of vulvar surgeries—especially surgeries on the clitoris—as "sexual enhancement" surgeries for women, designed to help them achieve their "proper role" as sexual partners. Indeed, these surgeries go back more than a hundred years. This book traces that history.

While some may be aware physicians removed the hood of the clitoris (circumcision) or the entire clitoris (clitoridectomy) in the late nineteenth and early twentieth centuries to cure women and girls of masturbation, masturbation was not the only sexual disorder doctors treated through clitoral surgery during this time, and circumcision and clitoridectomy were not the only operations on the clitoris physicians performed to treat sexual disorders. Since the second half of the nineteenth century, doctors have also removed smegma (material secreted from the glans of the foreskin and the labia minora) and separated adhesions (abnormal bands that bound the clitoris to its hood) between the clitoral hood and the clitoris, and they performed these clitoral surgeries along with female circumcision not just as therapies for masturbation but also for a lack of sexual response in the marital bed. Physicians' approach to clitoral surgery, at least as revealed in published medical works, has often been a cautious one that respected the importance of clitoral stimulation for healthy sexuality while simultaneously recognizing its role as cause and symptom in cases of medically, and socially, perceived unhealthy sexual expression.

My examination of these four clitoral surgeries (I am using this term broadly to simplify discussion) beginning in the second half of the nineteenth century and extending to the early twenty-first century illustrates doctors' knowledge of the organ and its role in female sexual pleasure, although what doctors regarded as a healthy organ and healthy sexual behavior were narrowly defined. Over the course of the last 150 years, physicians performed—and some women, their spouses, and parents of girls sought out—clitoral surgeries to maintain or conform to the sexual behavior deemed culturally appropriate for women. These procedures mirror medical and cultural beliefs about appropriate female sexual behavior, and these beliefs are embodied in medical ideas regarding the clitoris. Whether the operations were performed to curb the act of masturbation (a solitary sexual act and therefore not procreative) or to more easily produce an orgasm from a woman having sexual relations with her husband (promoting sexual harmony between spouses) or to curb a woman's hypersexuality or sexual attraction to other women ("masculine" traits), each occurred with the underlying goal of directing female sexual behavior to married, heterosexual, vaginal intercourse.

In tracing this out, we learn a lot more than the origins of modern female genital cosmetic surgeries. We learn that each generation of feminists and doctors seems almost to rediscover the clitoris as a sexually important organ. We also learn that a lot of people have paid a lot of attention to the clitoris and that women were active participants in surgeries designed to normalize them into a particular heterosexual ideal. We learn that what might have been a somewhat offhand remark by Sigmund Freud ended up in a major dispute as well as in many women getting the message that they were sexually deviant or immature. And we learn how vulnerable women have been in the face of a combination of heterosexist culture combined with doctors who think surgical quick fixes are prowoman.

I am by no means the first to examine the history of female circumcision and clitoridectomy in the United States. Indeed, more than fifty years ago, the historian John Duffy looked at the use of clitoridectomy to cure masturbation in the nineteenth century. But Duffy, like other historians after him, often confused clitoridectomy, the removal of the organ, with another one of the procedures. For example, in the case he cites toward the end of his article, Duffy noted how a physician "liberated" the clitoris.[9] Liberation, however, was not necessarily removal; here the physician could have meant removing the hood, or, perhaps more likely, breaking up the adhesions between the clitoris and the hood.

In addition to Duffy, other historians have made—largely cursory—mention of clitoral surgeries in the United States, though most often in a context of (male) medicine's hostility to female bodies.[10] Feminist scholars, too, at times (briefly) brought forth clitoridectomy and female circumcision as examples of misogynistic medicine.[11] My interest here, though, is to not only correct older misreadings of clitoral surgeries and move beyond simplistic histories that view the procedures as examples of misogynistic medicine, but also to consider the surgeries as an indication of doctors' understanding of the clitoris and female sexuality since the second half of the nineteenth century. By doing so I am adding to the modest amount of work conducted by others on the history of the clitoris.[12] For all that I agree (and disagree) with these histories, what is missing is an exploration of doctors' understanding of the clitoris and its sexual function and how some physicians redirected female sexual behavior by surgically altering the organ they understood to be responsible for healthy sexual response. Though at least one casual observer of female circumcision and clitoridectomy considered these procedures "isolated oddit[ies]," by reexamining their history and placing them in the context of the medical and popular understandings of the clitoris and of female sexual arousal, I seek to show how we should in fact view their occurrence in the United States as neither isolated nor odd.[13]

The Clitoris, Female Sexuality, and American Medicine

During the 150 years I cover here, women's sexual behavior outside the confines of married heterosexual intercourse was widely regarded as deviant, abnormal, and unhealthy, particularly for women who were white, native born, and middle to upper class. When presented with women labeled as sexually abnormal, some doctors observed the physical state of the clitoris and sometimes surgically changed the organ to help a woman respond more appropriately. Doctors related abnormal sexual behavior, whether it was masturbation or lack of orgasm during marital intercourse, to the state of the clitoris. This, then, implies that there was a medical understanding of what constituted a normative and healthy clitoris.

To frame the history of female circumcision and clitoridectomy in the United States as therapy for various forms of errant female sexual expression, it is essential to understand what standard medical knowledge of the clitoris entailed. Medical ideas about the clitoris have been fairly consistent since the late nineteenth century in two sources where one would expect to find information about the organ: anatomy and gynecology texts. In these texts, the clitoris has, since the late nineteenth century, often been regarded both implicitly and explicitly as a sexual organ.[14] While I realize not all physicians would have agreed with these texts and that there was then (as today) a difference between textbook-recommended practice and actual clinical practice, I am using these texts as a proxy for accepted medical understanding of the clitoris.[15]

Anatomy as a discipline is primarily concerned with how the body is constituted and with the participation between structures, not just the structures themselves. Clinicians used anatomy texts or atlases (the latter concentrate more on visual than verbal representations of anatomy) to verify anatomical information relevant to clinical questions.[16] Like anatomy texts, gynecology texts were used in a similar manner—to confirm information relevant to clinical questions. A physician may have consulted an anatomy text when presented with a consideration of the clitoris and its condition. Or because he (more rarely she) was treating a woman, an attending physician may have consulted a gynecology text when considering therapeutic interventions upon the female body. Both texts, though, reflected accepted ideas about the female body, including the clitoris, and even if a physician never consulted one of these medical texts, the information within them should be regarded as standard.[17]

The pioneer in anatomical representations of the clitoris as a sexual organ was Georg Kobelt. As historian Thomas Laqueur argued, once Kobelt published in 1844 his "massively documented" book, *The Male and Female Organs of Sexual Arousal in Man and Some Other Mammals*, "the anatomy of genital pleasure was firmly established." In this work, Kobelt concluded that the clitoris is the primary location of sexual arousal in women. He reached his conclusions by studying the organ's structure, noting the erectile tissues and blood and nerve supply. His drawings of the clitoris are intensely detailed. But though his book provided the most detail regarding the clitoris ever to be published to date, it did not, according to Laqueur, alter established views.[18] Kobelt's work may not have altered views regarding the organ, but it did illustrate those views.

Anatomy, as well as gynecology, texts published after Kobelt continued to refer to the clitoris, either implicitly or explicitly, as a sexual organ. Some scholars have argued that physicians and anatomists, in analogizing the clitoris to the penis, essentially read the female body as a lesser form of the male.[19]

While I do not disagree with this reading, there are additional ways to understand these texts. Though some texts explicitly labeled the clitoris as sexual, often information about the sexual nature of the clitoris was embedded within the textual references of the clitoris to the penis. As gynecologist Robert Latou Dickinson wrote in his 1949 *Atlas of Human Sex Anatomy*, the "general homology between the male and female genitalia" was "well known."[20]

References to the clitoris as homologous to the penis or as "comparable to the penis in the male," as Smout's 1962 *Basic Anatomy and Physiology* stated, were common in anatomy texts published during the twentieth century.[21] This comparison of the clitoris to the penis was typical, for doctors widely viewed the two organs as analogous.[22] For example, in the 1920 *Fundamentals of Human Anatomy*, the clitoris "corresponds to the penis in the male, on a diminutive scale."[23] A 1923 atlas described the clitoris as corresponding to the penis, but smaller, and the 1944 *A Method of Anatomy: Descriptive and Deductive* called the clitoris the "female penis," a description repeated in the 1948 and 1958 editions.[24] Texts published after the 1950s continued with this labeling; for example, a 1975 text described the clitoris as "homologous with the penis."[25] Like anatomy texts, gynecology texts also compared the clitoris to the penis: for example, the 1902 *Manual of Gynecology* described the clitoris as "analogous of the penis," a 1934 text labeled the clitoris "the homologue of the male penis," and the 1962 *Obstetrics and Gynaecology* described the clitoris as a "miniature" penis.[26]

This equation can be seen as a representation of the clitoris as a less significant organ, since anatomy texts compared the penis and the clitoris in only one direction.[27] But anatomy text authors acknowledged the two organs as homologous, and not just in origins, structure (save the urethra), and position, but also implicitly (I will discuss explicitly shortly) in sexual function by labeling the clitoris as a miniature penis, as equivalent to the penis, or most strikingly, as the female penis.[28] Anatomy texts were largely, though not exclusively, written by male physicians for largely, though again not entirely, men, as they dominated the practice of medicine through the 1970s. Male physicians, being male, possessed a penis, so the comparison of their organ to the corresponding female one may also be seen as indicating the importance of the clitoris to female sexual pleasure, by relying on the (assumed) reader's personal experience that the penis was the organ of male sexual pleasure. While the male body was the norm in anatomy texts and the female body was compared to the male body, such a comparison can also be read as giving an implicit equivalency between body parts—here the clitoris with the penis—and between both organs' sexual purpose.[29]

Anatomy and gynecology texts further implicitly called attention to the sexual purpose of the clitoris by noting it as sensitive and endowed with an ample amount of sensory nerve endings. For example, with the exception of the edition published in 1910, every American edition of Gray's *Anatomy* from 1859 through 1959 described the clitoris as highly or very sensitive.[30] Similarly, the 1954 *Basic Anatomy* described the clitoral glans as "highly sensitive," as did the 1960, 1963, 1969, and 1975 editions of *Anatomy: A Regional Study of Human Structure*.[31] Dawson's 1966 *Basic Human Anatomy* noted that the clitoris is "well supplied with sensory nerve endings" and the text *Synopsis of Gross Anatomy*, published the same year, also said the clitoris contains "abundant sensory nerve endings."[32] According to Dickinson in his 1949 *Human Sex Anatomy*, though the "female organ" is "minute compared with the male organ," the size and number of the clitoris's nerve endings is "demonstrably richer" than those in the penis; indeed, the clitoris, according to Dickinson, possesses perhaps "three to four times as large as the equivalent nerves of the penis."[33] Such descriptions also appeared in gynecology texts. A 1919 gynecology text, for example, labeled the clitoris as "well supplied with sensory nerves."[34] In addition, the 1934 *An Introduction to Gynecology* described the clitoris as "richly supplied with blood vessels and with nerves with special endings."[35] A 1959 text stated that the clitoral glans is "covered with mucous membrane containing many specialized nerve endings," and a 1977 text noted the clitoris is "generously supplied with nerve endings."[36] As a final example, a 1966 gynecology text described the organ as a "structure apart," having within it "special nerve endings which make the clitoris so sensitive."[37]

Further attesting to the implicit understanding of the clitoris as a sexual organ, many anatomy texts described the erectile tissue of the clitoris. For example, the 1939 *Anatomy and Physiology* stated that the clitoris is "composed of erectile tissue."[38] Additionally, the 1937 *Cunningham's Text-Book of Anatomy* described the glans of the clitoris as a "small mass of erectile tissue," as did the 1959 *Introduction to Human Anatomy*, while the 1975 *Essential Anatomy* called the clitoris "a small sensitive mass of erectile tissue."[39] Gynecology texts similarly described the clitoris as comprised of "erectile tissue" or having "erectile glans": an 1883 gynecology text described the clitoris as "erectile," the 1902 *Manual of Gynecology* labeled the clitoris "an erectile body analogous to the penis," the 1919 *Principles of Gynecology* described the clitoris as being "composed of erectile tissue," and in the 1934 *An Introduction to Gynecology* the clitoris contains "erectile tissue."[40]

These descriptions acknowledged the organ's capabilities for erection and engorgement, traits some anatomy and gynecology texts also included. For example, Morris's 1898 *Human Anatomy: A Compete Systematic Treatise* described the clitoris as "capable of erection."[41] Later, the 1960, 1963, 1969, and 1975 editions of *Anatomy: A Regional Study of Human Structure* all noted that the clitoris was "capable of enlargement as a result of engorgement with blood," and the 1978 *Human Anatomy* noted that the erectile tissue within the clitoris caused the organ "to become erected in response to erotic stimulation."[42] Descriptions of the organ's capability to become engorged appeared in gynecology texts as well: the 1870 *The Physiology of Woman and*

Her Disease from Infancy to Old Age noted that the clitoris is "capable of erection" and the 1883 *Diseases of Women* stated the clitoris "in its erect condition doubles its size."[43] Later texts reiterated this belief, as illustrated by a 1944 gynecology text describing the clitoris as a "small erectile organ richly supplied with blood and nerves" that, "during sexual excitement" fills "with blood and becomes swollen and firmer."[44]

Like this 1944 gynecology text, some anatomy and gynecology texts noted in their descriptions of the sensitivity, erectile tissue, and engorgement capabilities of the clitoris that the organ became erect in response to erotic stimulation, a description that explicitly defined the sexual purpose of the organ. To illustrate, the 1979 *Human Anatomy and Physiology* described the clitoris as "very sensitive to touch, becoming engorged with blood and erect when stimulated and contributing to the sexual arousal of the woman," and the 1967 *Structure of the Human Body* stated that the clitoris is "extremely sensitive to touch and in conditions of sexual excitement becomes filled with blood."[45] But such descriptions began prior to the 1960s: the 1939 *Anatomy and Physiology*, for example, called the clitoris "the organ of sensation of the female genitalia."[46] Like anatomy texts, gynecology texts also sometimes included information about the clitoris as a sexually sensitive organ before the 1960s. The 1870 *Physiology of Woman and Her Disease from Infancy to Old Age* described the clitoris as "endowed with intense erotic sensibility."[47] Doctors writing about the clitoris referred to it as the "principal seat of sexual orgasm in the female," as *May's Diseases of Women* did in 1890.[48] Such statements continued through the first part of the twentieth century: the 1934 *An Introduction to Gynecology* noted that "stimulation of the clitoris is supposed to induce" sexual excitement, and in the 1944 and 1953 editions of *Diseases of Women*, the authors asserted that the clitoris "is supposed to be the most sensitive of all the genital organs to sexual contact."[49] Likewise, the 1973 *Gynecology: Principles and Practice* stated that the "function of the clitoris seems to be that of a 'nerve-center' for coitus," repeating this statement in the 1979 edition.[50] *Principals of Gynaecology* in 1967 labeled the clitoris as "the most erotically sensitive part of the vulva."[51] And the clinician's edition of *My Body, My Health* stated that, "highly responsive to tactile sensations," the clitoris swells "with blood during sexual arousal and is a woman's primary orgasmic focus." The only "function of the clitoris is sexual responsiveness," this 1979 text concluded.[52]

Not all gynecology and anatomy text published since the late nineteenth century described the clitoris using this language. But while many anatomy and gynecology texts implicitly or explicitly acknowledged the sexual purpose of the clitoris by labeling it as homologous to the penis, erectile, and highly sensitive, this does not mean that these texts embraced the organ as enabling an independent female sexuality. Nor does it even mean that these texts, while acknowledging the organ's sexual purpose, did not also assert that the organ was not necessary for female sexual pleasure. In their 1977 *Synopsis of Gynecology*, for example, Daniel Beacham and Woodward Beacham noted that, during "sexual stimulation the clitoris fills with blood, becoming larger and firmer." But, they continued, though the organ is "richly supplied with nerves," it is not "essential for orgasm if the patient has developed a normal sexual reaction pattern."[53]

How, then, to understand this apparent contradiction: an acceptance of the sexual purpose of the clitoris and the belief that it was not essential for "normal" female orgasm? Beacham and Beacham's reasoning could have developed from the idea that "the nerve endings seen in the clitoris vary from patient to patient," according to the 1977 *Scientific Foundations of Obstetrics and Gynaecology*, meaning not every woman's clitoris is as sensitive as another's and that for some women the clitoris may not be the most sexually sensitive part of her body.[54] But Beacham and Beacham's belief that the clitoris is not necessary for female orgasm could also have stemmed from the continued regard of female heterosexuality as primarily vaginal. For while regarding the clitoris as the primary female sexual organ, they described clitoral stimulation in terms of vaginal intercourse.[55]

This continued focus on the vaginal model of sex, despite an understanding of the clitoris as the principal sexual organ for women, underscores the long-standing penetration bias in medical ideas about heterosexual sex. As Elisabeth Lloyd documented in her critique of twentieth-century studies of female sexual response, a male-centered penetration bias and background assumptions about female orgasm maintained ideas about the primacy of vaginal sex within these (supposedly) unbiased scientific studies. Lloyd examined the thirty-two studies conducted over the course of the twentieth century about female sexual response that included information on female orgasm frequency from intercourse, including studies by Robert Latou Dickinson in 1931, Alfred Kinsey et al. in 1953, and Shere Hite in 1976.[56] The majority of these studies took at face value women's reports of orgasm, not questioning, or even defining, what orgasm with intercourse meant. For example, did orgasm with intercourse count if the woman received manual stimulation of her clitoris before or during intercourse? As both Kinsey and Hite found, most women needed direct stimulation of the clitoris to reach orgasm, something most women did not receive from penetrative sex alone. Almost none of the studies, however, drew a distinction between assisted and unassisted orgasm during penetrative intercourse. Central to Lloyd's point was that the majority of these studies saw female sexual capacity through the lens of penetrative sex, a view Hite in 1976 called "backwards." Instead, Lloyd, echoing Hite, wrote that studies on female sexuality should examine "when and how women have orgasms first, and to view their sexuality in those terms."[57]

The studies, then, meant to uncover female sexual response, posited this response in terms contrary to how most women said they reached orgasm: not solely through penetration but through the stimulation of their clitoris. Though women may enjoy penetrative sex, vaginal intercourse alone rarely results in orgasm for women. Male heterosexual response, with its focus on penetration, however, was seen as normative. Thus the presumption was that women would follow this model, and studies on the sexual response of women were set up under the assumption that women did (or should) respond sexually like men and receive sexual stimulation from vaginal intercourse.[58]

Though seemingly paradoxical, surgical procedures on the clitoris helped maintain this belief in penetrative sex as normative heterosexual sex. Surgery on the clitoris, be it female circumcision, clitoridectomy, the removal of smegma, or the breaking up of clitoral adhesions, all underscored a medical understanding of the clitoris as sexual but in need of correction to maintain the primacy of the vaginal sex model. Through the use of these procedures, physicians sought to adapt the clitoris—and female orgasm—to fit the penetrative sex model. Physicians performed clitoral surgery by directing and, they believed, enabling female sexual response within this model.[59]

The History of Clitoral Surgery in the United States

The four procedures I explore here fit into a larger cultural history of the changing perceptions of female sexuality, medical ideas of the clitoris in female sexual fulfillment, and the enforcement of heterosexual married vaginal-penile sex—by both the women who sought the procedures and the doctors who performed them—as the only culturally and medically normal sexual behavior. In turn, I also argue that if we are to truly understand the history of female circumcision and clitoridectomy in the United States, this history must be one where the operations are seen as reflections of the larger history of medical and cultural ideas of what constitutes normal female sexual behavior.

Thus, these procedures can be seen as intricately woven into cultural and medical ideas regarding the clitoris and its relation to female sexual behavior: doctors viewed the clitoris as an important though at times unhealthy and unnecessary component of female sexuality. Physicians writing in medical publications that concerned female circumcision and clitoridectomy expressed a patriarchal concern with directing sexual behavior to what was considered normal (something that seems to have been a response to as well as a part of the changes in gender and sexual roles in society at large during the nineteenth and twentieth centuries) combined with a concern for the patient's health. The benefits of surgery were often seen not just by the physician but also by the patient's family or by the patient herself. While the bulk of my primary sources come from physicians, the patient's voice (or sometimes her parents') is often heard through these articles.[60] Unfortunately, the unfiltered voices of those whose clitorises were removed or reduced are largely unavailable until the late twentieth century (and they remain few and far between).

These surgeries were used primarily for three objectives: to stop masturbation, to enhance female capacity for orgasm within heterosexual vaginal intercourse, and to "correct" homosexuality or hypersexuality. I have framed this book around the purposes for the surgery, structuring a section around each reason for its use, and then weaving into this framework the medical and cultural ideas regarding healthy and appropriate female sexual behavior. By using this framework I hope to show that, far from being examples of misogyny or aberrations in medical practice, female circumcision and clitoridectomy were and remain intimately part of American culture.

In the first two chapters, I examine masturbation as the primary reason for the surgical treatment of the clitoris since the late nineteenth century. During this time, American physicians who removed all or part of a clitoris from a patient who obsessively manipulated it did so with the belief that they removed an unhealthy organ to prevent the further deterioration of their patient's health. Physicians who removed smegma or adhesions between the clitoris and its hood, removed the hood, or removed the entire organ, did so because they linked the ill health of their patients to a nervous irritability, the origin of which was an irritated, abnormal clitoris that provoked the women and girls into the medically and socially unhealthy behavior of masturbation. While perhaps not all physicians (or lay people) believed female masturbation to be a problem, some within both groups regarded the act as fundamentally improper socially and unhealthy physically because it focused sexual energy to the self and away from productive, constructive sexual relations (future or current) with the husband. In these two chapters, I argue that doctors performed one of these surgeries, quite often at the request of the girl's parents or by adult women themselves, to realign them with what both the medical and the nonmedical communities regarded as the only appropriate and healthy sexual behavior for middle-class white girls and women. They accomplished this by surgically treating a perceived physically abnormal clitoris. In the first chapter I examine clitoral surgeries on women as a treatment to correct adult female sexuality toward its only healthy direction: ardor for the husband. In the second chapter I build upon this by examining how clitoral surgeries were performed on female infants and children both to treat what were considered the immediate health implications of masturbation and to ensure that the child reached adulthood as sexually healthy.

In chapter 3 I examine how some medical authorities saw the atypically large clitoris as a physical manifestation of sexual behavior regarded as socially deviant and medically unhealthy from the middle of the nineteenth century to the early 1940s. The state of the clitoris—its size, color, whether it appeared swollen—revealed to doctors the practice of nonnormative sexual behavior. As in the first two chapters, signs of sexual ill health and social deviancy were read on the body. A red or enlarged clitoris indicated sexual deviancy, be it masturbation or homosexuality—the first often seen as a precursor to the second, and both regarded as forms of hypersexuality in women. Though physicians discussed whether the enlarged clitoris was either a cause for or the result of masturbation, two groups were seen as more likely, perhaps even expected, to have atypically sized clitorises: women of color and lesbians. I first turn to African American women and how some medical authorities believed that African American women in particular were inherently hypersexual and that this hypersexuality was inscribed on their bodies in the form of enlarged genitalia, including an atypically sized clitoris. I then turn to women who had sex with other women. Once so identified, physicians sometimes believed they were physically marked for such behavior by enlarged clitorises.

Physicians also blamed the clitoris for a woman's failed response in the marital bed. For just as the clitoris was seen as responsible for a woman's inappropriate sexual instinct when it manifested as masturbation, hypersexuality, or homosexuality, the organ was also blamed for their lack of sexual response. In the final four chapters, I explore the use of female circumcision as a method of increasing female sexual response to marital heterosexual sex from the late nineteenth through the late twentieth centuries. By removing the clitoral foreskin, some doctors and lay people thought the clitoris would be more exposed to, and would thus receive direct stimulation from, the penis during penetrative intercourse, thereby increasing female orgasmic potential.

These four chapters are broken into several decades. While these breaks are not definitive beginning or end dates in medical and popular attitudes of the clitoris and clitoral surgery, they do provide benchmarks of change. Chapter 4 deals with the use of female circumcision as a treatment for married women who wanted—or whose husbands wanted their wives to have—orgasms during marital sex before the popular acceptance of Freud's vaginal orgasm theory, roughly the late nineteenth century through the mid-1940s. In chapter 5 I turn to looking at how, even during the height of the Freudian vaginal orgasm theory, from roughly the 1940s until the mid-1960s, women continued to undergo circumcision as a sexual enhancement surgery. In chapter 6 I examine the roles the sexual revolution and the feminist health movement played in the practice and acceptance of circumcision. Building directly off chapter 6, the final chapter analyzes the work of gynecologist James Burt, probably one of the most prolific—and notorious—practitioners of female circumcision in the United States. Burt called himself the "love surgeon," and he practiced in Ohio from the late 1960s through the 1980s. Though he performed most of his love surgeries—a surgery that included circumcision—on women who apparently did not consent to it, he also marketed love surgery during the 1970s directly to women as a sexual enhancement surgery. As this book examines, from treating masturbation in the 1890s to love surgery in the 1970s to female genital cosmetic surgeries today, surgical attention to the clitoris has long been a part of medical, sexual, and cultural fashions in the United States.[61]

Chapter One

Women, Masturbation, and Clitoral Surgery, 1862–1945

In the early fall of 1896, John O. Polak, a doctor in Brooklyn, New York, examined Lizzie B., a twenty-nine-year-old single woman, who, until her nineteenth birthday, appeared to her family to be in exceptionally good health. Around this time, however, the young woman became morose and spent much of her time alone. She would, reported the doctor, "sit alone for hours masturbating," though she also masturbated "in the presence of friends and relatives." When Lizzie's father finally took his daughter to see Polak, the doctor described Lizzie as "pale and emaciated," and he learned she masturbated from twenty to forty times a day. Polak's physical examination of Lizzie revealed a somewhat larger than normal clitoris. Though Polak tried to explain to the distraught father that surgical intervention might not help his daughter, the father "insisted that something radical must be done, and assumed all responsibility." Polak reluctantly consented to operate, and, nearly two weeks after first examining Lizzie, he performed a clitoridectomy. The doctor concluded his report by writing that three months after the operation, Lizzie "has shown no desire to return to her former habits; she seems happier, and her mental condition clearer."[1] He believed his removal of her clitoris cured her of masturbating.

Contrary to prior accounts of female circumcision or clitoridectomy, Polak's and other physicians' approach to clitoral surgery, at least as revealed in published medical works, represented a cautious one that respected the importance of clitoral stimulation for healthy sexuality while simultaneously recognizing its role as cause and symptom in cases of insanity and ill health that were tied to masturbation. In addition to removing the foreskin or the entire organ, doctors during the late nineteenth century through the early twentieth century removed smegma and separated adhesions between the clitoral hood and the clitoris as therapies for masturbation. Physicians who performed these surgeries did so with the belief that the removal of all or parts of the clitoris corrected an unhealthy organ and thereby prevented the further deterioration of their patient's health from the vile effects of masturbation. Physicians who practiced circumcision or clitoridectomy, or who removed smegma or broke up adhesions, linked their patients' ill health to a nervous irritability, the origin of which was an irritated, abnormal clitoris. The irritated, abnormal clitoris was believed to provoke women into what was considered the medically and socially unhealthy behavior of masturbation. Doctors performed one of the four surgeries that fall under female circumcision and clitoridectomy quite often at the request of the young women's parents, or of women themselves, to treat masturbation.

Examination of these four clitoral surgeries illuminates doctors' knowledge of the organ and its role in female sexual pleasure, although what doctors regarded as a healthy organ and healthy sexual behavior were narrowly defined. During the period examined in this chapter, there was one kind of female orgasm, and it was clitoral; there was also only one kind of healthy sexual behavior for women, and it was linked to penetrative (hopefully procreative) sex with their husbands.[2] When women behaved outside of this normality by masturbating, their sexual instinct was seen as impaired and disordered. If healthy women, then, were believed to be sexual only within the marital embrace, what better way to explain these errant behaviors than by blaming the clitoris, an organ seen as key to female sexual expression? And so what better way for doctors to cure women of their sexual disorder than by surgically correcting this organ?

This discussion focuses on the use of these four practices to treat masturbation beginning in 1862, the year of the first American publication dealing with this treatment, and ending in 1945, the (approximate) year when psychoanalysis and the concept of the vaginal orgasm as the healthy orgasm for women began to be seen in the mainstream. While these are not arbitrary dates, neither should they be seen as absolute boundaries for when physicians surgically altered the clitoris as treatment for masturbation in women. During this time, within medical journal articles and within medical texts, physicians commented on individual cases such as Lizzie's and also spoke of the practice in general. Some of the articles were the published speeches of doctors to various medical associations in New York, Dallas, Chicago, Philadelphia, and Cleveland, to name a few. Although it is difficult to gauge how often the procedures were performed or the exact number upon whom they were performed, the appearance of the surgeries in standard gynecology texts, in medical journals, and as presented at medical society meetings, suggests at least that knowledge of the procedures was extensive and geographically diverse.

Though journal articles discussing female circumcision and clitoridectomy were published starting around the mid-nineteenth century in the United States, the bulk of articles appeared between 1880 and 1920, reflecting other changes occurring in medical practice during this time. First, Lizzie's case reveals the shift of masturbation from the category of sin needing religious redemption to that of an affliction needing medical intervention.[3] While masturbation had commonly been treated during the nineteenth century through noninterventionist techniques such as diet and hydrotherapy, as well as by medical appliances placed on the body designed to prevent masturbation, by the latter half of the century, surgical procedures directed at a physical cause, such as the clitoris, became more common.[4]

Second, that in 1896 Lizzie's father took her to a physician to be treated, that the physician agreed that masturbation was a problem he could treat, and that, though at first hesitant, he treated her through surgery illustrates the newly wrought authority Americans placed in doctors' hands.[5] By the late nineteenth century, Americans increasingly sought medical attention, attention that more often now meant surgery. Polak's use of surgery to treat Lizzie's condition, and indeed Lizzie's father's request for such an intervention, points to this increase, in part due to a wide acceptance of anesthesia, which also enhanced the appeal of surgery to patients and their families with the promise of a painless and permanent cure.[6] So while physicians were the ones being asked for treatment, parents and patients were still able to refuse it if it was not the therapy they had in mind or if they believed it would be ineffective. Though her work on the rise of surgeries between 1890 and 1910 focuses on Great Britain, New Zealand, and Australia, historian Sally Wilde's argument that submitting to surgeries during this time should not be taken as a sign of medical authority's dominance holds true in the United States as well.[7] Women patients—as well as at least in one instance the father of a female patient—valued the benefits of surgery and placed pressure on physicians such as Polak to enact surgical solutions.[8]

Finally, in addition to the rise in the use of surgery, by the late nineteenth century there occurred a similarly rapid rise in the division of medicine into specializations, including gynecology. While I am uncertain whether Polak understood himself to be a gynecologist, certainly if he was a general practitioner he would have at least been competing for female patients with this emerging specialty that regarded women's bodies as distinct from male bodies; indeed, gynecology, like other areas of science in the late nineteenth century, nearly uniformly regarded the female body, mind, and temperament as inferior to that of the male, a position that both reflected and helped maintain the larger cultural subordination of women.[9] The professional growth of gynecology during these decades undoubtedly contributed to the publication about clitoral surgeries to treat masturbation, if not their actual use.

That clitoral surgeries most frequently appeared in medical journals in the United States between 1880 and 1920 reflects the larger changes going on in American medicine during this time: changes in therapeutics; changes in the perceived power of medicine and in the power of medical authority; changes in treatment with the rise of surgery; and changes in the profession of medicine with the rise of specialization, in particular here gynecology.

With all of this came an interest in surgically treating the female body and in publishing about such treatment. Notably, it is not that surgical correction of the clitoris for sexual health went away after 1920; rather, it is that clitoral surgery became routine and thus less worthy of journal publication.

Before I continue, a few clarifications need to be made to help the reader better situate my analysis. First of all, though some of these women reportedly exhibited behavior that would still be looked askance upon today—such as Lizzie's masturbating forty times a day, including in front of others—I do not try to determine their "real" medical problem, if indeed they had one, nor do I claim that these women were not mentally or physically ill. Rather, the cases of clitoral surgery to treat masturbation reveal how doctors, women, and their family members, understood certain expressions of sexual behavior as problematic socially and unhealthy physically.[10] Additionally, because the women who patronized doctors during this time were largely white, middle to upper class, and native born, they are the women I discuss in this chapter. When they were not white or native born, physicians during this time tended to note this in their publications. Finally, though I am discussing the history of women and sexual behavior, the voices of women are not heard here without the filter of doctors. As other historians have observed, few people during this time left a written record of sexual behavior regarded as normative, let alone behavior deemed medically unhealthy or culturally inappropriate.

A Normal Clitoris and Healthy Sexual Behavior

Dr. Polak's examination of Lizzie's clitoris, an organ he described as a bit larger than normal, suggests he knew enough about the organ to recognize an atypical one when he saw it. Polak was not alone in his knowledge of the clitoris. Indeed, many doctors were quite detailed in their descriptions of the organ. A. S. Waiss, a professor of gynecology in Chicago, described the "glans clitoridis" as a "small, rounded tubercle, consisting of spongy erectile tissue and highly sensitive, a diminutive, but a true counterpart of the glans penis."[11] H. E. Beebe, giving a talk to fellow doctors in Ohio in 1897, described the clitoris as a "small elongated organ, composed of erectile tissue and located in the front part of the vulva," where it was "concealed by the fold of the nymphae." The body of the clitoris "was a full inch long" and, like the penis, possessed a hood, though unlike the penis, the prepuce of the clitoris did not surround the organ, rather it served "as a hood or top covering," a "gabled roof" for the clitoris.[12]

As I explored in the introduction, physicians during this time commonly believed that the clitoris, while not necessary to the function of procreation like the penis or the vagina, was the physiological source of sexual pleasure in women; according to Beebe, "in proportion to its size, and also being composed of erectile tissue, the clitoris is furnished with five times as many nerve endings as the penis."[13] Similarly, in an article published in 1900, Byron Robinson, a professor of gynecology at the Illinois Medical College, called the clitoris "an electric bell," the most "important and sensitive erectile tissue in the female organs" and the "chief seat of sexual excitement."[14]

Some lay texts—such as marriage guides and women's health prescription books—similarly described the clitoris as a sexual organ. For example, the 1890 *Ladies' New Medical Guide* noted the clitoris was "richly endowed with nerves" and became "erect during coition, and is the principal seat of the thrill or voluptuous sensation in the female." In the 1901 *Perfect Womanhood for Maidens-Wives-Mothers*, the clitoris was described as "the seat of special sensation, and becomes somewhat enlarged and hardened when the passions are excited."[15] These kinds of depictions of the clitoris as an organ of arousal illustrate the information available to nonmedical women (and men).

Healthy, white, middle-class women, however, were only supposed to experience sexual excitement during intercourse with their husbands. Nineteenth and early twentieth century marriage manuals implicitly argued for the importance of sex in marriage but couched the argument in terms of control and regulation, with some skepticism about the depth of female sexual needs.[16] While some advisors recommended that sex remain within the confines of a desire for children, others saw limited amounts of sex where procreation was prevented as a part of a healthy marriage.[17]

Overall, many late nineteenth-century physicians writing on the subject embraced a view of sex within marriage that accepted the act in moderate, controlled amounts. In his book *Physiology of Marriage*, published in 1866, physician William Alcott recommended married couples' "maximum frequency of sexual commerce" be once a month.[18] Though he believed it should be controlled and limited, Alcott considered it healthy. Similarly, in his 1907 book, physician Henry Guernsey called sexuality "ordained by God" and the sexual act "a special avowal of their relation to one another, and so often as it is repeated it is a renewal of their obligations to be faithful to each other."[19] Healthy white middle-class women were expected to enjoy sex, but only with their husbands during penetrative intercourse.

Some women, however, took orgasm into their own hands. Women masturbated, and doctors knew that they did so through "clitoridian manipulation," achieving orgasm on their own by touching that most important and sensitive organ.[20] Doctors noted the "simple titillation, or friction of the clitoris by the hand" as the most "prevalent form of the solitary vice," though some women were also able to achieve orgasm through "peculiar movements of the body, often calculated for this end" to accomplish "the same titillation of the clitoris."[21] Such peculiar movements included women crossing their "thighs and rubbing them at the same time" to produce "the desired result."[22]

Though Lizzie was "caught" masturbating, her larger than normal clitoris would have been seen by doctors as giving away her indulgence in the practice even had it been solitary, for an engorged clitoris was one of the most important visible signs doctors looked for. Wallace Abbott, a Chicago doctor, in 1904 described the clitoris of a woman who practiced masturbation as "red and swollen," the prepuce thick, "red and loose," with both the prepuce as well as the clitoris enlarged.[23] Joseph Howe, in his 1883 treatise on excessive venery and masturbation, wrote that "the local changes in the female genital organs always demonstrate plainly enough the results of masturbation, even when the patient denies the habit." These changes included an "elongated and thicker" clitoris than the healthy one of a woman who refrained from handling it.[24] This view did not end in the nineteenth century. In 1903, physician E. H. Smith described the signs of masturbation as including "a flattening of the upper portion of the labia minora, which gives the clitoris an unusually prominent appearance."[25] And University of Minnesota professor of gynecology Rae Thornton La Vake in 1928 considered "redness" of the prepuce and clitoris a sign of "onanism."[26] When doctors found the clitoris in such a state in an unmarried woman, "we are suspicious of masturbation," declared physician H. E. Beebe in 1897.[27]

The Disease of Masturbation

The rubbing together of thighs, the hand upon the clitoris—these acts concerned doctors, as well as family members and possibly the women who practiced them, because masturbation was generally regarded as unhealthy. Considered incapacitating since at least the time of Hippocrates, masturbation was not widely accepted as a disease, however, until around 1700.[28] During the nineteenth century, the practice was seen as a health issue linked to madness, idiocy, and epilepsy, as well as a variety of other psychological and behavioral problems.[29] To understand why masturbation was believed to be a dangerous disease with physical signs and symptoms and why masturbation was so feared, one needs to think of disease not just as an entity but rather as an example of how what counts as disease (or as health) is influenced by what is valued—both by the larger culture as well as by medical practitioners.[30] Sexual behavior like masturbation was understood to be problematic because it routed sex away from procreation and instead spent sexual energy recklessly.[31]

But concern about masturbation was not confined to its health risks, for it was also regarded as an inappropriate social act. Lizzie spent hours alone. Many during this time regarded masturbation as the ultimate secret addiction, what historian Thomas Laqueur called the crack cocaine of sexuality. According to Laqueur, those concerned with solitary sex saw the act as unnatural, and three things made it so: the object of desire was not real but rather a product of the imagination, masturbation was not socially engaged, and the desire and ability to masturbate was potentially endless.[32] Among women, solitary sex was at its most secret, and its most suspect, because healthy women were not thought of as independent sexual beings without the promptings of their husbands.

Additionally, the solitary act of masturbation was regarded as socially and medically unhealthy because it involved no chance of pregnancy. And this was a grave social problem, historians Carroll Smith-Rosenberg and Charles Rosenberg asserted, because many believed that a white woman's "willingness and capacity to bear children was a duty she owed not only to God and her husband but to her 'race' as well." By the second half of the nineteenth century, white Protestant Americans became more accepting of the view that regarded racial identity as fundamental, and thus an increase in white Protestant birthrates became imperative. Some argued that white women who failed to produce offspring were contributing to the race's suicide. Moreover, this belief in an impending race suicide was not laid equally at the feet of all parents but specifically at women's. It was "America's potential mothers, not its fathers, who were primarily responsible for the impending social cataclysm," argued Smith-Rosenberg and Rosenberg.[33] Though by and large these fears were aimed at women who practiced birth control, the problem extended to those who masturbated, for in both cases the women avoided pregnancy and failed to live up to their social and biological role as mothers.

That women masturbated and that doctors knew how women masturbated, however, suggests physicians understood women as capable of sexual response outside of penetrative vaginal sex.[34] While many doctors noted that women possessed an organ whose purpose was sexual pleasure, most simultaneously believed that women—at least respectable, healthy, middle class white women—ought to desire sex only when prompted by a husband's erotic desire.[35] Moreover, the only sex a woman wanted (or was supposed to want) with her husband was vaginal. While there existed a diverse range of medical opinions on the extent of women's ability to experience sexual pleasure, physicians did not question either the vaginal model of sex nor that such sex be engaged in between spouses.[36] Even though they possessed an organ with great sexual sensitivity, one that they could titillate themselves, women, or at least healthy women, needed a husband to awaken it. When a woman masturbated, especially excessively, physicians saw a clear indication that a woman had lost her normal sexual instinct.

When physicians determined that a woman's masturbation was due to a correctable condition of the clitoris, doctors treated the clitoris by cleaning the smegma, breaking up adhesions, or circumcising the clitoris—all methods that left the organ itself—to restore a woman to her normal sexual instinct. Based on their understanding of the importance of the clitoris to female sexual response, doctors used these procedures to retain their patient's ability for sexual response through clitoral stimulation but surgically redirected to its healthy form as stimulated during vaginal intercourse. Surgical intervention treated a physical problem. Still basing their decision on the physical condition of the clitoris, doctors performed clitoridectomy in cases where they deemed the woman's health at too great a risk from continued masturbation to not perform the most extreme of the procedures. Doctors, however, saw little value in clitoridectomy when they concluded that the basis of a woman's masturbation was psychological and not physiological, when masturbation was a symptom of a mental condition, not of a condition of the clitoris, as I show below.

Clitoral Surgery to Restore Sexual Health

As one doctor told a group of his peers in the late nineteenth century, "from the origin of the word, clitoris signifies to titillate, hence it must have long ago been deemed overly sensitive to irritation."[37] Just as doctors believed that a woman's clitoris was keenly sexually responsive, some also believed that an abnormal physical condition of the clitoris due to a local irritant caused a reflex action that prompted a woman to manipulate her clitoris to quell the irritation. Many cases of masturbation, New Orleans physician A. J. Bloch wrote in 1894, depended upon "a phimosis of the glans clitoridis, which were entirely relieved by removing the cause." Bloch stressed to his fellow physicians the importance of examining the genitals to reveal whether the troubles were of what he called a "reflex origin."[38] The pathogenesis of masturbation, then, was a physiological one: excessive nervous stimulation.[39]

The underlying theory, known as reflex neurosis, pictured the body as a nervous web intricately wired together, and many diseases, including masturbation, were attributed to it.[40] Reflex neurosis theory came into vogue around 1800 and continued in favorable standing through the late nineteenth century.[41] Under this theory, a woman's irritated clitoris instigated her actions: a clitoris became irritated; a woman touched herself to quell the irritation; the clitoris became perpetually aroused, erect, and inflamed. If the woman continued to try to stop the irritation by handling her clitoris, she further risked eroding her physical and mental health. Masturbation was thus not a willful action but rather a physical response to an unhealthy and abnormal condition of the clitoris caused by an irritation, compelling "the hand to go to the genitals," physician Wallace C. Abbott wrote in 1904.[42]

As historian Nancy Theriot argued in her examination of women and diagnoses of nervousness or insanity, if a patient's symptoms were unfeminine behaviors with causes regarded as within the body, a physical treatment was required.[43] Reflex neurosis provided a physiological explanation for problematic behavior.

In 1905, Robert Taylor, in his *Practical Treatise on Sexual Disorders of the Male and Female*, recommended that in "all cases of confirmed masturbation," the condition of the clitoris had to be carefully examined.[44] Believing, as Johns Hopkins University gynecologist Howard Kelly did, that masturbation was caused by an "irritation from lack of cleanliness," doctors sought to remove the irritation from the clitoris while saving the organ in one of three ways: removing the smegma from between the clitoris and the hood, separating adhesions between the glans and the hood, or removing the hood.[45] According to reflex theory, smegma—material secreted from the glans of the foreskin and the labia minora—built up between the glans of the clitoris and the clitoral hood and caused irritation, "particularly in careless" and unclean women. When doctors found smegma, they were advised to clean it out carefully, and place "a little tuft of absorbent cotton soaked with leadwater . . . over its parts."[46] Byron Robinson advised that all smegma between the clitoris and hood be removed "so that all physical irritations of the genitals may be removed."[47] When the "glans of the clitoris cannot be freely uncovered" because of a "constriction or narrowing of the foreskin," the condition gave rise to smegma or other secretion accumulating between the clitoris and the clitoral foreskin, causing "inflammation, itching and nervous irritation."[48] The smegma, according to a 1934 gynecology textbook, "may cause irritation which can result in masturbation."[49] After referring to the inflammation of the organ upon its accumulation of smegma as the "most common" disorder of the clitoris, a 1903 text described the removal of smegma: peel back the prepuce, wipe off "all filth" with a cotton cloth dosed in boric-acid solution, then dry the surface and apply Vaseline. Such a treatment was to be given for several days in order to prove effective.[50] Removing the smegma removed the irritation and thus, it was believed, the compulsion to touch the genitals.

But sometimes just cleaning the area around the clitoris was not enough, for an adherent prepuce could, according to another physician, bind down the clitoris and imprison "smegma thrown out by secreting glands."[51] According to one doctor, "adhesions of the prepuce in the female may have a pathological significance," acting as an "irritant" that leads to masturbation.[52] Because the clitoris is so very sensitive, it requires attention; Chicago gynecologist Byron Robinson stressed to his fellow physicians that it was "very important that all adhesions between [the clitoris] and the prepuce should be broken up so that the patient's attention may not be attracted to it, enticing masturbation."[53] Such a state, gynecologists Howard Kelly and

Charles Noble wrote in 1907, is "very common" and requires the clitoris to be freed and "all secretion removed."[54] In addition, Charles Reed, a gynecology professor at the University of Cincinnati, recommended in 1913 that physicians and nurses should always examine the clitoris for adhesions when given the opportunity and that, if found, they should be broken up under anesthesia.[55] Gynecologist E. C. Dudley believed physicians needed to "separate that prepuce from the glans either by breaking up the adhesions or by incision," thus explaining Reed's recommendation for anesthesia.[56]

In September 1891, a mother took her nineteen-year-old daughter to see J. M. Sligh, a physician in the neighboring town of Granite, Montana. Sligh described the daughter as "well developed," having "always enjoyed good health," until eleven months prior, when her appetite changed, her color left, she suffered from frequent headaches, and menstruation became painful and irregular. Additionally, the young woman often suffered from backaches as well as an "aching pain in the groins" and a sense of "utter worthlessness that prompted in her a desire for death." The doctor informed the worried mother that her daughter's problems lay "probably with the genital organs" and he asked for permission to examine them. The mother reluctantly agreed, "on condition that it should be under chloroform." Upon examination, Sligh found the clitoris bound down by adhesions, which he proceeded to "free" by using a probe and his fingernails. On the following day, Miss O. seemed remarkably improved, and she admitted to the doctor she masturbated, "probably impelled thereto by the irritation produced by the adherent prepuce and imprisoned smegma," Sligh reasoned. The doctor met with Miss O. several times over the following months, and "her quick restoration to perfect health astonished me as much as it pleased the patient and her mother."[57]

This case, along with another Sligh similarly treated, impressed upon the doctor the importance of preputial adhesions in the female. He advised his fellow physicians that when a "young neurotic patient" came seeking their aid who exhibited such symptoms as headaches, pickiness regarding food, the shunning of society, or listlessness, they should not "let the symptoms continue until catalepsy, epilepsy, confirmed hysteria, melancholia, or actual uterine or ovarian disease" set in before examining the clitoris. While Sligh did not believe a clitoris bound down by an adherent prepuce "responsible for all the ills that human femininity is subject to," he advised his fellow medical practitioners of the necessity to examine this organ as a source of the problems, for "a great many women who have heretofore sought relief in vain."[58]

But sometimes even cleaning the clitoris of smegma or removing adhesions that bound the clitoris down within the foreskin failed to completely or permanently remove the irritation. Doctors then opted for the third therapy, circumcision. Though Howard Kelly believed cleaning the prepuce of smegma "desirable" whenever the accumulation was "considerable" in order to treat masturbation, he also considered circumcision necessary when "accumulation persistently recurs."[59] Edwin Hale believed his fellow physicians needed to look for malformations of the female prepuce, as he saw many cases where the prepuce was "too long, or too tight, causing compression of the clitoris and allowing an accumulation of irritating smegma around that organ."[60] Conditions where the clitoral hood was "elongated or hypertrophied" were ripe for trapping the smegma, thus promoting a constant irritation and necessitating removal.[61] Physicians discussed this procedure among themselves in medical journals and texts and at medical society meetings. But women, too, apparently had some knowledge of it; in 1900, a twenty-six-year-old woman proposed the removal of her clitoral hood to a physician in Chicago, who performed the procedure.[62]

Doctors circumcised the clitoris by drawing the hood up between their thumb and forefinger in a manner that caused the glans to extrude, and then, especially when they regarded the hood as long, "a narrow strip of skin and mucous membrane was removed with scissors, the wound closed in with a fine continuous catgut structure, and this covered with a thin layer of flexible collodion," and finally the "clitoris was covered with sterilized Vaseline."[63] According to S. L. Kistler, a physician in Los Angeles, female circumcision was easier than male circumcision, and he believed male circumcision so easy a man could perform his own with the use of a phimosis clamp, "provided he did not become faint-hearted." In an article that appeared in the *Journal of the American Medical Association* (*JAMA*) in 1910, Kistler directed that on women, the clamp needed to be applied to the elongated or hypertrophied part of the clitoris. Once applied, the ligatures were inserted, the part excised, the upper blades removed, and the ligatures tied "without necessity of pulling loops." The physician then removed the clamp and applied dressing. Kistler believed this simple operation performed with this tool reduced the likelihood of masturbation.[64]

Cleaning out smegma, liberating the hood, removing the hood—these were all procedures designed to keep the clitoris and the possibility of clitoral stimulation, although not through masturbation. In cases where doctors determined that a woman's masturbation was due to a correctable condition of the clitoris, doctors treated the condition and preserved the clitoris in an effort to restore a woman to her normal sexual instinct. One doctor, who believed in the necessity of cleaning smegma and sometimes removing the hood, called the removal of the entire organ "burning a house to roast a pig." Though relief could sometimes be found when clitoridectomy was performed, this doctor thought that "much harm" results "by a destruction of all the normal sexual instincts, and occasionally insanity was the result."[65] Knowing the importance of the clitoris for those "normal sexual instincts," doctors sought surgical remedies that removed the irritation while maintaining the organ.

Clitoral Surgery as Desperation Surgery

There were cases such as Lizzie's, however, when some doctors believed the clitoris should be removed. Clitoridectomy, the removal of the entire organ, was performed when doctors diagnosed a woman's sexual disorder as past the point of regaining her sexual health through surgery. The fear of continued deteriorating health from masturbation thus necessitated the organ's removal. While under less extreme conditions doctors sought to treat but retain the organ to restore a woman to her sexual balance, in cases like Lizzie's, physicians determined that saving the woman necessitated the destruction of all—healthy and unhealthy—sexual instincts by removing the clitoris. And they did this because, as physician E. S. Cooper wrote, even death was "infinitely preferable to insanity" from masturbation.[66]

When it came to surgically correcting the problem of masturbation by removing the entire organ, it appears that doctors were most likely to intervene when the solitary act, as in Lizzie's case, was neither solitary nor infrequent, both indicators that the woman uncontrollably suffered from an unhealthy sexual instinct. As Robert Taylor wrote in his treatise on sexual disorders of men and women, in "cases in which females indulge excessively in masturbation," there was cause for great concern because the act results in "deterioration in the health of the patient" unless she obtains "proper hygienic care" and ceased "to indulge in the bad habit."[67] It was when masturbation was performed repeatedly or in front of family, friends, even strangers that family members or the woman herself sought medical assistance and doctors most radically intervened to help her.

Most doctors who performed clitoridectomy reserved it for extreme cases, which some physicians labeled nymphomania, a condition from which there was believed to be no chance of restoring healthy sexual instinct. In her study of the disease of nymphomania, historian Carol Groneman asserted that while physical causes were seen as reasons for the condition, nymphomania was both a medical and a social problem consisting of inappropriate and unmanageable sexuality. The disease illustrates how doctors, patients, and the larger culture viewed certain forms of female sexual behavior not just as inappropriate but also as diseased.[68]

G. R. Southwick, a professor of obstetrics at Boston University's School of Medicine in the 1890s, wrote that nymphomania was "fortunately not a common complaint" and a woman suffering from it "should be pitied, and not at all [held] responsible for her words or actions."[69] But though some physicians did not think the complaint common, it was still of concern. Joseph Howe in the 1880s described a nymphomaniac as having "an uncontrollable appetite for lascivious pleasures, exhibited (in its worst forms) in public and private, without regard to time, place, or surroundings," while Robert Taylor in 1905 described nymphomania as "a very infrequent form of masturbation," one "observed in degenerate sexual perverts."[70] These women, Taylor further stated, "suffer from inordinate and excessive sexual desire, and many of them are frequently guilty of great foulness and lewdness of speech and action," including exposing their genitals to men and women and masturbating in public. Because of such behavior, "cases of nymphomania," Taylor wrote, "are very distressing."[71] Indeed, in his 1871 book, *Satan in Society,* physician and morality crusader Nicholas Cooke described the onset of nymphomania as transforming a timid woman into "a termagant, and the most delicate modesty to a furious audacity which even the effrontery of prostitution does not approach."[72] In these cases, doctors assumed removing the center of a woman's sexual sensitivity better than allowing the disease to destroy her.

But before performing clitoridectomy doctors stressed the necessity of confirming the basis of the disorder in an unhealthy condition of the clitoris. Doctors acknowledged the seriousness of removing the entire organ, for when "full excision of the clitoris (clitoridectomy) may be performed" to cure the patient of her extremely unhealthy sexual behavior, the "surgeon should seek consultation with one or two expert colleagues" and "the nervous condition of these patients should be fully and carefully considered and treated" to ensure that such radical treatment would be effective, according to Robert Taylor in 1905.[73] In 1872, physician William Goodell in Philadelphia sought the advice of his peers before operating upon a woman who had "earnestly begged him to amputate her clitoris," as she saw this organ as the basis for "her whole trouble," masturbation. Though another physician in Baltimore had removed a portion of her clitoris (perhaps the foreskin, though this is unclear), she now sought the organ's entire removal. During discussion of the case at a Philadelphia Obstetrical Society meeting in the early 1870s, a fellow physician asked "whether the root of the trouble was in the clitoris," while two others suggested using lupulin (a sticky yellow substance derived from hops formerly used as both an antispasmodic and a sedative) instead of removing the organ. The physician who recommended lupulin stressed that the removal of the clitoris would not work "unless the mind of the person had been directed to that organ as the one causing the desire."[74]

The Influence of Dr. Isaac Baker Brown

Perhaps some physicians' caution in using clitoridectomy was because they were familiar with one of their British peer's overuse of it; indeed, in the above meeting, the physicians ended their discussion noting the surgery as performed by Isaac Backer Brown.[75] Others referenced Brown's work too; during his 1893 speech before the Cleveland Medical Society, Alvin Eyer

referred to the British surgeon. Regarded by many on both sides of the
Atlantic as the man who popularized the removal of the clitoris as therapy,
Brown was called by Eyer one of "the most distinguished English surgeons,"
who "through lack of appreciation and acceptance of his work" died "bro-
ken-hearted." However, Eyer believed Brown erred, as his "enthusiasm" for
clitoridectomy prompted him to choose cases indiscriminately; indeed, cases
of "epilepsy, catalepsy, hysteria, insanity, and idiocy soon recurred" after clitoridectomy.[76] Though Eyer believed Brown mis- and overused clitoridectomy, he still considered the operation useful in certain cases.[77]

Like Eyer and the Philadelphia physicians, several American doctors who
reported trying clitoridectomy commented on the infamous British physician's attempts.[78] And while they perhaps considered him a good surgeon,
they too tended to think he overused the operation. Brown did not invent
clitoridectomy, nor was he the first to use it to cure masturbation or nymphomania. Clitoridectomy, according to historian Edward Shorter, is one
of the oldest operations in the history of medicine and was performed in
ancient Rome to cure nymphomania. Late in the eighteenth century and
in the early nineteenth the clitoris was removed occasionally for masturbation.[79] In 1825, for example, British doctors removed the clitoris of a four-
teen-year-old girl who masturbated.[80] And Brown was not the only one of his
countrymen in the 1860s to perform it.[81] He was and is, however, the most
notorious of its nineteenth-century practitioners.[82]

In 1854 Brown published his first book, *Surgical Diseases of Women*, a book
that established him as something of a celebrity. In 1865, he was elected
president of the Medical Society of London, and the following year published his second book, *On the Curability of Some Forms of Insanity, Epilepsy, and
Hysteria in Females*, where he outlined his use of clitoridectomy.[83] Brown documented forty-eight cases where he removed women's clitorises. He claimed
to have cured forty-five of these women (two received no relief and what happened to the other is uncertain). He operated on married, single, and widowed women, though most frequently on single women. The oldest woman
who lost her clitoris to Brown's scissors was fifty-seven, the youngest sixteen.
He first amputated a clitoris in 1859. Operating as both a private practitioner and as senior surgeon at the London Surgical Home, Brown noted that
the operation had been "observed by numerous medical men" and many
became "firm converts" to the utility of clitoridectomy. He believed the clitoris played a central role in the inception of various female ailments, including hysteria and epilepsy, all of which originated in the manipulation of the
clitoris during masturbation.[84]

According to Brown, clitoridectomy was to be performed with a patient
"placed completely under the influence of chloroform." Brown then
excised the clitoris "freely" with either a knife or scissors. The wound was
then "plugged with graduated compress lint and a pad, well secured by a

T bandage." The woman was put to bed and watched by a nurse to make sure no "injurious results" were incurred through hemorrhage. The patient received bed rest for a month, time enough for the "perfect healing of the wound, at the end of which time it is difficult for the uninformed, or non-medical, to discover any trace of an operation."[85]

Shortly after the appearance of *Curability*, the *British Medical Journal* (*BMJ*) published a three-page scathing review. Letters to the editor arrived frequently following the review and the controversy raged in the *BMJ* through the spring of 1867.[86] The debate in part concerned the way Brown interacted with his patients and whether he obtained consent from them (or consent from their husbands, fathers, or friends).[87] But physicians also charged Brown with incorrectly using the operation. Forbes Winslow wrote in a letter published by the *BMJ* on December 22, 1866, that, by performing clitoridectomy to treat insanity, Brown "begins his treatment of these cases at the wrong end" when the source of the affliction lay in their heads.[88]

In April 1867, with the controversy heated, the Obstetrical Society of London voted 194 to 38 to remove Brown.[89] His expulsion from the Obstetrical Society ruined his career; his health soon deteriorated and he died in poverty in 1873.[90] Americans followed this debate through the medical press. In February 1867, two months before Brown's expulsion from the Obstetrical Society, an editorial in the *Southern Journal of the Medical Sciences* noted that the "mass of opinion is wholly adverse to the views of Mr. Brown, and his operation is unqualifiedly condemned."[91] In July 1867, the *Chicago Medical Examiner* noted that the "celebrated Dr. Brown has recently been expelled from the Obstetrical Society of London, for unprofessional conduct, in connection with his operations of clitoridectomy."[92] Some of the American physicians who referred to Brown noted, as Joseph Howe did, that "Mr. Brown incurred the enmity of his professional brethren for a too free use of the operation."[93] George Engelmann said that Brown's "enthusiasm carried him too far, and led to such unprofessional practices that he received the just censure of the profession."[94]

American physicians who mentioned Brown in their work tended to argue that Brown's expulsion was the result of his overzealous use of the operation, not a full rejection of the operation itself. Most agreed with Brown in the suitability of the operation but believed he chose his patients too broadly. For example, Engelmann, while believing Brown deserved his censure, noted, "It cannot be denied that there are certain cases in which it is a justifiable procedure."[95] In 1867, vice president of the American Medical Association (AMA) Horatio R. Storer agreed that Brown used the operation too frequently, but there was no doubt in Storer's mind that, when used for "certain exceptional cases," clitoridectomy benefited the patient.[96]

Physicians like Storer who believed that in "certain exceptional cases" clitoridectomy was necessary stressed the importance of carefully examining the condition of the clitoris in "all cases of confirmed masturbation" to verify that it was indeed the cause of the sexual disorder.[97] W. Gill Wylie, at a 1901 New York Women's Hospital Society meeting, stressed the need to look for an irritated clitoris when examining patients afflicted with masturbation. Physicians, he believed, often assumed that such patients came to them with "some disease or abnormal condition of the brain or nervous system causing trouble, instead of there being an imperfect development of the generative organs resulting in reflex nervous disturbances."[98] C. C. Frederick also supported this reasoning, saying that, so long as the patient possessed "no hereditary predisposition, no neuropathic taint in the individual, removal of the local cause or causes would generally effect a cure."[99] Physicians tended to agree with this sentiment; in his 1880 text, William B. Atkinson considered clitoridectomy to be "justifiable when other means fail, and the cause appears to be local irritation."[100] When the basis of masturbation was found to be a physiological imbalance in the condition of the clitoris, doctors saw good reason to operate on the organ or remove it entirely to treat the disorder. But doctors stressed the need to examine the clitoris of "confirmed" masturbators because masturbation was also considered a symptom of a mental disorder.

When Clitoral Surgery Proved Futile

Recall that Polak removed Lizzie's clitoris, but he did so only after hesitating, perhaps unsure of the etiology of her masturbation: Was it physiological or psychological? Doctors who removed the smegma, separated adhesions from between the clitoral hood and the glans, removed the hood, or removed the entire clitoris did so when they believed that this physical intervention would quell the physical problem. Proceeding on a case-by-case basis, doctors noted that these procedures did not work when the problem was not physiological. When physicians found masturbation to be primarily a symptom of a psychological disorder, they believed operating on the clitoris did not work. Charles Mills, a neurologist at the Philadelphia Hospital, told fellow Philadelphia physicians in 1885 that, when masturbation was "intrinsically nervous or mental," the operative procedure of clitoridectomy failed to "radically cure the patient." According to Mills, the "condition which causes the symptoms in many of these cases is in some defect or change in the nervous system of the individual which cannot be removed by mere operation."[101]

Coexisting with the reflex theory was the theory that masturbation was a symptom not of a problem with the physiological state of the clitoris but of the psychological state of the mind. One doctor wrote that women who suffered from nymphomania had "marked cerebral disease."[102] During the late nineteenth and into the early twentieth centuries, nymphomania and masturbation were considered to be disorders with one of two origins, physiological or psychological. Alongside the reflex theory existed the theory of an organic disease of the brain itself. According to this theory, if patients became hysterical or psychotic, with masturbation as a symptom, it lay not in an irritated clitoris but rather in an inherited nervous condition that affected their minds.[103] A condition of the brain, physicians who advanced this theory believed, could not be treated through surgery on the body.

St. Louis physician George Engelmann discovered this after he removed the clitoris of Mrs. M., of Herman, Missouri, to end her masturbation habits in 1918. Mrs. M. resumed her preoperative activity soon after the removal of her clitoris, something Engelmann attributed to Mrs. M.'s "nervous disturbance," a psychological condition he realized he failed to take into account before operating and that physical intervention could not cure.[104] Likewise, Paul Munde, a professor of gynecology at Dartmouth College and a gynecologist at Mount Sinai Hospital in New York City, cautioned his fellow practitioners to evaluate carefully before operating. In a paper he read before the Woman's Hospital Society in November 1897, Munde noted how tempting it was to ascribe a female patient's masturbation to an irritated clitoris and to recommend an operation, but he thought study of such cases necessary and believed that his fellow practitioners should "draw the line pretty closely when advising operations on the genital organs of a female for apparently entirely unrelated and independent mental disturbances." He strongly advised against removing the clitoris to cure insanity.[105]

In one of the few statements made by a woman regarding her uncontrollable sexual instinct—with the caveat that it was provided to us through a physician—a twenty-nine-year-old woman described to neurologist Charles Mills her years of suffering from a "mental trouble" that compelled her to masturbate and her various treatments to cure her disorder, including clitoridectomy. According to the young woman's description of her progression to nymphomania, even "getting into a bath or merely washing the parts would often bring it [orgasm] on," and, by that point in her life, "the weakness began to settle in the nerve-centres of different organs,—first the heart, then the uterus and brain, causing pain and a kind of stoppage in their regular action."[106]

In this remarkable story, both Mills and the woman describe her disease as nymphomania, showing that she, along with her doctors, understood her sexual feelings as excessive. Conscious of her fall from normal sexual instincts, her narrative echoed the terror she must have felt.[107] But, in addition to her (filtered) voice, one also hears Mills, and, read together, they describe the confusion of both doctors and patients on how to treat disordered female sexual instinct, treatments that ranged from nerve tonics to institutionalization to clitoridectomy when there was confusion as to the origins of the disorder. Mills, who entered the story after all of these treatment options had been tried, pointed out that clitoridectomy failed because this particular patient's nymphomania was mental in origin. And Mills, like many of his peers, believed that when masturbation did not originate in a condition of the clitoris, operating on or removing it altogether failed to provide a cure.

Doctors knew the clitoris to be a unique and powerfully sensitive sexual organ, the "electric bell" of female sexual instinct. But they also believed—and some reinforced this belief through surgery—that women should only have use for that organ when their husbands aroused it through vaginal sex. When a woman masturbated, especially when she did so frequently or in front of others, her sexual instinct was manifesting itself in an unhealthy manner, and doctors looked for a problem with the condition of the clitoris or of the mind to explain her behavior—the condition of her clitoris or her mind compelled her to handle the organ. Treating the unhealthy condition of the clitoris gave the woman (and her family) a medical explanation, a medical out, for her socially inappropriate sexual behavior. Masturbation may have been considered the crack cocaine of venery, but rather than concede a willful addiction, some physicians, women, or perhaps their families, based the proclivity as a result of either a physiological or a psychological imbalance.[108]

Chapter Two

Children, Masturbation, and Clitoral Surgery since 1890

During a December 1893 speech before the Cleveland Medical Society, physician Alvin Eyer stated that the only cure for masturbation was either marriage or amputation of the clitoris. Eyer then described his removal of the clitoris of a seven-year-old girl, referred to by the initials M.E.H., who had been adopted the previous year. The mother told Eyer how she caught her daughter "gratifying her passions as often as four or five times a day" and that the child confessed to masturbating in the orphanage. Upon examination, the doctor found her clitoris "much developed for one her age" and then proceeded to bury the clitoris within the folds of the child's labia to hide it from her touch. M.E.H, however, would not be so thwarted, and Eyer decided to remove the organ entirely. Nearly six weeks after the operation, the mother reported that her daughter confessed to trying to masturbate again but had told her mother: "you know there is nothing there now, so, of course, I could do nothing."[1]

M.E.H.'s mother was concerned about her daughter's health as a result of masturbation, and her view of the physical problems masturbation wrought on children were reflected in the medical literature at the turn of the twentieth century. According to a 1905 pediatric textbook, masturbation made children "languid," and they suffered from headaches, "palpitations, mental and physical relaxation, anemia, emaciation, and a change in demeanor." Moreover, masturbating children became "bashful," and "shy" as well as potentially "hysterical."[2] Fears of such immediate health repercussions often prompted parents to seek medical attention—indeed, one physician recommended in his 1923 *Nursery Guide for Mothers and Nurses* that parents inform their physician as soon as they discovered their child masturbating.[3] Though M.E.H.'s mother was concerned enough she sought medical treatment, she, along with Eyer and the other physicians who treated girls with one of the four clitoral surgeries, also regarded masturbation as an abnormal and unhealthy sexual behavior, a behavior that could manifest itself into a variety of physical and mental health problems.[4] But among physicians this early abnormal sexual behavior was believed to impact the child's future sexual health as well.

Physicians removed smegma, broke up adhesions, circumcised the clitoris, and, at the most extreme, removed the clitoris of women to surgically redirect sexual instinct to what was considered physically healthy and socially acceptable: vaginal sex, prompted by a husband. When physicians used one of the four clitoral surgeries on female infants and girls, they also did so with the intention of directing their patient's future sexual instinct and behavior. Concerns about youthful masturbation reflected the idea that the only healthy sex for females was marital and responsive to their husbands when they were adults. Thus, the use of one of the four clitoral surgeries as therapy for masturbation in children should be seen as based on a medical concern for the future health of female infants and girls as often as it was about the immediate ill-effects of masturbation.

The Means to Correct It at Once

If the only cures for masturbation were either marriage or amputation of the clitoris, when it came to children, surgery of some sort was really the only option. As historians R. Danielle Egan and Gail Hawkes noted, "Discourses about childhood sexuality were, for the most part, not really about children; rather they were emblematic of the anxieties surrounding larger social instabilities and the need to bring them under control."[5] Physicians often noted that masturbation was quite common in children of both sexes, with some arguing the practice was more common in young girls.[6] Moreover, though medical as well as lay ideas about the immediate and long-term implications of masturbation changed during the late nineteenth to the mid-twentieth centuries, concern for masturbation as a behavior to be stopped remained. During the late nineteenth century, masturbation was considered by many medical practitioners as a practice with grave outcomes, though increasingly in the early twentieth century physicians came to regard it more as an "evil habit" akin to thumb sucking than as a disease per se, but still the "most serious" of the bad habits, one which required parents to seek medical assistance for its correction. Such was the advice of Le Grand Kerr, a Brooklyn physician, who instructed parents in his 1910 *The Care and Training of Children* that it was "of prime importance that parents detect the very first signs of the habit and take means to correct it at once."[7]

Physicians knew how female infants and girls masturbated and that the clitoris was the principal organ used in the practice. "In the adolescent girl," like in the woman, New York neurologist John F. W. Meagher wrote in the 1920s, "the clitoris chiefly, and next the labia minora, are used for the purposes of masturbation."[8] Infants and girls under age one were considered by physicians to be the easiest for parents to discover in the actual act of masturbating. Often infants masturbated "by means of thigh rubbing," a practice which was "not very uncommon in female babies under one year of age."[9] In older children, thigh rubbing was only one of many means. In his 1915 book for mothers and children's nurses, L. Emmett Holt described childhood masturbation as "the habit of rubbing the genital organs with the hands, with the clothing, against the bed, or rubbing the thighs together." Additionally, some children sat "upon the floor" with their legs crossed and rocked backward and forward. "Many of these things are passed over lightly and are regarded for months as simply a 'queer trick' of the child" by mothers or caregivers. But Holt, a professor of diseases of children at Columbia University medical school, recommended quick action upon discovery. "Masturbation," he told mothers, was "the most injurious of all the bad habits, and should be broken up just as early as possible."[10]

Though sometimes parents noticed an infant or young child masturbating, an older, more active child was often harder for parents to detect. However, when parents suspected their child masturbated, physicians could look for certain telling symptoms, such as "dark rings round the eyes, peevishness, languor, and perhaps a lack of healthy interest in the games and pleasures of childhood," according to a 1910 pediatric text.[11] In addition, a girl who lost her "freshness and beauty," whose color had left her complexion, and who developed a "sad expression, dry cough, oppression and panting on the least exertion," showed signs of masturbation.[12] As illustrated in these warning signs, masturbation adversely affected a child's "bodily and mental health," both immediately and in the future.[13]

Though physicians were concerned about the effects of masturbation on a child's immediate well-being, underlying the treatment of masturbation was also a deep concern for the future child's ability to blossom into a sexually healthy woman. The alternative was, as James Frederic Goodhart and George Frederic Still wrote in their 1910 pediatric textbook, that the masturbating child would grow up to be "the wretched sexual hypochondriac with whom every medical man is only too familiar."[14] For a girl to avoid such a fate, she needed to not masturbate; having a healthy clitoris helped.

The Importance of a Healthy Clitoris for Future Healthy Womanhood

For girls to grow into healthy women with normalized sexual responsiveness to their husbands, physicians needed to be aware of the condition of the clitoris and examine it for any abnormalities. Physician Edwin Hale believed that "involuntary masturbation is common in children," even at young ages, "if the clitoris is in an abnormal condition; otherwise it rarely occurs."[15] Like in women, girls were compelled to touch the genitals because of an abnormal state of the clitoris; the reflex theory applied, regardless of the age of the patient. An irritated clitoris was often the cause of an abnormality, and both smegma and clitoral adhesions caused irritations. "Even the slightest irritation of adhesions may call the attention of the girl to those organs and induce masturbation," stated De Forest Willard in his 1910 book on childhood surgery. In all cases where adhesions existed, the doctor continued, every source of the irritation should be removed.[16]

Girls were not seen as masturbating for the physical pleasure of it but were rather compelled to do so to alleviate irritation. Historian R. P. Neuman, in an examination of the condition labeled as "masturbatory insanity" by physicians in the late nineteenth century through World War I, argued that, by labeling the condition, physicians provided a medical diagnosis, and thus treatment, for the social problem of childhood sexuality. In their visualization of childhood as asexual and adolescence as sexually controlled, middle-class parents were disturbed by masturbation, a practice that challenged this belief. By both naming masturbation as a condition and as providing its basis in physiology—smegma, an adherent clitoris—physicians provided, as they did with women, a physiological reason for the problematic behavior, with subsequent physical treatment.[17]

Sometimes a lack of cleanliness was credited as the causal factor in the creation of irritations to the clitoral area prompting the hand to go the genitals.[18] A 1940 text recommended that, after separating clitoral adhesions, the area should be cleaned regularly.[19] New York physician Charles Gilmore Kerley wrote in 1907 that to prevent masturbation, girls needed to have their genitals kept clean and powdered daily.[20] This advice went beyond physicians informing their peers; doctors also educated parents about the necessity of keeping their daughter's genitals clean. Richard Smith, a professor of pediatrics at Harvard Medical School, told parents in his 1921 book, *The Baby's First Two Years*, that a "lack of cleanliness" was perhaps a cause of masturbation.[21] This focus on cleanliness (or lack thereof) makes sense in the early twentieth century, when there was a strong emphasis from physicians and public health reformers for homes to be "antiseptically clean" to be clear of germs and to prevent disease; the performance of both household and personal cleanliness took on, as historian Nancy Tomes documented, a gospel-like adherence.[22]

In addition to bodily irritants on the clitoris, physicians also believed girls masturbated because of external irritations to the clitoris. Indeed, according to Wallace Abbott, "half the girls who masturbate would not do so were there no irritation of the clitoris," irritants that included "the heat of clothing or bedding."[23] G. Stanley Hall, in his 1905 two-volume study of adolescence, considered one of the causes of masturbation in children to be local irritants.[24] Speaking before the Federation of Child Study on February 18, 1915, A. A. Brill, a lecturer on psychoanalysis and abnormal physiology at New York University, stated, "Any external irritation of the genitals, such as pin worms or tight clothes, may bring about masturbation in children."[25] A girl would not touch her clitoris, in other words, unless she was prompted to do so because of an external irritant or an abnormality with the organ such as smegma or an adherent clitoral prepuce.

Physicians noted that, in the case of a masturbating child, they should pay attention to the physical state of the clitoris and correct it if the organ was in an unhealthy state. When the problem could be traced to an accumulation of smegma, which physicians like gynecologist William R. Pryor believed to be the cause of masturbation in children, then the smegma had to be removed.[26] Similarly, in his 1936 book New York City physician Louis Fischer instructed his peers as well as mothers and nurses to remove the "cheese-like deposit around the clitoris" to forestall masturbation in small children.[27]

Of particular concern to physicians, or at least of concern enough to warrant many printed references to it, were clitoral adhesions that could "bind down the prepuce so closely that no part" of the glans clitoridis could be seen.[28] A clitoris so bound down, New York physician Egbert H. Grandin believed, caused "neurosis."[29] Breaking up these adhesions was important not just to the immediate health of a child but also her future sexual health. In 1906, Alfred Cleveland Cotton, a professor of pediatrics at Rush medical school in Chicago, wrote that if an adherent clitoral prepuce persisted throughout a child's life, it would interfere with the circulation and result not just in masturbation habits of the child but also perhaps "result in hypererethism [abnormally acute sensitivity] with erotic tendencies, or in extreme sexual apathy in later life." As neither a strong sensitivity nor sexual apathy was considered healthy for women, Cotton recommended that physicians be alert for a tight prepuce in girls and remove adhesions under and loosen a tight prepuce to facilitate the "normal growth" of the organ.[30] Ten years later, in his textbook on the diseases of children, Philadelphia pediatrician Edwin E. Graham repeated this contention, writing that if an adherent prepuce in girls was "allowed to persist, the result will be hypererethism or sexual apathy in later life."[31]

Sidney Wilcox, a physician in New York City, described to the February 1906 meeting of the New York State Homeopathic Medical Society how to go about breaking up clitoral adhesions. Wilcox described the "ordinary method of separating the hood from the clitoris and then trying to prevent readhesions by tucking in bits of gauze, applying ointments, etc.," as "completely unsatisfactory." Instead, he recommended a new operation, though one he cautioned as being "very painful." Regardless of it being, as he wrote, "cruel" to perform on a "delicate little girl," he began by noting that adhesions should be broken up with a "blunt instrument—never a sharp one." Using a "piece of sterilized rubber tissue" backed with "a little roll of iodoform gauze" used to "prevent the suture cutting through the rubber tissue," he then held the hood of the clitoris with forceps while the needles are passed through the hood at the base of the gland, about one-third of an inch apart. The ends are then tied over a fold of gauze in a single bowknot. As the threads are pulled up the rubber tissue is drawn down between the clitoris and its hood, thus effectually separating them for as long a time as the operator thinks necessary. The smooth rubber is unirritating, and it does not stick to the tissues like glue, and allows the mucous membrane to return to a normal condition in which readhesion is not likely to occur.

The child, noted Wilcox, should "of course" be kept "quiet and the parts carefully cleansed." He recommended leaving the rubber in place for a week to ten days.[32]

Though not all physicians saw the therapeutic value in "loosening adhesions or freeing the clitoris," a practice New York physician Henry Koplik regarded in 1910 as "unwarranted," most physicians who discussed adhesions believed they merited breaking up.[33] In 1934, Wilburt Davison, a pediatrician at the Duke University School of Medicine, regarded an adherent prepuce, though rare, as an indication of masturbation, something relieved by the manual or surgical separation of the prepuce from the organ.[34] This belief existed throughout the course of the first half of the twentieth century: in 1927, William Palmer Lucas, a professor of pediatrics at the University of California, San Francisco, Medical School, recommended removing irritants in cases of masturbating children and the 1947 multivolume textbook *Therapeutics of Infancy and Childhood* recommended removing irritants such as adhesions of the clitoris.[35]

As with women patients, some physicians first tried the treatment of either removing the smegma or breaking up adhesions in girls. But, as in older patients, these two therapies at times did not work or did not work completely. Rowland Godfrey Freeman, a physician practicing at Bellevue Hospital in New York, noted in his 1917 *Elements of Pediatrics for Medical Students* that the impetus for masturbation was "adhesions of the prepuce to the clitoris and irritation of the enclosed smegma." Physicians should first "promptly" free the clitoris from smegma or adhesions, but in some cases adhesions "quickly re-form, unless a circumcision is done." According to Freeman, "All masturbating infants should, I believe, be put under anesthesia and be well circumcised by some surgeon accustomed to perform this operation."[36]

Others agreed with this protocol. E. C. Dudley, in his 1898, 1902, and 1908 gynecology texts, recommended circumcision for girls in cases where irritants could not be removed effectively.[37] Sidney Wilcox, the New York City physician who described his method of breaking up adhesions, stated at the end of his article that "the complete removal of the hood in many cases might be less bothersome and quite as satisfactory" in ending a child's masturbation.[38] In 1915, Charles Green, a Harvard Medical School professor of obstetrics and gynecology, published his account of a two-year-old girl who, while in "perfect health, . . . was observed several times a day to become quiet while at play, and lie or sit rubbing the thighs together for a time." Though the mother had attempted to end the habit, the child continued, and she took her child to see Green. Upon examination, the prepuce appeared "tightly adherent" to the clitoris and "somewhat enlarged and reddened." Breaking up the adhesions proved only partly successful, "and as the habit of thigh-rubbing persisted circumcision was advised." Following circumcision, the child stopped masturbating, according to Green's report.[39]

Not all physicians agreed with this progressively more interventionist therapy. W. J. Hawkes, a physician in Los Angeles, wrote an article in 1909 in "protest" of circumcision. He advocated and performed only the breaking up of adhesions. Indeed, Hawkes found it to be "almost criminal" to remove a clitoral hood. Nature, he wrote, put the hood there "for a good purpose, and nature usually knows what she is about."[40]

In addition to first trying the "milder" treatments of smegma removal and the breaking up of adhesions, some physicians initially recommended physical restraint of the child to prevent her from touching herself. To prevent masturbation, a child could be put in "braces" or a "knee crutch" to wear at night to prevent her from handling her genitals.[41] In addition, parents could purchase "preventative undergarments."[42] Some physicians, even those who did not believe in physical restraints for older children, still saw them as effective for infants and very young children; in a 1947 pediatric textbook, the age given for when mechanical restraints were no longer effective was three.[43] Parents were told to give mechanical restraints a few weeks or even months to see whether such devices ended the practice.[44] But while physicians may first have recommended physical restraints such as "elbow splints or separation of legs at night," if this did not work, then some physicians recommended circumcision to end masturbation, as J. P. Crozer Griffith and A. Graeme Mitchell did in the 1927 and 1934 editions of their pediatric textbook.[45] Similarly, in his 1942 book, Louis Sauer also advised that the removal of the clitoral hood was indicated if physical restraints failed.[46]

What Is Good for Boys Is Good for Girls

Mechanical restraints to stop a child from masturbating were not applied only to girls; boys also had devices placed upon their bodies to prevent their hands from going to their genitals. Similarly, a handful of medical practitioners extended the popular medical advice of routinely circumcising boys to girls. By the end of the nineteenth century, circumcision was advocated by some doctors as a standard preventive measure for all infant boys, with some even likening it to a vaccination against future problems, including masturbation, a measure they pressed upon parents.[47] By the early years of the twentieth century, circumcision for infant males moved toward becoming a standard practice in the United States; following World War II, at least half of all male infants were circumcised at birth.[48]

Some physicians noted the success of male circumcision and sought to extend the preventive benefits of early circumcision to female infants. "The value of circumcision in boys in many diseased conditions is very well known to most physicians," J. A. Burnett, a physician in Brawley, Arkansas, noted in 1903. "But strange to say the same operation on girls is sadly overlooked and almost wholly unknown to physicians."[49] Other doctors argued, as Burnett did, that both infant boys and girls should be circumcised as part of standard practice. In 1896 a Chicago physician, C. B. Walls, called the circumcision of both boys and girls as infants as "applying preventive medicine."[50] Another Chicago area doctor in 1900 contended that every obstetrician who failed to at least examine the clitoral foreskin, if not circumcise the organ, of infant girls "submits them in many cases to disease and nervous phenomena as a handicap to their physical and mental development at the very outset of their existence."[51] Robert T. Morris, a professor of surgery at the New York Post-Graduate Medical School, wrote in 1912 that girls "apparently require circumcision as often as boys do and for the same general reasons."[52] M. Margaret Hassler, a doctor in Pennsylvania, told members of the state's Homeopathic Medical Society in 1897 that it was their duty as physicians to "not only restore the lost, but to prevent the destruction and save our girls from the gradual invalidism to which so many are heirs to at puberty or soon thereafter" by removing the hood of the clitoris of their young female patients.[53]

Belle Eskridge of Houston agreed with the idea of circumcising all girls at birth, and in 1917 read a paper before the State Medical Association of Texas arguing for the necessity of circumcising both boys and girls as infants. Eskridge, a clinician at a children's home in Houston, circumcised all children in her care and found that girls responded to its effects more than boys. Describing female circumcision as "a very simple surgical procedure," she described her method to her fellow doctors. Separating the prepuce from the clitoris by gently pulling it with the thumb and index finger covered with gauze, the physician seized the prepuce with forceps and lifted it free from the clitoris. Then, using "a pair of sharp scissors," Eskridge described removing "a V-shaped piece, extending upward large enough to uncover the glans well back." According to Eskridge, "the skin and mucous membrane are then united as in the operation of the male." Finally, she covered the united edges with compound tincture benzoin and instructed the attending nurse to "keep it clean and pushed back twice a day until healed." While Eskridge did not consider circumcision for the female a "cure-all," she insisted that "the female genital organs should receive as careful attention at birth as those of the male-child."[54]

Benjamin Dawson, a physician practicing in Kansas City, MO, in the early twentieth century, similarly believed girls had been "sadly neglected." He felt compelled to make a plea on their behalf and "cry out against the shameful neglect of the clitoris and hood."[55] Likewise, Edwin Harley Pratt, a surgeon in Chicago, was a strong advocate for circumcising girls as well as boys at birth. Writing in 1898, Pratt stated that girls had been "neglected" and though they had "a hood corresponding to the foreskin of the male and just as sorely in need of attention, and just as prolific of mischief when neglected as the corresponding parts of the males, have been permitted to suffer on in silence." Girls, he argued, should have as "fair a start in life as the boys." He called on his fellow practitioners to let both sexes have an equal beginning in life and be "entirely freed from the sexual self-consciousness which inevitably comes from impinged terminal nerve fibres about the clitoris and its hood, as well as the glans penis and its foreskin."[56]

Many of those who advocated for preventive circumcision for infant boys and girls seem to have been associated with the American Association of Orificial Surgeons. Walls and Costain, for example, published their articles in the journal of this organization, and both Pratt and Dawson were members of this small group, which formed in 1888.[57] Orificial surgeons were largely nonregular practitioners such as homeopaths and eclectics; Benjamin Dawson, for instance, was president of the Eclectic Medical University. As nonregular practitioners in the early twentieth century, they were already on the fringes of medical practice in the United States and, indeed, were considered on the extreme by those who practiced homeopathy.[58] Membership in the association was never very large, and the group did not exist for long; in 1894 the association had just over two hundred members, and it existed formally only until the mid-1920s.[59] But regardless of their small membership, they were not unknown by regular medical practitioners, as evidenced by speech given by John F. W. Meagher, a neurologist, on October 3, 1922, before the Italian Medical Society of Brooklyn. Meagher called orificial practitioners members of a cult who practiced "quackery" and who were "especially dangerous to the health of women patients."[60]

Though physicians who associated themselves with the orificial society were on the extreme, their ideas regarding the condition of the clitoris and the sexual health of girls (who would someday grow to be women) were accepted beyond their membership. A central difference between those who advocated for routine circumcision and those who did not was an issue of scale; while it seems a small number of physicians advocated for routine female circumcision, it appears that more physicians, like William Easterly Ashton, believed in its limited and specific use. Ashton wrote in 1910 that a problematic clitoral foreskin, one he described as a "large, flabby, redundant prepuce" was only "occasionally met in children." But when doctors encountered such a condition, he recommended "excision of the redundant skin" to prevent the habit of masturbation.[61] So while some physicians recommended routine circumcision for girls, others who believed in the surgery thought it needed to be patient specific. This was particularly true when the therapy under consideration was clitoridectomy.

The Removal of a Child's External Organ

Though by far the most contentious of the four clitoral surgical therapies, with physicians like Harvard Medical School professor of pediatrics John Lovett Morse calling it in 1913 "absolutely unjustifiable," clitoridectomy was, as he also noted, still "sometimes recommended."[62] One of those who sometimes recommended the surgery was E. C. Dudley, who wrote that the operation of the "brilliant and blighted Baker Brown" had "very restricted" indications for use.[63]

Physicians in their published work seemed to reflect Dudley's opinion and indicate that the removal of the clitoris should be done only in extreme conditions, those where perhaps the other three therapies proved useless. In 1862, an "almost frantic" mother who wanted him to cure her daughter of masturbation approached E. S. Cooper, a professor of anatomy and surgery at the University of the Pacific in San Francisco. The mother of this thirteen-year-old had "abandoned all hope of saving her from a permanent residence in the Lunatic Asylum." The distraught mother "implored" Cooper to "do everything, to try every experiment that offered the least probability of cure." Cooper must have recommended clitoridectomy, for this is the therapy he noted the mother consented to having her daughter undergo.[64]

In a similar case in 1889, a woman in Indiana called upon J. A. Sutcliffe, a professor of surgery at the Central College of Physicians in Indianapolis, to treat her seven-year-old daughter. Sutcliffe called the girl "a bright, beautiful blonde," who "appeared to be in perfect health, with the exception of an intense morbid desire to manipulate the clitoris." The child caused her parents constant "distress." The mother prayed for her daughter's "recovery or her death, and begged that something be done, regardless of any risk, to save her child from a life of disgrace." Sutcliffe examined the child and decided nothing "short of removing the clitoris would be of any service."[65] Did Sutcliffe and Cooper first mention another treatment, perhaps one of the other clitoral surgeries? Or were both physicians convinced that of greater necessity was stopping a further decline in the child' health, and so the removal of the organ appeared as the best therapy to be provided? We do not know; regardless, the mother who took her daughter to Sutcliffe "cheerfully consented" to the removal of her daughter's clitoris, and he performed the operation.[66]

For these mothers, the removal of their daughters' clitoris was more important than correcting the organ and enabling its healthy functioning when their children were adults. As these cases attest, the choice between the unhealthy and abnormal behavior of masturbation and the removal of the clitoris was no choice at all for these parents; whether they "cheerfully" consented is, while perhaps telling (or perhaps an overstatement on the part of the attending physician), not as important as the fact that they consented to it at all. Parents, however, did not always agree with physicians about any of these treatments. In 1897, C. D. W. Colby, a physician in Jackson, Michigan, examined a seven-year-old "unusually precocious" girl who learned the "habit of vicious children" at a country house two years earlier. The parents tried to stop their child from masturbating by making her sleep in sheepskin pants and top, "with her hands tied to a collar about her neck" and feet "tied to the footboard" so that she could not "slide down in bed and use her heels." After trying this physical restraint, they took their child to Colby. On examination, Colby found the child's clitoris bound down with smegma and with a problematic clitoral hood. Colby must have suggested the removal of the child's clitoris, for he notes that the parents "objected to a clitoridectomy."[67] Though the parents obviously desired their daughter end her habit, they would not go so far as to accept the doctor's recommendation for the removal of one of her organs. This is the only case I found where a physician published the refusal of the patient or the patient's parents to a clitoral surgery.

The refusal of these parents and the consent of the mothers in the cases brought forth by Cooper and Sutcliffe illustrate the dialogue between physicians and parents concerning the use of clitoral surgeries. Regardless of what prompted the parents who initially sought Colby's care for their daughter to refuse consent, that the parents did object reveals that a dialogue between the parents and the physician occurred about both the medical problem of the child's masturbation and the proposed course of treatment. Similarly, the mother who "implored" Cooper also engaged with him in a dialogue about treatment possibilities—apparently any he could offer. The parents in all of these cases, like the physicians they went to for treatment of their daughters, accepted the idea that a condition of the clitoris lay at the basis of the inappropriate and unhealthy behavior. Though perhaps to modern readers the concept of a conversation between parents and physicians about whether to pursue clitoridectomy (or one of the other three surgeries) to cure masturbation seems appalling, this event illustrates—like Lizzie's desperate father who pushed Polak to operate in the story that began chapter 1—that parents negotiated for treatment they wanted.

The End of Clitoral Surgery to Treat Masturbation

In his 1910 book, *The Diseases of Infancy and Childhood, Designed for the Use of Students and Practitioners of Medicine*, New York physician Henry Koplik stated that the "operative treatment" on the clitoris for masturbation "seems to me unwarranted."[68] His opposition to such surgeries was probably not an isolated one, but while in the nineteenth and early twentieth centuries there were physicians who opposed surgeries to the clitoris as a treatment for masturbation, by the early twentieth century some physicians began noting that such treatments were on the decline or even absent from available therapies. In 1908, E. C. Dudley wrote that he believed the clinical use of clitoridectomy to be "almost obsolete."[69] In 1928, New York City surgeon Richard Walker Bolling asserted that while adhesions and smegma may result in an irritated clitoris, this was not the cause of masturbation and the "amputation of the prepuce of the clitoris is never indicated."[70] In his 1929 book on masturbation, neurologist John F. W. Meagher labeled "operations on the external genitals" of females as "apt to be harmful" and "condemned by most authorities."[71] In 1942, in his textbook *Pediatric Gynecology*, Goodrich Schauffler called clitoridectomy a "relic of barbarism" with no "legitimate indication short of malignant disease or irremediable trauma."[72] And Lyman Mason of the University of Colorado School of Medicine, argued in 1933 that "much harm had been done in the past" by operations such as circumcision and clitoridectomy, "for such indications as masturbation and other complaints which are dependent more upon mental factors than upon anatomical states."[73]

The decline in the use of two of the surgeries—breaking up of clitoral adhesions and female circumcision—to treat masturbation in children can be seen by following their presence in one of the standard pediatric textbooks of the early twentieth century, L. Emmett Holt's *Diseases of Infancy and Childhood*. In the fourth edition, published in 1908, Holt noted that physicians sometimes saw improvement in girls "if a dorsal slit is made in the prepuce" of the clitoris following the separation of the hood from the clitoris under anesthesia. If this, however, did not prevent adhesions from reforming, "complete circumcision is sometimes done with advantage, and in very obstinate cases the clitoris can be cauterized." This advice, with the exception of the dorsal slit recommendation, was repeated in the seventh edition of the text, published in 1916. By the tenth edition in 1933, however, Holt first recommended breaking up adhesions and then, with seeming hesitation, noted that "even circumcision or cauterization of the clitoris have all been tried, but as a rule which has exceptions these measures accomplish little." By the 1940 edition, a revised edition now authored by L. Emmett Holt Jr., clitoral adhesions are no longer "regarded as causes per se" of masturbation and "circumcision should not be performed except for the usual indications," indications Holt Jr. does not provide. Circumcision, however, as a "psychotherapeutic procedure is contra indicted."[74]

These changes in the advice regarding the therapy of female circumcision and the removal of clitoral adhesions were in response to changes in medical understandings about masturbation and about how the body functioned. By the late nineteenth century, the reflex theory began to wane, and by 1900 it was no longer accepted as a dominant medical model of nervous disease. A growing disbelief among medical practitioners as well as the expanding science of physiology, including the discovery of the endocrine system, led to a decline in the reflex theory, thus eliminating one of the reasons for performing these procedures.[75]

Additionally, the idea that masturbation was a health problem that directly led to insanity began to lessen. In her 1919 book aimed at educating young people about sex, Mary Ware Dennett told her readers that though "for generations this habit has been considered wrong and dangerous," scientists now believed the "chief harm has come from the worry caused by" masturbation, not the act itself.[76] Historian R. P. Neuman argued the decline occurred in part because doctors increasingly found it difficult to accept at face value "the notion that mental 'illnesses' like masturbatory insanity were directly linked to physical causes." He put the climax of such beliefs before the First World War.[77] And historian Thomas Laqueur contended that the concerns over the health implications of masturbation declined because a wide range of disciplines, from anthropology to zoology, found masturbation was nearly universal among the young. Psychologists provided these observations with psychological significance, with the father of psychoanalysis Sigmund Freud arguing that masturbation formed the basis of sexual expression.[78]

Certainly the public stance of the professions of medicine and psychology accepted this view of masturbation, as reflected in some pediatric textbooks. In the 1940 edition of Holt's *Diseases of Infancy and Childhood*, for example, masturbation was regarded as common and no longer considered harmful, so long as it did not preoccupy the child.[79] Similarly, a 1945 pediatric textbook stated that the only harm from masturbation was from the "guilt" it induced.[80] And in 1942, pediatrician Goodrich Schauffler said it was "fortunate that the trends of intelligent opinion is definitely away from the deep concern which was formerly felt in relation to masturbation, except in exaggerated instances."[81] Physicians communicated such information to parents. For example, best-selling author and pediatrician Benjamin Spock soothed worried parents' fears over the practice by telling them in his 1945 book, *The Common Sense Book of Baby and Child Care*, that a mild early interest in sex was natural; curious children touched themselves.[82]

It is, however, the latter part of Schauffler's sentence quoted above that is worth paying more attention to, for while this Portland, Oregon, pediatrician applauded the reconsideration of masturbation, he also removed clitoral hoods of girls for this very indication. In his 1942 *Pediatric Gynecology*, Schauffler first advocated breaking up adhesions when the foreskin was adherent, but he also advised circumcision as a "more permanent" solution

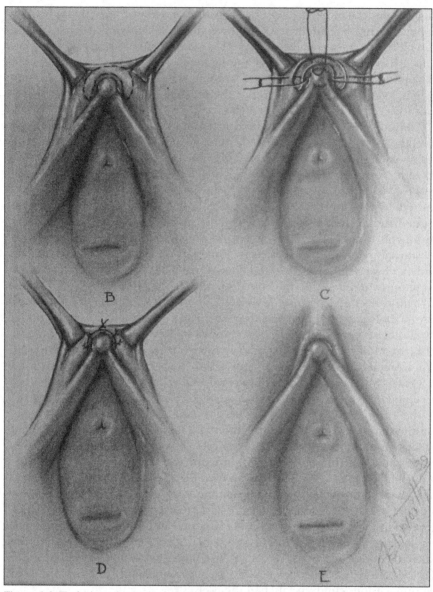

Figure 1.1. Technique for performing female circumcision, frontal view. Image caption reads: "*B*, foreskin retracted, incision outlined; *C*, sutures in place—mattress in midline; *D*, sutures tied; *E*, correct plastic result." Goodrich C. Schauffler, *Pediatric Gynecology* (Chicago: Year Book, 1942), 54. Reproduced with permission from Elsevier.

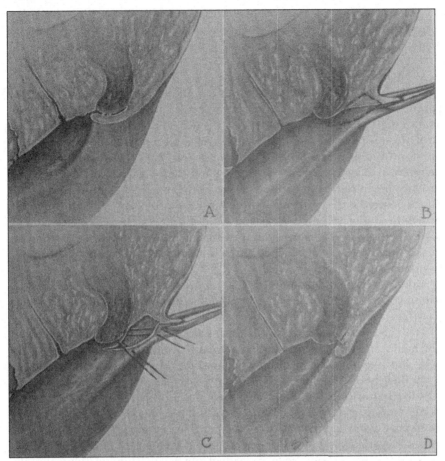

Figure 1.2. Technique for performing female circumcision, side view. Image caption reads: "*A*, redundant, adherent foreskin in situ; *B*, foreskin retracted, wedge incision outlined; *C*, sutures in place; *D*, sutures tied—immediate plastic result." Goodrich C. Schauffler, *Pediatric Gynecology* (Chicago: Year Book, 1942), 55. Reproduced with permission from Elsevier.

if breaking up adhesions failed. Schauffler disagreed with those who thought the procedure not necessary; indeed, he believed that in girls afflicted with repeated bouts of trapped smegma and an adherent prepuce that produce itching and attracts "the child's attention to her genitalia," circumcision often helped. But he also warned that it was not a cure-all—that circumcision was only "helpful" in cases where the cause lay in the irritated organ and that some placed too much optimism in the operation.[83]

Others similarly were mixed in their assessment on the use of clitoral surgeries to treat masturbation; in the 1945 text I cited just before Schauffler's, the *Textbook of Pediatrics*, the authors recommended circumcision for girls, though noting it was rarely indicated.[84] Similarly, Waldo Nelson, a professor of pediatrics at the Temple University School of Medicine, noted in 1945 that "rarely circumcision of clitoris may be indicated" to treat masturbation.[85] What constituted such an indication? Parents.

Though in both the medical literature and in standard texts written for parents by physicians such as Benjamin Spock masturbation was described as no longer a medical concern, the practice still troubled parents. In an effort to illustrate the ways parents worried too much over masturbation, Spock provided an example: in his *Common Sense Book of Baby and Child Care*, he referred to an adolescent boy whose parents were so worried he may masturbate they hired a companion to stay with him around the clock. This, Spock pointed out, only provided the boy with a constant reminder of masturbation "and gave him a monstrous fear of it."[86] Parents, then, continued to fear the effects of masturbation on their children's current and future health well after masturbatory insanity stopped being an acceptable diagnosis in mainstream medicine.

Moreover, while medicine in the larger sense stopped regarding masturbation as a medical problem necessitating intervention, some individual physicians continued to regard the practice as unhealthy. In a 1959 survey of graduates and faculty at five medical schools in Philadelphia, for example, half of the students believed masturbation frequently caused mental illness, and one in five of the faulty believed so.[87] Indeed, though Goodrich Schauffler noted that he was "often embarrassed by lay acceptance" of female circumcision as a treatment, "such misinformation" remained "prevalent" among gynecologists "out of touch with medical progress." Such physicians made "poorly worded statements" to parents.[88] So the medical profession's disavowal of the connection between masturbation and insanity does not necessarily mean individual physicians stopped removing all or part of a girl's clitoris to appease a concerned parent. Schauffler related such a case in 1927 when a mother persuaded a fellow physician to "excise the clitoris" of her child to stop her daughter from masturbating—masturbating that had been brought on, the physician believed, by irritation from the mother cleaning the child's genitals three times a day.[89]

By the 1930s and increasingly in the 1940s, physicians writing in pediatric textbooks noted the problem of masturbation was really a problem of educating parents about the practice's lack of health implications. "Parents," wrote Abraham Levinson, a Northwestern University professor of pediatrics, "are usually unduly alarmed over the pernicious effects of this habit."[90] Indeed, pediatrician L. Emmett Holt Jr. labeled masturbation as "the most common sex complaint for which the physician is consulted."[91] Though physicians were telling parents that masturbation was common and that the "usual symptoms of neurosis, hysteria, mental deficiency, and sexual perversions supposed to be due to masturbation are more cause than effect," they also informed parents that the children most likely to masturbate were "mentally defective or neurotic," according to a 1947 pediatric textbook.[92] A 1945 textbook listed masturbation as only a problem when the habit was "excessive." However, the textbook also said that masturbation might indicate a "marked neurotic disposition" or "feeblemindedness" that resulted in a "predisposing cause" of the common habit of masturbation; it was then that "it becomes a matter of serious consequence." Additionally, the text listed nymphomania as a result, not a cause, of masturbation.[93] But nymphomania—excessive sexuality—was also a socially problematic behavior, outside the parameters of healthy adult behavior and definitely those of a child. While stating that there was "no evidence of harm from masturbation," L. Emmett Holt Jr. noted that "it is surprising to what lengths parents will go to force a child to stop it at once."[94] Perhaps this should not be surprising; confronted with such confusing information, fearful parents no doubt wondered what "excessive" masturbation meant, and whether their daughter was merely engaging in a "common" practice or whether her masturbation indicated something more alarming, that their daughter was "mentally defective," "neurotic," or destined to be a nymphomaniac. Parents perhaps, then, cannot be blamed for their confusion and resultant alarm.

Nor should they be blamed for seeking medical attention. Although many physicians by the 1930s began calling masturbation common in children, even in infants, it was still something that some believed should and could be "cured," often by "raising the health mentally and physically" of the girl but also by "removing local irritants," according to a 1954 pediatric textbook.[95] Much easier, perhaps, and more immediate for parents to push physicians to try an interventionist "cure."

When clitoral surgeries as a treatment for masturbation began appearing in medical publications in the United States in the mid-nineteenth century, American medicine was undergoing profound changes: changes in therapeutics; changes in the perceived power of medicine and in the power of medical authority; changes in treatment with the rise of surgery; and changes in the profession of medicine with the rise of specialization, in particular here gynecology and pediatrics. With all of this came an interest in surgically treating the female body and in publishing about such treatment. By the early twentieth century, the surgeries had become routine—not routine in the manner advocated by those who believed all female infants should be circumcised but routine in the sense they apparently no longer merited having a published conversation about them. Neither the surgeries nor their results were novel; they were, instead, procedures quickly performed in a clinician's office. What I am suggesting, then, is that though after the early twentieth century the surgeries became less worthy of journal publication, they did not become less worthy of use—hence why they continued to be mentioned in pediatric and gynecology textbooks. Their continued existence in medical textbooks hints that clitoral surgeries had become accepted and normalized into clinical practice.[96]

How accepted and normalized? One man, whose mother lost her clitoris when she was five in 1916 as a treatment for masturbation, recalled that during a conversation in the 1950s with a "second-generation gynecologist then in his eighties," he was told that the practice of clitoridectomy and female circumcision "had been a lucrative industry in the United States from 1867 until at least 1927, and possibly much later—a thriving business few people spoke about afterward."[97] In a 2000 article in *Ms.* magazine, a woman interviewed stated she had lost her clitoris in 1944 when a child as treatment for masturbation.[98] Patricia Robinett wrote about her struggles to understand why she had had her clitoris removed when she was seven in the 1950s, reasons she was sure concerned masturbation.[99] The handful of published articles documenting physicians' experiences with clitoral surgeries as treatment for masturbation that appeared after 1950 indicate that such surgeries remained a treatment option for some: in 1958, C. F. McDonald recounted how he removed the clitoral prepuce to stop girls from masturbating; LeMon Clark noted how he removed the hood of a five-year-old girl's clitoris to stop her from masturbating in 1963; and Warren Johnson, a professor of health education at the University of Maryland, in 1963 advised two women students of his to ignore the advice given by another physician who suggested removing the clitoris of their daughters to stop them from masturbating.[100] Finally, as late as 1995, the Council for Scientific Affairs for the American Medical Association noted that, "currently, clitoridectomies of US women and girls are infrequent, but in rare instances they are inappropriately prescribed as treatment for controlling masturbation."[101] Regarded as inappropriate therapy or not, both the anecdotes and the published accounts by physicians provide a hint that some physicians remained willing to remove smegma, break up clitoral adhesions, or perform female circumcision or clitoridectomy to alleviate parental concerns over masturbation— or perhaps because individual physicians, too, still considered masturbation problematic for girls, long after medical beliefs about the practice's damaging health effects had been abandoned.

Chapter Three

Female Sexual Degeneracy and the Enlarged Clitoris, 1850–1941

In a 1921 article discussing sexual "degenerates," Perry M. Lichtenstein, a physician with the New York City prison system, noted that "both white and colored women indulge in the practice" of obtaining "sexual satisfaction from association with other females." Lichtenstein noted that, upon examining such women, "in practically every instance" one would find "an abnormally prominent clitoris, . . . particularly so in colored women."[1] While according to Lichtenstein an atypically large clitoris was common in women who had sex with other women regardless of race, his belief that this was especially true of women of color was based not just on their sexual relationships with other women: as E. Heinrich Kisch wrote in his 1910 book, *The Sexual Life of Woman*, the "congenital enlargement of the clitoris" was commonly found to exist in "certain African races" to such a degree the organ was "an obstacle to coitus" with men.[2] African American women, according to some American medical authorities, were inherently hypersexual, with the physical evidence found in their supposedly enlarged clitorises.

Physicians recognized the clitoris as homologous to the penis. Therefore, as Margaret Gibson pointed out in her essay on medical constructions of female homosexuality in the late nineteenth century, if the penis and clitoris were mostly differentiated by size, an enlarged clitoris illustrated sexual activity and thus masculinity to physicians.[3] It illustrated, then, a feminine body that was other than a normative feminine body, for a woman who possessed a clitoris deemed overly large was labeled by many medical practitioners as acting in ways that were, if not masculine, at the very least as not appropriately feminine. Women who had sex with other women or women who were overly sexually active with men or with themselves were often regarded as hypersexual. And some physicians looked for physiological manifestations of these nonnormative sexual behaviors by looking at the size of the clitoris. But though many physicians believed all women's bodies held evidence of their nonnormative sexual behaviors in the form of an enlarged clitoris, it was in particular women of color and lesbians regardless of color who were most often regarded as inherently hypersexual. They were often seen as inherently sexually nonnormative, degenerate, or sexually underdeveloped, beliefs that were reflected in the perception that these women "commonly" had an enlarged clitoris.

In an era when the body was believed to reveal behaviors as well as character traits, some looked to the clitoris as an area for revelation. Beliefs that nonnormative bodies showed signs of difference and inferiority from "normal" (white, heterosexual) bodies were fairly well accepted in medicine during the second half of the nineteenth century. Using vital statistics, many physicians sought to support ideas about the inferiority of African Americans by reading for marked differences between white and black bodies.[4] But such beliefs also held sway in the social sciences such as anthropology and criminology. Cesare Lombroso, an Italian criminal anthropologist, examined female offenders' bodies for signs (including clitoral measurements) that would differentiate them from normal women.[5] Lombroso's anthropometric measurements, designed to calibrate character traits through body measurements, were adopted by others, including Alphonse Bertillon, a Paris police official, who developed eleven anthropometric measurements to be used to identify criminals.[6] Others measured the ears and facial contours of those labeled as perverts in an effort to identify the traits of deviants.[7]

Lombroso was not the only one, however, who read the size of the clitoris as marking women outside norms of femininity. The state of the clitoris— its size, color, whether it appeared swollen—apparently was regarded as evidence for some doctors of the practice of nonnormative sexual behavior.[8] Like a red clitoris, the enlarged clitoris also indicated sexual deviancy, be it masturbation or homosexuality, the first often seen as a precursor to the second, and both regarded as forms of hypersexuality in women. Though this chapter concerns clitorises that were regarded as atypically large, it will not address those who were labeled hermaphrodites.[9] Instead, I concentrate on how some physicians read the body for physiological signs to help them differentiate "normal" female bodies and feminine sexual behavior from "degenerate" female bodies and behavior. Physicians' efforts to demarcate female bodies through bodily signs, however, also revealed those very demarcations as being fluid, unstable, and ultimately unreliable.[10]

Size as an Indicator of Self-Abuse

As seen in the first two chapters, the condition of the clitoris "revealed" to physicians examining it the sexual practices of the female to whom it was attached, even if the woman or girl being examined denied the sexual practice. In the case of masturbation, this physical evidence often included a reddened or engorged clitoris, but it also could include an enlarged organ. In 1884, William Goodell, a professor of gynecology at the University of

Pennsylvania, claimed that "evidences of masturbation" included redness and enlargement of the clitoris.[11] The physical condition of the clitoris was often a telltale sign for physicians in determining whether masturbation lay behind the patient's health problems, and an inflamed clitoris even had various terms. In the 1854 edition of *Medical Lexicon: A Dictionary of Medical Science,* "clitorism" was defined as "a word, invented to express the abuse made of the clitoris" as well as an "unusually large clitoris."[12] Appearing in the 1900 edition, the word's meaning became more explicit, and in addition to repeating that the word meant "an unusually large clitoris," the dictionary further stated that "clitorism" meant "the abuse made of the clitoris to satisfy an unnatural sexual desire."[13] Similarly, the 1897 *Lippincott's Medical Dictionary* defined "clitorism" as a "morbid enlargement of the clitoris."[14]

Thus, doctors considered an enlarged clitoris as both a sign and a result of abnormal sexual behavior. Upon examination, a sixteen-year-old girl with an "enlargement of the nymphae and clitoris" reportedly "confessed" to having "been in the habit of self-pollution almost daily for six months," resulting in enlarged genitals, according to this 1842 case report.[15] W. Penn Buck, a Philadelphia physician, reported in the early 1870s of a case from London where the "elephantine development of the clitoris" was the "result of masturbation."[16] Physicians George Gould and Walter Pyle noted in 1897 that self-abuse "brought on" the enlarged clitoris of a masturbating patient.[17] H. E. Beebe told fellow doctors at a Homeopathic Medical Society of Ohio meeting in the spring of 1897 that both the clitoris and the labia were often hypertrophied by masturbation.[18] Indeed, as late as it 1959 edition, the *Mitchell-Nelson Textbook of Pediatrics* noted that manifestations of extreme cases of masturbation could be a larger than normal clitoris and labia.[19]

But though some doctors believed masturbation led to enlargement, others thought it was the reverse: a large clitoris prompted a woman to engage in masturbation. Horatio Bigelow noted that one of the reasons for masturbation among women was the irritation of an "elongated clitoris."[20] Samuel Ashwell said so in 1855, noting he had seen a clitoris as large as four inches.[21] Whether the clitoris prompted or resulted from masturbation, however, an enlarged clitoris informed the examining physician that the patient engaged in the practice. An 1841 case of a twenty-nine-year-old farmer's daughter suspected of nymphomania was confirmed to the doctor by the revelation she had an eight-inch long clitoris.[22] In 1905, Robert Taylor wrote of a case of "enormous hypertrophy of the clitoris," describing the organ at its base "as large as a small male index finger" and "fully three inches in length." Taylor, a retired professor of genitourinary diseases at Columbia University's College of Physicians and Surgeons in New York, believed that the "great enlargement of the clitoris" was a direct result of masturbating. The degree of hypertrophy depended, according to the doctor, "on how long the manipulation is practiced, how often, and over how long a time the patient has been addicted to the vice."[23] Joseph Howe agreed. In his 1883 book, the doctor stated that the "local changes in the female genital organs always demonstrate plainly enough the results of masturbation, even when the patient denies the habit," because the clitoris looked elongated and "thicker than in health."[24] In his 1886 treatise against masturbation, a practice he called a "loathsome ulcer," physician and later cereal baron J. H. Kellogg warned that continued masturbation led to "marked hypertrophy" of the clitoris.[25]

Not all physicians shared in the idea that an enlarged clitoris was a sign of masturbation. W. B. Platt wrote in 1885 that the belief that masturbation enlarged the clitoris was "quite unfounded."[26] Alfred Lewis Gallabin wrote in 1882 that "hypertrophy of the clitoris" was "not usually connected to masturbation."[27] F. Winckel, whose book was translated from the German and published in the United States in 1887, called the belief that masturbation caused hypertrophy in women a "mistake," since this did not happen in men who masturbated.[28] And Robert Latou Dickinson, a New York gynecologist, wrote in a paper published in 1902 that though a patient claimed her clitoris "began to grow large at 14, when she was given to much rubbing," he thought that while "it may have been developed in this way," it seemed to him "far more probable" that the clitoris was "congenitally large."[29]

Moreover, many physicians did not regard every case of an enlarged clitoris as evidence of sexually abnormal behavior, for in some cases the enlarged organ was seen as a result of syphilis, a cyst, or a tumor.[30] Forty-three-year-old Martha M., for example, was seen for "hypertrophy of the clitoris." Married with four children, she had contracted syphilis seven years prior, though the attending physician was uncertain whether the syphilis had caused the hypertrophy.[31] When the problem was suspected as a result of syphilis or a tumor, physicians readily recommended removal of the organ, for fear of the suspected cause of the enlargement spreading.[32]

Removal of the clitoris was also considered when masturbation was regarded as the etiology of the enlarged organ, though this treatment option, like its diagnosis, was not unanimously held as appropriate. In 1896, John Keating wrote that though the clitoris could become enlarged by masturbation, he called the amputation of the organ to stop the practice a "discredit to gynecology."[33] Similarly, E. C. Dudley, a gynecology professor at Northwestern University, wrote in his 1908 text that though "acquired enlargement is associated usually with masturbation," excision of the clitoris "unfortunately . . . usually" failed to "put an end to the habit."[34]

Though Dudley may have been inclined to remove the atypical organ, he saw no benefit in doing so; he did not see masturbation ceasing as a result. Others, however, were not so opposed as Keating to amputation of an enlarged clitoris as a means to end the habit. When a patient's clitoris was considerably enlarged and when the typically reliable and efficient treatment of "cooling ablutions and a non-stimulating diet" failed, A. L. Clark in 1881 wrote that amputation of the clitoris "often [produced] beneficial results."[35] J. William Ballantyne told his fellow doctors when encountering a large clitoris brought on by masturbation, "it may be necessary to amputate the clitoris."[36] In 1891, doctors removed the clitoris of a married woman because it interfered with coitus; part of the diagnosis and reason for its removal was that it was regarded as overly large.[37] Thomas More Madden wrote that when an overly large clitoris caused "erotic troubles" it should be removed. Such cases, however, Madden believed to be "very rare, and in the course of a tolerably long experience I have only once found it necessary to amputate a clitoris for this reason."[38] Physicians who advocated for the removal of an enlarged clitoris, at least as revealed in their published medical documents, did so on a case-by-case basis, and such cases, according to Madden, rare.

Normative Clitoral Size

The labeling of a clitoris as "overly large" or even as "enormous" means there must have been awareness of a "normal" size. In their descriptions of the clitoris, physicians only sometimes mentioned size. Actual measurements physicians gave for a normal clitoris varied from the late nineteenth through the mid-twentieth centuries. For example, in his 1938 *Textbook of Gynecology*, Arthur Hale Curtis stated that "the body of the clitoris," meaning the external visible portion, measured from "2 to 3 cm. in length."[39] A measurement of two centimeters was given in the 1934 *Introduction of Gynecology*.[40] Other texts gave more descriptive rather than numerical measurements: an 1883 text labeled the organ as a "miniature penis," and two texts published in 1944 simply described the size as "small."[41] But though some physicians and gynecology texts noted that there was a normal size for the clitoris, a precise size was not important for all gynecologists; Lawson Tait, in his 1879 *Diseases of Women*, wrote that the "size of this organ varies very much, for in some women it is represented only by a depression in the anterior commissure, whilst in a few it is found to be really erectile, and representing in miniature the appearance of a penis."[42] In the 1919 *Guide to Gynecology in General Practice*, the authors noted that the "size of the labia and the clitoris varies within normal limits."[43] And in an article published in 1902, E. H. Smith stressed the diversity of size for female genitals; indeed, Smith stated that there was "as much variation in the normal appearance of the genitals as there is in the normal mouth, nose, or eyes."[44]

One of the most prolific chroniclers of female genitals was gynecologist Robert Latou Dickinson, who appears to have been motivated to do so for what he termed the "missing facts" about "exact genital measurements" of women.[45] Dickinson, a practicing gynecologist in the late nineteenth through early twentieth centuries, made hundreds of drawings of his patients' genitals.[46] But his concern with obtaining "exact measurements" did not mean that the New York City gynecologist failed to note how women's genitals varied in sizes and in shapes. In a speech he gave before the AMA's Section on Obstetrics, Gynecology, and Abdominal Surgery in 1925 and published later that year in *JAMA*, Dickinson estimated that 75 percent of women fell within a normal size range: their clitoris measured between 2.5 and 6.5 millimeters. Five percent of women, according to Dickinson, had small clitorises, measuring between 1 and 2.5 millimeters, while twenty per cent of women had large organs, measuring between 6.5 and 15 millimeters.[47] Twenty-four years later, in his *Human Sex Anatomy*, Dickinson wrote that, based on his studies, the "clitoris varies considerably" in size. Dickinson delineated these sizes with the following groupings: "*intersex, large, average* or normal, and *small.*"[48]

According to Dickinson, "anatomists are loose in their statements" regarding "what constituted a normal or average clitoris." As listed by Dickinson, various anatomists measured the average clitoris as between 5.6 to 8 millimeters, although Dickinson considered 4 millimeters the most common size.[49] A few anatomy texts gave approximation on the typical size of the organ, with the 1939 text, *Gross Anatomy*, noting the organ was "frequently about one inch in length," though this text also noted that the clitoris was "variable in size."[50] Sometimes, however, all that was noted in reference to size was that the organ was "small," the manner in which it was labeled, for example, in the 1893 edition of *Gray's Anatomy, Descriptive and Surgical* and the 1909 *Anatomy and Physiology of the Female Generative Organs and of Pregnancy*.[51] The size of the clitoris was also referred to frequently as "miniature" compared to the penis in anatomy texts.[52]

Warm Climates, Large Genitals

Returning to Gibson's question, what did it mean to medical practitioners when women had a clitoris above the range of typical variation? In some women, an enlarged clitoris was perceived by certain physicians not as a sign of masturbation but as physiological evidence of an inherent sexual difference between them and normal women. This was true for three types of women. First were women whom physician William Tod Helmuth described in 1876 as having "small breasts and muscular development," those who may (or may not) be considered to have congenital differences of sex development today.[53] Second were women who had sex with other women. And third were African American women or women from "warm climates."

During the nineteenth and into the early twentieth century, gynecology texts occasionally noted the seeming prevalence of enlarged clitorises among women from warm or tropical climates—terms used by imperial countries to differentiate European and other parts of the temperate world from culturally alien parts of the world.[54] An enlarged clitoris, William P. Dewees, a professor of midwifery at the University of Pennsylvania, noted in his 1831 book, "occurs most frequently in hot climates."[55] A gynecology text from 1881 stated that "excessive enlargements of the clitoris are most common in warm climates."[56] Another doctor noted in 1887 that a hypertrophied clitoris was "larger in the tropics than in the northern and temperate latitudes."[57] Northwestern University professor of gynecology E. C. Dudley noted in his 1908 text, *The Principles and Practice of Gynecology*, that he believed an enlarged clitoris and labia occurred "more frequently in the tropics than in temperate zones."[58] Johns Hopkins University gynecologist Howard A. Kelly and Women's Medical College gynecologist Charles P. Noble in their 1907 gynecology text wrote that hypertrophied clitorises were "rare in temperate climates," implying such clitoral sizes were not rare in tropical ones.[59] British physician John Knott, writing in the *Medical Press and Circular* in 1890, noted that a "degree of hypertrophy of the clitoris" had been observed "among the female inhabitants of tropical climates." Indeed, Knott wrote, "the general rule appears to be that the clitoris is much more prominent and highly developed among the females of inter-tropical climes than with those of the extra-tropical."[60] And in 1906 physician J. Wesley Bovee noted that in prostitutes, "and in some savage races," a large clitoris was often found. Bovee believed that "perversion and excessive coitus" were probably directly related, "though this statement is by no means a fact, but rather a logical deduction."[61] Geography mattered when differentiating female bodies.[62]

What, then, if anything, did physicians recommend by way of treating the enlarged clitoris among women from tropical climates? W. Penn Buck, a physician in Philadelphia, quoting from a surgical text in his 1872 essay, noted that hypertrophy of the clitoris, sometimes congenitally acquired, often reached "immense" size in women from "Persia, Turkey, and Egypt." The immense clitoris, he continued, was "generally caused by protracted irritation." Whether congenital or acquired, when the clitoris attained "a large bulk, the only remedy is excision."[63] E. C. Dudley, like Buck, believed that congenital enlargement of the clitoris occurred more frequently "in the tropics than in temperate zones." Such a clitoris, he then argued, was "an indication for removal (clitoridectomy)."[64] J. Wesley Bovee further agreed, stating that although an enlarged clitoris "usually causes no trouble," should the organ "prevent coitus or become irritated, or the seat of inflammation, as is frequent from friction against clothing, amputation or resection may become imperative."[65]

Of the handful of physicians who made the brief comments regarding the genital size of women from warmer climates, few then spoke of treatment suggestions to ameliorate it. Perhaps this was because women from tropical climates—in particular women of African heritage—were seen as inherently hypersexual. In that sense, both noting the supposed commonality of the enlarged clitoris in women of color and its treatment are almost throw-away comments, made simply to point out, and reinforce, gender and racial hierarchies among women. As with a white woman presenting for masturbation, if the etiology of the condition was found in the mind, removal of the clitoris was seen as having no discernible benefit. So perhaps the removal of all or part of the clitoris did not make therapeutic sense, either, for treating "inherently" hypersexual black women.

Evolution and the Clitoris

In his 1895 article, "Is Evolution Trying to Do Away with the Clitoris?" gynecologist Robert T. Morris hypothesized that the clitoris was larger among women in tropical climates while disappearing from civilized (meaning white, middle-class) women. Working from his observation of three hundred patients over the course of a year, Morris wrote that about 80 percent of "Aryan-American women" possessed preputial adhesions to such a degree that the adhesions bound the clitoris down so closely "that no part of the *glans clitoridis* is in sight." Ten "negresses" were among the women he examined, three of whom also had such adhesions, a trait Morris attributed to the likelihood that these three women "possessed an admixture of Caucasian blood."[66]

Morris and others in the nineteenth and early twentieth centuries believed that women of African heritage were uncivilized, primordial, even savage. And they perceived this savagery as written on their bodies via the size of their clitoris: as an 1896 gynecology text stated, "The clitoris is found hypertrophied in certain savage races."[67] Though such ideas certainly did not begin in the nineteenth century, it was during the nineteenth century that anatomical measurements between whites and blacks became a central method of differentiating, and arranging in a hierarchy, races; everything from skin color to hair to skull and genital sizes were measured to distinguish and determine racial types. For example, Rudolph Matas, a physician in New Orleans, stressed in the 1890s that "in addition to the differences" recognizable to the "most careless observer" between "typical individuals of the white and negro race" there were also "numerous characteristics" distinguishing "the negro from other races, which to the comparative anatomist, anthropologist, the evolutionist, and philosopher are profoundly interesting and significant."[68] These distinctions were commonly accepted among physicians through the end of the nineteenth century, according to historian John Haller Jr. Given the need to legitimize slavery, and later in the nineteenth century discrimination, the black body was theorized to be less developed and closer to animals, a distinction that then lead to presumptions about sexual behavior, intelligence, and even genital anatomy.[69] Commonly held racial myths of inferiority were buttressed by misrepresentations and distortions of evolutionary theory.[70]

As part of the larger acceptance of anthropometric measurements during this time, nonnormative sexual behavior was seen as inscribed upon "uncivilized" bodies in the form of exaggerated physical features, including and in particular enlarged genitals, in both men and women.[71] According to Haller, there was a "certain morbidness" in how American physicians emphasized African Americans' sexual behaviors, an emphasis reflected in medical interest in genital size. Physicians accepted as true that the penis of an average African American male was larger than a penis of an average white male, Haller argued.[72] Sexuality labeled as deviant was symbolized and represented through large genitals. According to a 1903 editorial in the *Atlanta Journal-Record of Medicine*, "Among the many points of difference that exist in the physical make-up of the white and black types of mankind, there are none so striking than those presented by the reproductive organs, especially those of the male." In particular, the editors wrote, it was "natural" for the penis to attain "excessive development," and "even before the age of puberty" a black boy's penis was "noted to exceed in size that of an average white man's."[73] But while the large penis racially differentiated black from white men and signified both hypersexuality and danger, as historian Paula Giddings argued, the codification of black male deviance was primarily linked to hypersexual black women. Just as white women were culturally seen as the foundation for white morality, black women were culturally seen as the foundation of black morality; if black women were presumed to be hypersexual (and by implication immoral), so were black men.[74] If "civilized" white women had sexed bodies, "savage" black women were differentiated by having hypersexed bodies.

European and American myths about African female hypersexuality, as theorist Beverly Guy-Sheftall noted, began with the implementation of slavery by whites on that continent, followed the women to America, and helped to justify their sexual exploitation both during slavery and after emancipation.[75] For example, in his study of the "anthropometric characteristics of the colored race as compared with the whites," Frederick Hoffman in 1896 found an "immense amount of prostitution" among African American women in American cities, a finding he regarded as supporting his belief that African American women had more frequent sexual relations outside of marriage.[76] Following emancipation, white men used rape, legal scholar Dorothy Roberts argued, as a method of ensuring white supremacy. The rape of a black woman rarely resulted in prosecution, because white authorities failed to see sexual assault as harmful because of her presumed hypersexuality. "Black women's sexual impropriety was contrasted with white women's sexual purity," according to Roberts; "while white wives were placed on pedestals of spotless morality, all black women were, by definition, whores." Though white women were affected by sexism and racism, Roberts asserted, they were not seen as "*inherently* licentious."[77] Recent work by Cynthia Greenlee-Donnell found similar rates of legal charges brought against white and black men for raping white and black girls in South Carolina in the late nineteenth and early twentieth centuries, which complicates this narrative, raising the interesting question of there perhaps being an age when this supposed inherent hypersexual trait began.[78] I will return to such a tension when I explore the disconnect between larger cultural perceptions and clinical assessment shortly, but for now I note that, on the larger cultural level, just as in the explicit (supposed) differentiation between the clitorises of white and black women, this (perceived) differentiation between the sexual behavior of European-heritage women and African-heritage women served to demarcate acceptable sexual behavior. And presumptions of nonnormative, hypersexual behavior of African American women were thought by some medical authorities to be inscribed on the body.

Contemporary feminist critique of the representation of the black female body within both medicine and culture as inherently hypersexual and of this hypersexuality as physically appearing on the body has often focused on the South African woman Sara (or Saartjie) Baartman.[79] This Khoisan woman was brought to England and France for public exhibition in the early nineteenth century as an example of both the "presumed ugliness and heightened sexuality of the African race during her era," noted Janell Hobson in her book on blackness and popular culture. Baartman's body, with "large" buttocks and vulva, was regarded as a visible manifestation of these presumptions. Upon death, her genitals were preserved at the Musée de l'Homme in Paris until the twenty-first century, when her remains were returned to her country of origin. Baartman is an icon for racist views of the black female body, and as Hobson argued, few rival her for overexposure.[80] Indeed, though Baartman was not the only woman so displayed in the nineteenth century, she is the most famous today. Evolutionary biologist, historian of science, and popular science writer Stephen Jay Gould and more recently feminist scholars have written about her and the way European, supposedly scientific, ideas about her both stood for and helped establish stereotypes of blackness as meaning sexual savagery and sexual deviance.[81] Coming from a group considered on a low rung of what Gould labeled "the racist ladder of human progress," French and British scientists assumed Baartman's body was a sign of her close relation to animals, and her sexuality was then bestial.[82]

As historian Sander Gilman argued about Baartman, black women came to represent sexual deviancy, both in art and in medicine. They were regarded as primitive, savage, and therefore less sexually developed, but such presumptions demanded evidence in the nineteenth century, evidence read upon the physiological differences found not just upon Baartman's body but more grandly between all white and black female bodies. Black women's genitals, iconized by Baartman, were regarded as generally larger than those of white women, with the hypothesis being that this was due to the warmer climate and more primitive culture.[83]

Sociologist Zine Magubane described Gilman's analysis of Baartman as "the genesis for a veritable theoretical industry"; his article made Baartman into an "academic and popular icon." But Gilman's analysis has not been without its critics, including Magubane, who stressed that Gilman, and others who have followed him, focused centrally on Baartman's bodily difference, thus scholars have uncritically accepted his assessment that by the eighteenth century, the black body became an icon for deviant sexuality. By doing so, Magubane contended, Gilman, and those who followed his lead, failed to take into account definitions of who was "black" and for whom this definition mattered in Baartman's historical context. Looking explicitly at Gilman, Magubane argued that the ethnicity to which Baartman belonged was not considered representative of all Africans. According to Magubane, though Gilman's intentional argument was that race was socially constructed, by focusing on Baartman's body, he actually stressed a physiological difference. Further, by arguing that not all Africans were considered to be Negroes nor were all Negroes considered to be black during Baartman's time, Magubane questioned Gilman's central, and most frequently cited, claim: that Baartman's genitalia were representational of the black female body throughout the nineteenth century.[84]

Were Baartman's "enlarged" genitals representational of how American physicians perceived black women's genital anatomy in the nineteenth century? Possibly because anatomy texts were concerned with the representation of normative bodies, of the forty-eight anatomy texts published between 1845 and 1945 I examined, none noted racial differences in the sections dealing with the clitoris.[85] While not expressed in these anatomy texts, Gilman's claim certainly seems reflected in gynecology texts that briefly noted women from warm climates had enlarged clitorises. But what did other published medical texts say about the size of African American women's genitals and sexual behavior?

Perhaps surprisingly, given the preponderance of racial, and racist, assumptions and attempts to differentiate white from black bodies, there appear to be only a few articles published in American medical journals specifically concerning the physical difference between the genitals of white and black women.[86] Of note, then, are the comments found in two articles with titles concerning genital anatomy. The first, the 1903 "Genital Peculiarities in the Negro," included the quotation above that asserted black men had much larger penises than white men. When it came to women, however, the same article stated, "Among women sexual difference are much less marked." The enlargement of the clitoris in particular was "no oftener seen among colored women than white, and when found is usually due to disease."[87] The second, a 1911 article that appeared in the *American Journal of Obstetrics* entitled "Observations on the Comparative Anatomy of the Female Genitalia," included no discussion of genitals or genital differences among women. Rather, the discussion compared the anatomies of human females to animal females. In the final section of this article, when human females were compared to female apes—an animal that, at times, had been used as a close link with African women to illustrate a racist assumption of a supposed lower order of development—there was no comparative discussion of race, or even of race at all.[88]

While not about the clitoris, an 1877 discussion in the pages of the *American Journal of Obstetrics* concerned racial differences in the location of the hymen. In an article in January 1877, Edward B. Turnispeed, a physician in Columbia, South Carolina, pondered whether it was "known to the scientific world that the hymen of the negro woman is not at the entrance of the vagina, as in the white woman, but from one and a half to two inches from its entrance in the interior." Turnispeed's estimate was based on having examined "a good many cases." He believed this difference was "one of many of the anatomical marks of non-unity of the races."[89] At the end of Turnispeed's article, however, the editor of the journal called for others to answer Turnispeed's claim, "either corroborating or refuting his observations, as to the correctness of which we ourselves, we confess, have not been able to overcome some doubts." Surely, the note from the editor continued, "there must be many physicians, both North and South, who are able to throw light on this, if true, certainly very remarkable anatomical feature in the negro race, which thus far would appear to have escaped scientific observation."[90]

Others may have answered this editorial doubt, but only two responses were published in the following volume three months later. H. Otis Hyatt, a physician in Kinston, North Carolina, responded to Turnispeed by first noting that he had much gynecological experience with black women and that, based on his clinical knowledge, he needed to "say that the doctor has fallen into error." As Hyatt wrote, "I have during the last eight years examined one thousand negro women for diseases of the sexual organs, and have never seen any marked difference between the vulva and vagina of negroes and that of whites, with the solitary exception that the labia minora or nymphae of negroes are generally larger and more prominent than those of white women." Hyatt concluded his article by again stressing that he had "never seen any marked difference between the sexual organs of the two races, and I have done a good deal of gynecological work for both."[91] So though Hyatt repeated what some gynecology texts stated—that African and African

American women's labia, for instance, were larger—he also contradicted himself by saying he had not noted any marked differences. Perhaps he was just speaking to Turnispeed's comment regarding the hymen. Regardless, the difference between the genitals was "not marked."

Following this letter, the editor of the journal again interjected an editorial note, writing, "Since the reception of Dr. Hyatt's paper, we have been studying the normal anatomy of the vulvo-vaginal orifice in a number of cases." Though the editor in this instance was concerned that Turnispeed was "in error" regarding the structure of female genitals, the editor concluded his interjection by stating there was "no doubt a great diversity" in the anatomy of the female vulva and, along with Hyatt, stressing the need for more careful study.[92]

But while Hyatt disagreed with Turnispeed on the location of the hymen in black women, the article following the editorial note supported Turnispeed. C. H. Fort, a physician in Adams Station, Tennessee, provided six clinical cases of African American women and noted that, although he could "give a few more such cases," his clinical observation was that "every hymen I have ever seen or examined in the negro or mulatto is placed farther within the vagina than any I ever saw or examined in the white race." Indeed, he so strongly believed in this anatomical "peculiarity," along with the "apparently greater density of the hymen in the negress," that any "practiced physician" could "distinguish the negro from the white race, even in the dark, by the aid of touch alone."[93]

What does this discussion of the placement of the hymen in black and white women mean in relation to medical ideas about the supposed anatomical differences of female genitals, especially the clitoris, with one race's supposedly inherent hypersexuality represented anatomically? To begin, the short debate in the 1877 *American Journal of Obstetrics* illustrates a diversity of opinion: physicians who examined black women and white women were not uniform in their assessment that African American women possessed different genitals—a hymen in a deeper place or a clitoris occupying more space—from European American women. Further, this debate was among clinicians—those who reported they saw black and white women in their gynecological practice—and they were using clinical knowledge to support their difference of opinions. Compare this with the statements of those who claimed difference in size of the clitoris was inherent between white women and black women: an enlarged clitoris "occurs most frequently in hot climates," "excessive enlargements of the clitoris are most common in warm climates," and the "congenital enlargement of the clitoris" existed in "certain African races." With the exception of Robert Morris, these latter comments were not part of cited cases from an obstetrical or gynecological practice; they were statements about abstract bodies, not clinical case reports concerning female patients.

Published case reports of African American women with enlarged clitorises or genitals frequently concerned either elephantiasis or syphilis; instead of being signs of inherent sexual degeneracy, they were signs of acquired disease. One of them—elephantiasis (filariasis)—was a disease brought over during the African slave trade that became endemic in parts of the American south. Carried by the mosquito, the adult worms intruded upon the human body in the lymphatic vessels and lymph nodes causing an inflammation, and over time their inhabitation closed off of circulation, resulting in the characteristic swelling of the affected body part, commonly the scrotum, labia, leg, or foot. Though cases were reported beginning in the eighteenth century across the American south, according to historian Todd Savitt, it became endemic in Charleston, South Carolina, and existed there until the 1930s, afflicting both white and black people. Cases reported in the medical literature often originated from or around this area, though it was not until the 1880s when routine blood examinations could confirm whether a case was truly filariasis.[94]

Prior to blood confirmation, Isaac Parrish, a Philadelphia physician, was asked by another physician in 1839 to examine a nineteen-year-old married and pregnant "negress," of "robust frame and healthy constitution," whom he suspected had a case of elephantiasis. Parrish agreed that the young woman's "large tumor of an oblong form," "found hanging between the thighs and extending almost to her knees," was likely the result of this infection. However, because she was "far advanced in pregnancy," they decided to hold off on surgery until after she gave birth.[95] Decades later, in an article published in 1887, Baltimore physicians William Moseley and Robert Morison wrote about a forty- to fifty-year-old "dark negro woman" who "presented herself" at their private dispensary for examination of her enlarged right labia, which the doctors measured to be "fully 7 inches in length, 4 inches in breadth, and 2½ inches in thickness." In addition to the uncomfortable size, the woman told the physicians of the "intolerable itching and burning"; they removed the afflicted area.[96] As a final example, Howard Kelly, a gynecologist at Johns Hopkins Hospital, published a case concerning "M.W., African, age 31, single," admitted in January 1890 with the diagnosis of elephantiasis of the clitoris. A day after he admitted her, he removed the enlarged organ.[97]

Kelly, Parrish, Moseley, and Morison, though describing black women with enlarged genitals, did not make any mention of relative size; there was no discussion about commonly perceived enlargement of genitals among African American women in their analysis. This is noteworthy, in particular because, in the Moseley and Morison article, the authors seemingly went out of their way to note "an item of some interest" revealing the "anatomical peculiarity of the male negro": as they wrote, "in spite of the decided obstruction to coitus offered by the enlarged external lips, this woman aborted only three months previous" to being seen in the dispensary, implying that they assumed the black male with whom she had sex had a stereotypical penis—the "anatomical peculiarity"—large enough to bypass the obstruction.[98]

Though elephantiasis was seen as a problem, some physicians believed sexually transmitted diseases to be endemic within the African American population. Citing statistics, Frederick Hoffman wrote in 1892, "Any physician who has practiced among colored people will bear me out" that "at least three fourths of the colored population are cursed with one kind or another of the many diseases classified as venereal." The reason for this was, Hoffman asserted, their "gross immorality."[99] Perhaps surprisingly, then, given syphilis's equation with sexual immorality, the presumption that the disease was widespread among African Americans because of their presumed hypersexual behavior, and the belief in the late nineteenth through early twentieth centuries that the disease manifested itself differently between blacks and whites, was William Tod Helmuth's discussion of a case of syphilis in an African American woman.[100] Helmuth in 1876 described a case involving a "colored woman, aged thirty years." Married, this woman had three children and had contracted syphilis from her husband, resulting, according to Helmuth, in her labia becoming swollen and enlarged and in her clitoris swelling to four and a half inches in length and three inches in circumference. "Strange to say," Helmuth wrote, "this woman earns her living at service, being obliged to stand upon her feet most of the time," a position which increased her pain. In addition to standing, walking irritated her swollen genitals, which as a result were "constantly bleeding," noted Helmuth. Along with syphilis, she had "painful external hemorrhoids" resulting in constipation, leaving her "in constant distress." Until she could be "received into the hospital," Helmuth "ordered" her to have "frequent sitz baths" among other therapies to treat her various problems. Though the treatments were effective in providing some relief, they did not reduce the swelling of her clitoris. When she was finally admitted, Helmuth "drew the organ forward and removed it with the ecraseur." The patient, he concluded his article by writing, "left the hospital cured."[101] Helmuth made no mention of this woman's genitals being reflective of other African American women's genitals; it is the disease of syphilis, not her race, that caused their enlargement. Nor was there any comment about what normal genitals, presumably enlarged, should look like on an African American woman.

As historian Christopher Crenner noted in his examination of the University of Kansas School of Medicine's free dispensary from 1906 until 1912, "though the historical literature on race and medicine is extensive, little work has been done using the evidence of routine clinical practice, where physicians shaped durable medical habits and rules of thumb." This dispensary, staffed by young white male medical students and supervising physicians, saw a racially diverse group of patients. Through his examination of routine clinical practice, Crenner found that race functioned often only implicitly, despite the pervasiveness of racial concepts in existence and acceptance during this time, including anatomical and physiological differences based on race. Beyond an initial categorization of a patient, the clinic medical staff avoided recording anatomical racial differences, even, Crenner noted, in the records of patients with a sexually transmitted disease—at a time when the dominant medical ideologies regarding venereal disease stressed the importance of racial differences. As Crenner wrote, "Given the climate of the times, it seemed almost inevitable that these white male students would note or at least hint at widely discussed racial features of black genitalia, such as the size of the penis or the length of the foreskin." However, according to Crenner, the records suggest the opposite was true at this clinic: "the students scattered remarks on the normality of black male genitals contradicted the majority opinion and suggested a restraint about matters of physical racial difference," something Crenner argued "certainly cuts against the grain of early twentieth-century medical literature on racial differences in venereal disease."[102]

This is not to say that African American men or women were treated equally in this clinic or in other clinics, for, as Crenner found, there were racial differences in treatment: African Americans tended to be given a local anesthetic rather than a general anesthesia, for example, compared to white patients.[103] In the late nineteenth century, especially in the south, African Americans were either barred directly from or segregated within majority hospitals and clinics.[104] Segregated medical facilities also existed in the north, where blacks had varying access to hospitals and clinics.[105] But what Crenner's findings do point to is a difference between these larger racial and racist structures and the treatment of individual patients and their bodies.

I tentatively considered the possibility that a reason for a lack of published suggestions for the treatment of an enlarged clitoris among African and African American women was that, like the removal of a white woman's clitoris for masturbation, if the etiology of the condition was found in the mind, the removal of the clitoris was seen as having no discernible benefit; an inherent condition could not be treated through surgery. But could there be a possibly coexisting, or even alternative, reason for a lack of published documentation for removing the (some assumed) larger clitorises of African and African American women—perhaps that ideas of the inherently hypersexual black woman and the visible manifestation of this hypersexuality in the form of a large clitoris was not uniformly accepted within medical discourse? Was the conception that the genitals were inherently larger in black women a normative medical idea in the United States? In a 1902 article, prominent gynecologist and prolific documenter of female genitals Robert Latou Dickinson called the "designation" of hypertrophied labia after "Hottentot" women wrong. In an article published in *American*

Gynecology, Dickinson stated that such hypertrophy was of no "racial peculiarity of the Bushman tribes, but common in Europe and America." Defining genital hypertrophy within one particular racial group was a "gross error" in his view. Women with labia one and a half to two inches long, as found in "three autopsies on women of Bushmen tribes" in the earlier nineteenth century, Dickinson wrote, was a "size not infrequently encountered in northern climates, and found among American whites and negroes."[106]

African and African American women were, according to some, inherently hypersexual and inherently sexually licentious; some, like Lichtenstein, thought such aberrant sexuality was marked upon the body. But this is only part of the narrative. As exemplified here by Dickinson, as stated in the article on "genital peculiarities" of African Americans and as hinted at in the case reports of African American women with syphilis or elephantiasis, medical ideas about what constituted normative female genitals for black women were not necessarily bound by size. Though statements about the size of genitals, including the clitoris, of women from "tropical" climates often both reflected and reinforced larger racial and racist ideas about black female sexuality, there appears to have been a diversity of opinion regarding the relative size of African and African American women's genitals—at least as expressed in published medical discourse—through the early part of the twentieth century.

Clitoral Size and Homosexuality in the Nineteenth Century

As historian Sander Gilman argued in his examination of representations of black female sexuality as embodied in the genitals, the enlargement of the genitals lead to excess, including an excess of love between women; according to Gilman, "the concupiscence of the black is thus associated with the sexuality of the lesbian."[107] It was from such a belief that Perry Lichtenstein, the New York City prison system physician, made his comment that an enlarged clitoris was particularly common among African American lesbians. Such an assertion, theorist Patricia Hill Collins noted, was based on the idea that if black women in general were constructed as inherently sexually deviant and degenerate, the black lesbian served as the foundation of this perceived deviancy.[108]

As other contemporary scholars have argued, the nineteenth century saw the rise of the classification of bodies, both in terms of race and sexuality. Scholar Siobhan Somerville stressed that theories regarding race and gender supported one another and such theories helped give shape to emerging conceptions of homosexuality. By characterizing African American women's bodies and lesbian women's bodies (regardless of color) as genitally different from normative white, heterosexual female bodies, the nonnormative bodies could be equated and seen as underdeveloped physically and morally.[109] Race and sex converged in the study by white male scientists of the so-called primitive female, beginning with conceptions of African women's bodies and then extending to the examinations of other deviant women in civilized societies, including, historian Jennifer Terry argued, women who desired or had sex with other women—women regarded as having sexual drives and desires similar to men.

By focusing on women considered to be inherently deviant (black or white), scientists in the nineteenth century reinforced the expected roles of civilized white women and supported the sexual double standard. The classification of homosexuality resembled racial classifications. As Terry asserted, "The racial logics at play in the initial naming of the homosexual as a distinct type involved more than merely drawing an analogy between homosexuals and racial Others, or, for that matter, between the concepts of sexuality and race. Indeed, the homosexual was viewed as having many of the same characteristics that distinguished 'primitive' races from their 'advanced' European heterosexual counterparts, namely, degeneracy, atavism, regression, and hypersexuality."[110] Women from tropical climates, then, were not the only ones subjected to preconceived ideas about the size of their genitals as a physiological manifestation of inherent sexual deviancy.

Other historians have argued that, beginning in the late eighteenth and extending through the early twentieth centuries, one of the most common medical assumptions and physical characterizations of a lesbian was that she possessed an atypically large clitoris.[111] Like masturbation, a behavior with which female homosexuality was often conflated and one some physicians often believed lead to female homosexuality, physical evidence existed upon the body in the state of the clitoris.[112] And, like masturbation, the treatment of homosexuality moved at this time into the purview of medicine and science. The medicalization of homosexuality, followed shortly by the medicalization of heterosexuality in the late nineteenth century, helped give rise to the invention of new categories of people. Though sexual relationships between people of the same sex existed well before the late nineteenth century, just as they had between people of the opposite sex, it was not until this time that the difference between these relationships were labeled. Prior to this date, homosexuality and heterosexuality were perceived as forms of sexual behavior, not as identities.[113] Several things converged for medicine to come into the authoritarian role regarding homosexuality, including the intimate proximity of doctor and patient, the professional organization of medicine during the late nineteenth century, and the authority they gained from this organization.[114] Homosexuals also entered classification as primitive and inherently degenerate alongside those who were poor or not white.[115] And, like white and black, male and female, homosexuality thus became the defining "other" for heterosexuality.

Once cast as a sin or crime committed by any individual, homosexuality began to be associated with certain types of people by the end of the nineteenth century. As historian Jennifer Terry argued in her history of homosexuality and medicine in America, when homosexuality moved from being considered a moral offense to a matter for medical consideration, efforts at decriminalization and social acceptance were minimalized in favor of medical intercession. American doctors worried homosexuality would erode the distinctions between the sexes. This concern reflected a conservative reaction to the changes going on in the larger society regarding women's roles and represented an effort to stem those changes by asserting what was normal and healthy. Some, then, concentrated on homosexuality because of its potential for upsetting distinctions between genders and the two-sex, one sexuality system.[116]

Doctors, as well as the public, often feared homosexuality because homosexuality seemed to further disrupt sex roles already being challenged by women entering the public sphere. J. Richardson Parke, formerly a physician with the military, wrote in 1909 that he believed there was an increase in "Sapphism" in America because of the "many influences at work to promote and foster its development," including "the domestic emancipation of women, the movement in favor of social equality and political rights" as well as "the fear of begetting children."[117] Doctors shifted their idea of female deviance from a rejection of motherhood, historian Carroll Smith-Rosenberg argued, to a rejection of men. The "New Woman" of the first decades of the twentieth century, unmarried and childless, active in her career and politics, challenged and upset gender classifications by combining male and female and thus embodying social disorder. Lesbianism was linked to the ultimate rejection of female roles, and as women gained an increasing amount of political power following the right to vote, the charge of lesbianism became a means to discredit women and the institutions they founded to challenge the social order.[118]

Beginning in the late nineteenth century, a variety of scientific studies sought to postulate in some manner a foundational connection between the body and homosexual desire. Discourse from 1869 until the 1920s presented complicated and often-contradictory explanations for homosexuality, but all, in some manner, viewed the "contrary sexual instinct" as rooted in the body.[119] Scientists, then, searched for bodily signs to differentiate homosexual bodies from heterosexual bodies, including variation in clitoral size. This assumed physiological difference was not new.[120] However, according to sociologist Darlaine Gardetto, a large clitoris in the seventeenth century often meant a woman was lustful toward men; by the late nineteenth century a large organ became a sign of lust for other women.[121] During the nineteenth century, many of the medical cases of lesbians commented on their physical features, including their genitals. Gynecologists, working alongside psychiatrists, used their knowledge of the female genitals to look for any visual differences, believing that lesbians would have markers on their bodies showing stunted development.[122] Late nineteenth-century British physician and sexual theorist Havelock Ellis, for example, believed homosexuals were like savages and criminals in that they too had failed to develop.[123]

In the 1880s, New York physicians found just such a marker on Lucy Ann Slater, who went by the name of Joseph Lobdell. She was committed to the Willard Asylum, an upstate institution for the clinically insane. Lobdell had been considered insane because she wore male attire, hunted, threatened violence to herself and others, and lived as though married with another woman, all regarded as masculine behaviors. She also had an enlarged clitoris, something doctors attributed in part to her masculine social traits and her sexual attraction to other women. According to a report published in 1883 by physician P. M. Wise, Lobdell apparently told the doctor "she made frequent attempts at sexual intercourse with her companion and believed them successful; that she believed herself to possess virility" of a man.[124]

Since nineteenth-century physicians understood sexuality and genitalia as connected, lesbians were viewed as masculine for two reasons, according to historian Margaret Gibson: first, because lesbians were active sexually with other women, and, second, because the clitoris of lesbians was believed to be larger than that of normal, that is, heterosexual, women. "An enlarged clitoris," Gibson explained, held the potential of penetrative sex with another woman and "indicated that the invert [i.e., homosexual] could not be considered truly female, and thus underlined her essential masculinity."[125]

Thus, Theophilus Parvin, a doctor in Philadelphia in the 1880s, wrote that some women practiced clitoral masturbation with another woman's "exceedingly large clitoris."[126] In popular culture, too, the large clitoris was often seen as an indicator of homosexual behavior. In an 1858 reproductive physiology and marriage guide, the author noted, "Occasionally we find cases where it [the clitoris] attains an unusual size, so much that it can even be used like the penis, with another female."[127]

Though these American texts illustrated the existence of anatomical explanations for lesbian sexual behavior, such ideas had lost favor within Continental Europe by the late nineteenth century. Havelock Ellis, for example, assumed that the body of someone he termed a "sexual invert" may be anatomically different and distinguishable from sexually normal people, but he did not believe that clitoral size was one such difference. While Ellis conceived of the body as a text that could be read and noted the assertion that an enlarged clitoris equated lesbianism, he argued against a connection between this anatomical marker and sexual behavior.[128]

While anatomical theories were not, perhaps, influential within Continental European theorists' discourses regarding same-sex desires, British gynecologists, as historian Chiara Beccalossi argued, continued to use anatomical explanations for female same-sex desires until at least the end of the nineteenth century, revealing the extent to which bodily signs remained important to medical discourse. So though Italian, German, and French medical literature regarding lesbians stated that their patients did not have abnormal genitals, British discourse remained interested in finding differences in the genital anatomy of women.[129]

Like their British peers, American physicians, both in the nineteenth and the first few decades of the twentieth century, continued to look for bodily signs of sexual activity between women and, as a result, often provided therapy upon the body in order to treat same-sex behavior and desire. Psychiatrists, with the help of gynecologists, examined the clitorises of their lesbian patients to discover any physical differences that could diagnose homosexuality. Once doctors found evidence, some recommended removing the organ. As Margaret Gibson claimed, "The interaction between clitoridectomy and masculinity in the case of the female invert suggests that some doctors viewed removing the clitoris as a way of 'feminizing' the patient."[130]

In 1882, Horatio Bigelow, a physician practicing in Washington, DC, published the case of Miss H., a twenty-two-year-old woman with an "unstable, nervous temperament," who came to him complaining of numerous bodily pains. Her list included a "pricking sensation in the clitoris, aggravated by contact with her drawers, or even by the sheet." Bigelow persuaded the young woman to allow him to look at her genitals, and he found her clitoris measured three inches. The examination, he noted, "was most embarrassing, as the least touch provoked the most intense orgasm that I have ever witnessed." He compared her response to an epileptic seizure and wrote that Miss H. "seemed lost of all sense of shame or decency, using her own hands to intensify the erethism." Miss H. began masturbating at age twelve and currently did so by using a "rubber imitation of the male penis" or "with the finger of a female friend," Bigelow reported Miss H. as telling him. Further, he reported that Miss H. and her female friend gratified each other several times a day and had "both lost all desire for men." In his article, Bigelow noted that a fellow physician recommended a "natural gratification of the sexual passion," namely marriage, and amputating the large organ, though Bigelow did not indicate to what extent he followed this advice.[131]

Freud and the Development of Female Sexuality

The anatomical marker of female homosexuality was eventually undermined when Sigmund Freud's theories about the development of sexuality became widely accepted in the twentieth century.[132] Freud recognized that the leading erotic area in girls was located in the clitoris, an organ that was homologous to the "masculine genital zone of the glans penis." Though as children they masturbate using their clitoris, Freud believed that to become a mature adult female, women need to move their sexual sensations to their vaginas. During puberty, young women put aside their "childish masculinity" to become feminine. An inability to do so was a chief determinant of many forms of neurosis and sexual perversions. According to Freud, as girls reached puberty, they needed in effect to deny their "male-like" clitoris and embrace the more feminine vagina during sex. In his 1905 "Three Essays on the Theory of Sexuality," Freud theorized that girls realize at a certain point in their development that they are missing an organ comparable with those their brothers possess and feel envious of the penis, symbolic of the cultural status and power given to males within society. Girls recognize the differences in their bodies and in little boys' bodies "immediately and are overcome by envy for the penis—an envy culminating in the wish, which is so important in its consequences, to be boys themselves," Freud wrote.[133] With the discovery that they do not possess the large and powerful penis, healthy women, Freud hypothesized, abandon their smaller organs (and thus clitoral masturbation) in favor of the passive sexuality embodied in their vaginas.[134]

The moment when girls discover they do not possess a penis is a "turning-point in the life of the girl," according to Freud. At this moment, three "lines of development diverge from it; one leads to sexual inhibition or to neurosis, the second to a modification of character in the sense of masculinity complex, and the third to normal femininity."[135] With three options, only one of which leads to healthy adulthood, what happened if en route to becoming women girls do not abandon clitoral masturbation following puberty? What if they maintained their sexual sensations in their clitoris, refusing to transfer all—or any—sexual feelings to the vagina? Those who retained sensitivity in their clitoris and directed their sexual desire in a "masculine" manner to attraction to other women had not matured into healthy adult women and were suffering from a sexual perversion, according to Freud. As theorist Barbara Creed argued, Freud believed lesbianism was a woman's desire to be a man because of her inability to relinquish clitoral (and thus phallic) sexuality. So while Freud did not seem to consider lesbianism as pathological—he does not, Creed pointed out, describe therapy for homosexuality—by emphasizing vaginal orgasm as providing the only healthy and real source of sexual pleasure for mature women, Freud made it clear he regarded sexual practices between women as unhealthy and immature.[136] Though others before him had made the argument, Freud largely popularized the idea that the clitoris signified women's erotic ability without men and outside of male control.[137]

As historian Jennifer Terry noted, Freud's ideas provided the means to question the etiology and embodiment of homosexuality that would challenge, if not entirely replace, the examination of the body. Freud's work presented a strong critique of the idea that anatomy could be read for same-sex sexual behavior, but some medical practitioners and scientists continued to search for such signs. Indeed, the link between a large clitoris and lesbianism continued through the mid-twentieth century.[138] A physician in Massachusetts, for example, wrote in 1933 that among the various lovemaking techniques lesbians used was when "one of the women is provided with an extraordinarily long clitoris, in which quite a degree of turgidity may be developed, and by which she can simulate the coital act with her partner."[139] And in 1954, physician Frank Caprio in his book on female homosexuality wrote, "Some lesbians with an unusually elongated clitoris have been known to insert the end of the clitoris into the vagina of their partner."[140] Such beliefs can also be seen as furthering the centrality of penetrative sex as normative for women—even among women who have sex with other women.

But while these physicians maintained their conviction that an enlarged clitoris was an anatomical commonality among lesbians, not all physicians in the early twentieth century agreed. G. Lombard Kelly, a professor of anatomy at the Medical Department of the University of Georgia in Augusta, believed that the "sexual organs of women inverts tend to be either normally feminine or to be infantile, or underdeveloped," a belief he attributed to his reading of Havelock Ellis.[141] By the early decades of the twentieth century, then, conceptions of the enlarged clitoris as physical evidence of female homosexuality were in flux.[142]

The Sex Variant Study

Though there was disagreement (or at minimum no agreement) within medical discourse on the size of the clitoris among lesbians during the first half of the twentieth century, it is worth turning attention to a significant study that purposefully looked for genital differences among heterosexual and homosexual women. Indeed, according to Jennifer Terry, "while other American research from the period combined psychological and physical examinations, the Sex Variant Study is perhaps the most thorough in its attention to the human body."[143]

Begun in the 1930s, the Sex Variant Study included forty men and forty women, largely from the New York City area. This study, unprecedented in scope and ambition in the United States, was undertaken by the newly formed Committee of the Study of Sex Variants with the aim of investigating diverse aspects of homosexuality. Part of the study involved a physical examination to see whether there were any measurable differences physically between homosexuals and heterosexuals. Though in a few cases men's genitals were measured, the researchers gave much more attention to women's, and drawings were made only of the women. Gynecologist L. Mary Moench conducted the exams on the women, and the text was written by, and compared with, work gynecologist Robert Latou Dickinson had conducted in his private clinic on, presumably, heterosexual women.[144] Dickinson's interest in studying lesbian women can be seen as an extension of his research interest regarding heterosexual female sexual satisfaction, marital adjustment, and maternal health, which he began in the 1890s. He believed that, just as frigidity and female sexual frustration could ruin a marriage, so could a history of lesbian relations.[145]

Dickinson was, of course, the gynecologist who wrote in 1902 that there were no uniform physiological differences between the genitals of white and black women. Nevertheless, Terry argued that he believed the female body could be read for sexual practices.[146] With this assumption going into the study, the gynecological exams resulted in ten anatomical characteristics of lesbians that differentiated them from "normal" heterosexual women.[147]

Comparing drawings of the lesbian women in the study with those made at his gynecological practice, Dickinson noted a "definite grouping of vulvar and vaginal conditions" among lesbian women. These conditions "had to do with certain marked enlargements and surface alterations, together with evidence of active erotic response," wrote Dickinson. Among the genital differences was a "clitoris of large size." Dickinson sometimes just noted clitoral measurements: Fannie E. had a "small" clitoris, four by three millimeters, as did Julia I. Mae C.'s clitoris, which measured two by four millimeters, fell into the small to average range for Dickinson, while Marvel W. had an "average" sized clitoris. Other women had larger clitorises: Pearl M., a "49 year old negro singer," had an erect clitoris measuring eleven by five millimeters, thus falling into the large range; similarly, Molly N. also had a "large" clitoris, measuring nine by six millimeters, and so did Nora M., at eleven by six millimeters; Rose S. had a "long" clitoris, nine by four millimeters, while Rowena K.'s was "large but not excessively developed." The size of Alberta I.'s clitoris, however, was "very unusual," with "diameters as 17 by 8 mm." Such a size was twice as wide and more than three times as long as Dickinson's average, longer than any clitoris among the 1,087 he had drawn from measurements, except the four he labeled as "intersex."[148]

But it was the women who claimed to have such large clitorises that they could penetrate other women who fascinated and concerned Dickinson.[149] Susan N. declared her "clitoris enlarged is three inches, though it can actually be drawn out but 1½ inches." Such a claim was, Dickinson noted, "the second instance in the series claiming a clitoris so large as to permit entry into the passage of the lover 'about one inch.'" While Susan N. was not identified with a racial category, the other woman Dickinson referred to was: Myrtle K., a "thirty-year old negress," claimed her "clitoris is two inches long" and, "enlarged, it's three inches, and the thickness of a little finger." Wrote Dickinson, "she is able, she declares, to 'insert the clitoris in the vagina,' and produce orgasms in other women in a most desired fashion.'" Measurements taken by both Dickinson and the female gynecologist, found the clitoris to be ten by eight millimeters (when measured by Dickinson) and twenty-five by nine millimeters when erect (measured by the female physician).[150]

In addition to descriptions in the text, Dickinson provided drawings of genitals, including one depicting the differences between "average" and typical "sex variant," with the latter being about 1.5 mm longer. Some of the women Dickinson discussed appeared in these drawings. One drawing showed Susan N.'s clitoris with the erection length noted, while on a later page her clitoris was labeled as one of a "negress" and as "large," showing a projected angle of it erect. Alberta's "large" clitoris was also drawn, though her race (African American) did not appear on this page.[151] As Jennifer Terry wrote in her critique of this study, the sketches featured particular women:

> Elongated clitorises were noted in several of the African American women as well as some of the white women, perhaps because a few of them boasted about how their lovers really liked them for this fact. Some gynecological sketches noted the race of the subject ("negress") next to what was seen to be an unusually long clitoris, recalling the lesbian counterpart to the stereotypical savage with an unusually long penis. Here, as in other representations combining racial difference and sexual deviance, we find a link in the medical imagination between blackness and hypersexuality, this time through a clinical reading of lesbian masculinity in female genitals.[152]

Terry also critiqued the study's tendency to refer to the African American participants as promiscuous.[153] However, neither the study's general editor, George Henry, nor Dickinson argued, as Lichtenstein did, that African American women were inherently hypersexual or more likely to have enlarged genitals. This was possibly because, as historian Elazar Barkan argued, between the two world wars, racism, while still present, ceased to command respectability in part because of the removal of scientific "evidence" of difference to bolster racial claims: the defense of racism moved from biological to cultural claims.[154]

In closing, I want to turn to Terry's argument that Dickinson read individual women's genitals as evidence of masculine sexual behavior, experiences, and desires. A large clitoris or labia for Dickinson was evidence, according to Terry, of masturbation or homosexual behaviors. But stimulation of the clitoris and other parts of the vulva could also occur during heterosexual sex, something Dickinson knew and even advocated to his married patients and their husbands, "and this is precisely where the logic of the gynecological examinations began to unravel," asserted Terry. In the Sex Variant Study, Dickinson believed that evidence of clitoral stimulation was a reliable sign of lesbianism—even though many of the women in the study had at one time had sex with men, or were having sex with men and with women, or were masturbating—complicating the means of acquiring the reliable sign. According to Terry, "Dickinson appeared unaware of this contradiction in his own thinking."[155]

Were genitals a reliable sign? According to Dickinson, the clitoris of "sex variants averaged *over one-third larger*" than his clinic (presumably heterosexual) patients; however, "like most of our comparisons, this statement is based on very small numbers in either case; namely, 23 measured in sex variants; 109 in ordinary gynecological practice." For Dickinson, the possible genital difference between lesbian and heterosexual women was not conclusive; as he wrote, "the local group of findings above emphasized *point to, but do not in and of themselves, enable the examiner to make a definite diagnosis* of homosexual practices." When a clinician saw a larger than usual clitoris, Dickinson said the examiner should "bear in mind the possibility of homosexual methods of considerable duration and frequency."[156] The larger than usual clitoris, then, was a *possible* sign, but not a stable one, something Terry noted when she argued that after the study concluded both Dickinson and Henry realized they could not determine who was a homosexual by only looking at the body.[157] By the early 1940s, then, the usefulness of clitoris size as a reliable mark of sexual difference proved too elusive to be clinically tenable.

Chapter Four

Female Circumcision to Promote Clitoral Orgasm, 1890–1945

In 1896, Eugene P. Bernardy, a physician in Philadelphia, wrote about a young blonde woman who came to him complaining of an "absence of sexual feeling." Married for two years, with three pregnancies and two living children, it was during her most recent lying-in that the eighteen-year-old woman complained she had "never experienced" the "pleasure I hear so much about." Indeed, she told Bernardy, "the approaches of my husband I abhor." Shortly after, her husband came to Bernardy with a case of gonorrhea. Bernardy lectured him on how he had come to acquire the disease, but in explaining his dalliances the straying husband told the physician he had "no pleasure with [his] wife," comparing her to a "piece of marble." Convinced the wife's lack of sexual desire lay in the condition of her clitoris, Bernardy decided to examine it; her lying-in state made "an easy excuse" to do so. Bernardy found the prepuce adherent to the glans, and, by "catching the margin of the prepuce with a pair of dressing forceps," he separated the adhesions. He then bathed the glans in carbolized cosmoline until the raw edges "were completely healed." A year later, Bernardy saw the husband again, who "informed [him] that everything was satisfactory."[1] Bernardy, I think it safe to say, believed the removal of the clitoral adhesions responsible for the couple's now satisfactory sexual relationship.

Bernardy published his account of breaking up clitoral adhesions in 1896—the same year Polak published his report on removing a woman's clitoris to treat her masturbation. As seen in the first chapter, doctors based their decisions on when to use—or not to use—one of the clitoral surgical procedures on what they deemed to be the origins of masturbation. But masturbation was not the only sexual disorder to be treated through clitoral surgery because it was not the only imbalance in women's sexual instinct seen as having its origins in the condition of the clitoris. For, just as the clitoris was seen as responsible for a woman's inappropriate sexual instinct when it manifested as masturbation, hypersexuality, or homosexuality, the organ was also blamed when a woman failed to respond in the marital bed. As Bernardy stated, though "aneroticism" may arise from "numerous causes," he believed the "condition of the clitoris and its cover" was the reason for "many, if not the majority, of the cases."[2] Women, it seems, suffered from an abnormal sexual instinct when they lacked sexual response in marriage. And, like when women masturbated, when women did not experience sexual pleasure in the marital bed, the physiological problem was suspected to lie in the condition of the clitoris.

From the 1890s through the mid-1940s, some physicians treated women for both masturbation and aneroticism with two of the same surgeries— the removal of clitoral adhesions or the removal of the clitoral hood.[3] This seems paradoxical: the same procedures used to promote different ends, preventing masturbation and promoting orgasm. Indeed, physicians noted this seemingly conflicting use of two clitoral therapies at the time. Goodrich Schauffler, a Portland, Oregon, physician who believed in the merits of circumcision in girls to treat masturbation, wrote in 1942 about this seeming paradox. When circumcision was used on men and girls, it was to "diminish the sensibility of the glans," whereas in "the adult female" the "scientific intention of circumcision is the exact opposite; in other words, to untent the clitoris is thought to increase the woman's sensitiveness to sexual contact."[4] Though Schauffler does not say so explicitly, the difference in the purpose of female circumcision to treat the clitoris were age and relationship dependent; the clitoris of a young unmarried girl who masturbated was regarded as unhealthy, as was the clitoris of a married woman who did not have an orgasm with her husband.

Physicians' use of the surgeries illustrates their understanding of the importance of the clitoris to female sexual pleasure, an understanding that supported the diagnosis that the clitoris had to be in an unhealthy state when a woman had an orgasm on her own or when she failed to have one with her husband. While many doctors noted that women possessed an organ whose purpose was sexual pleasure, most simultaneously believed respectable, healthy, middle-class white women were only sexual when prompted by a husband's erotic desire.[5] Thus, physicians reflected and reinforced the cultural norm of heterosexual marital sex as penetrative sex. But this does not mean that they denied the role of the clitoris; instead, they sought to adapt the organ to maintain the penetrative sex model.

Changes in the Expectations of Marriage

To understand why some physicians proposed and performed—and why some women agreed to undergo—surgery on the clitoris to enable marital orgasm, we need to understand what those who were white and middle class anticipated from marriage. In particular we need to appreciate the increasingly nonprocreative role of sex in marriage and the expectation that women would respond to sex with orgasm within the context of marriage. During the late nineteenth and early twentieth centuries, popular attitudes about sexuality and domesticity reshaped how Americans regarded and experienced marriage. Marriage as based in love lost its negative connotations of recklessness and emerged as the only legitimate basis of intimacy for men and women.[6] Marriage also came to be increasingly viewed as an intimate union between a man and a woman that was to promote the happiness of both and was no longer regarded simply as a duty.[7] Many white middle-class couples came to see marriage as a state of comradeship, wherein two people came together and made a happy life. By 1910, books such as *Little Problems of Married Life: The Baedeker Guide to Matrimony* provided couples with a guide to the "fortune" of "success, prosperity and happiness" that could be "earned by their united effort."[8]

By the late nineteenth century, marriage was increasingly seen as a pivotal experience for men and women, one that was to be mutually satisfying socially and, increasingly, sexually. While some in the late nineteenth century continued to debate the extent and necessity of female passion, by the early twentieth, wives were expected to embrace passion, for sex was the physical expression of married love.[9] Attitudes toward sex were complicated and diverse, but by the end of the nineteenth century sex began to be regarded as a healthy and necessary part of marriage for both men and women outside of its reproductive possibilities.[10] By the 1920s this change in cultural attitudes was largely complete.[11]

Physicians like Henry Guernsey, a retired homeopathic professor of obstetrics, endorsed sex as healthy when the act served to unite a married couple. According to Guernsey in 1907, "well-regulated sexual intercourse is just as necessary to the married couple as are the functional demands of all other organs of the body." And though Guernsey believed sex should result in pregnancy, he also considered sex itself a necessary component of a healthy marriage.[12] Guernsey expressed a growing medical opinion that moderate amounts of sexual expression were healthy for men as well as women within marriage.[13] But it was also one both should enjoy. Physician James Kent in 1879 argued that all sexual embraces should include orgasm for both parties, for the lack of such a response on the part of the wife "is very detrimental and causes disease."[14] Ralph Perry, a physician in Farmington, Minnesota, wrote in 1899 that women "had just as much right to enjoy sexual life as a man" within marriage.[15] A Chicago physician argued in 1905 that "sexual excitement not brought to its natural climax and reaction leaves a woman in a very disagreeable condition, and repeated occurrences of this kind may even lead to general nervous disturbances."[16] Twenty-five years earlier, Rufus Griswold, a physician practicing in Connecticut, wrote that a woman should not simply be the "passive slave for the sensual gratification of her husband" and that she should receive "reciprocal sensation."[17] But while physicians may have recognized that healthy women enjoyed, even needed, sexual release, physicians believed it was healthy for women to do so only with their husbands.[18] Physicians and society described female sexuality as secondary to male sexuality; as the passive partner, women needed to be aroused into sex by their husbands and only by their husbands.[19] Once prompted, women were expected to be engaged, interested, and responsive to sex with their spouses.

The companionate marriage, which came to be seen as the model marriage by the 1920s, based marriage in love and satisfying sexual relations. As marriage counselor Ernest Groves wrote in the 1920s, "No desire is more universal nor more strongly felt among young people than the wish to be happily married."[20] Though Groves was responding to what was perceived as a marriage crisis, Americans' desire for strong, supportive, and sexually satisfying marriages prompted, and was encouraged by, the flowering of marital work exploring, teaching, and publishing advice on ways to achieve them.[21]

Joseph Collins, in his 1929 book, *The Doctor Looks at Marriage and Medicine*, called sex the "the keelson of the ship of marriage."[22] As such, physicians increasingly called for premarital counseling for couples, partly to provide them with information about sexual intercourse. S. Bernard Wortis, a physician in New York City, told his peers that a premarital consultation should be "in the nature of a friendly interview" and should include information on "an adequate and satisfactory sexual adjustment." Wortis noted the importance of explaining to a couple "that it often (but not always) took months or even a year or two for completely satisfactory sexual timing and orgasm to occur" and that both must work to achieve "mutual adjustment."[23]

The importance placed on education about these needs in marriage, including the importance of sex, was not confined to physicians recommending premarital consultations; such concern also prompted the creation of college and university courses in marital relations across the United States beginning in the 1920s. By 1948, more than five hundred higher education institutions had courses on family relations, courses that covered "every phase of the physical and emotional aspects of marriage."[24] As part of the curriculum, courses covered sex; at the State University of Iowa in Iowa City, for instance, an entire class period centered on "sex adjustment" in marriage. Iowans wrote to the university in reaction to the course, which began in the mid-1930s, but of all the letters received from "Iowa farmers, from ministers, judges, editors, lawyers, physicians in the state, there was no hostile criticism of the course," according to Moses Jung, an educator at the university, in 1939.[25]

For those not attending college, courses were offered at other institutions, such as the Young Women's Christian Association (YWCA) in Chicago. In 1929, the YWCA offered a ten-week class, attended by secretarial workers, which included a session on the "physiological" aspects of marriage.[26]

Additionally, marriage consultation centers began forming around the country beginning in the 1920s, typically run by community organizations or church groups.[27] Women more often than men went to these centers for advice. The Marriage Counsel of Philadelphia, for example, noted that women dominated their clientele and that most had been married fewer than five years. Some came after hearing about the program from a friend, while physicians referred others to the center. Though the women went to the center for a variety of marital concerns, "sexual maladjustments" was one of the more common.[28] In addition, the seven hundred Planned Parenthood centers across the country all had a marriage counseling component because women who went to the centers for birth control information also often asked questions about sexual concerns and problems.[29] Some marital counselors considered knowledge about sex as a "factor making for marital stability."[30] By 1940, according to one list made by the director of the Marriage Counsel of Philadelphia, there were at least twenty-three centers in the United States dedicated solely to marriage counseling.[31]

While university marriage classes were popular and marital consultation clinics were increasing in numbers, marriage manuals arguably were, after the advice of a family member, the most common form of advancing information about sex. In a study published in 1929 on the sex lives of women, 57 percent of respondents who regarded their married lives as happy received some sex instruction. The women who responded to the survey most commonly cited their mother as their source for sex information, with books and pamphlets a close second.[32] In a 1920s study of two hundred married spouses, twenty-two of the one hundred women had "read about" sex.[33]

Though marriage manuals were published before the early twentieth century, by the 1920s, like child rearing and etiquette guides, they gave married couples guidance and often even detailed instructions. But although we cannot take their advice as being more than prescriptive, they are still useful to understand expectations of sexual norms.[34] As historian Ronald Walters noted, marriage and sex manuals cannot tell us how individuals actually behaved, though they do tell a great deal about how they were expected to behave.[35]

Historian Jessamyn Neuhaus's examination of marriage manuals informs my discussion here. Neuhaus argued that the manuals of the 1920s and 1930s, though largely written with the idea that men "awakened" women to sexual pleasure, held female orgasm as central to "successful" sex. Marriage manuals sought to provide instruction to men on their technique to enable their wives to reach orgasm. For example, in his 1917 book, *Married Life: A Family Handbook*, physician Reinhold Willman told married couples that the wife "more often than the husband is lacking in amorous excitement" and that the "husband should endeavor by acts of endearment and caressing, [to] induce excitement" so that the "act may be agreeable to her."[36] In 1923

C. W. Malchow, a medical professor in Minnesota, reiterated this by noting an old saying: "the youth spontaneously becomes a man; but the maiden must be kissed into a woman."[37]

One of the most widely read manuals during the 1930s was Theodore H. van de Velde's *Ideal Marriage: Its Physiology and Technique*, published in the United States in 1930. Translated from the original Danish, Van de Velde's book, like those written by Americans, stressed the need for men to acquire sexual skills for women, who had different needs than they, to be stimulated. One could read this as men having control over a woman's right to sexual pleasure. But as Neuhaus stressed, this is an oversimplification of these manuals; these authors' concern about a wife's sexual pleasure and the husband's fundamental role for providing that pleasure is an example of larger social constructions of middle-class sexuality that recognized women's gains politically while at the same time reasserting male power. The manuals were not simply about reasserting patriarchal privilege.[38] Similarly, in her examination of marriage and female sexuality in the early twentieth century, historian Christina Simmons also noted this stress within marriage manuals. Marital sexual advice books often contained "contradictory messages," Simmons argued, by attempting to reinforce and reassure male power in marriage while also trying to reshape the sexual lives of women as being culturally important, albeit important still primarily in regard to men and reproduction while "at least partly belonging to women themselves."[39]

The manuals encouraged men to be patient and compassionate in opening up their wives to sexual desire and provided husbands with instructions on how to best produce pleasure for their wives.[40] Some marriage manuals, such as one by physician H. W. Long, were sexually explicit. The audience for Long's book, because it was published in 1919, was largely fellow physicians and patients to whom physicians passed it along. By the 1930s, with a series of court cases challenging and overturning the Comstock law (which had forbidden sexually explicit materials in the US mail, thus effectively restricting their use), more sexually explicit books became available to Americans who were not physicians.[41] These details were important, for as Theodore van de Velde wrote, "most married people do not know the A B Cs of sex."[42] Many of these manuals remained popular for decades after their original publication date, with some continuing to be published into the 1960s.[43]

As physician M. J. Exner wrote in his 1932 book, *The Sexual Side of Marriage*, the "basis for a harmonious, mutually satisfying sex adjustment in marriage" was an understanding of the "anatomical structure and the functions of the woman's sex mechanism" by both the husband and the wife. In the anatomical drawings that appeared in his book, Exner pointed out the location of the clitoris as well as the hood of the organ. He also provided information on its location in his narrative, describing the clitoris as being "just above the junction of the inner lips," a location "roughly represented by the knob of the wishbone, above the junction of the two wings." While referring to the clitoris as a "miniature penis," he furthered noted the two organs each had erectile tissue and that when erect the clitoris was "about the size and shape of a pea or a small bean." Exner further described the organ as "supplied with highly sensitive nerves which respond to sexual stimulation"; indeed, the clitoris was the "center of erotic response," the location from which "sexual feeling radiates to the other areas in the vulva and vagina."[44] Similarly, in their book meant for use as a marriage course text, Evelyn Millis Duvall, the secretary of the National Conference on Family Relations, and Iowa State University sociology professor Reuben Hill identified the clitoris on a drawing of a woman. They further described the organ's purpose in their narrative, stating that the clitoris was "usually the seat of woman's first localized *erotic* (sex) response, and its manipulation usually leads to sexual excitement."[45]

Many marriage manuals stressed the importance of foreplay for women, encouraging husbands to gently caress or kiss the nipples, and they told husbands to pay particular attention to the clitoris. Exner described the clitoris as the "principal organ of sex feeling" in women, an area husbands should especially stimulate during foreplay.[46] Van de Velde told husbands they "cannot miss the most sensitive spot of all" and that stroking the clitoris "is acutely delightful to the wife and increases her desire, incalculably."[47] The emphasis on a husband's stimulation of the clitoris was quite common and explicit in the manuals.[48] And husbands were encouraged to use more than just their fingers on the clitoris. Van de Velde noted the stimulation of the organ through the "genital kiss, by gentle and soothing caresses with lips and tongue," an act that provided the added benefit of lubrication.[49] The "caress known as the 'genital kiss'" helped in the "necessity of lubricating the female organs in order to assist penetration," noted two doctors in their 1940 book, *Encyclopedia of Sexual Knowledge.*[50]

Although oral sex was encouraged, it was regarded as foreplay; penetration was the ultimate sexual goal for married couples, according to the manuals. While they stressed the importance of the clitoris and the importance of orgasm to both husband and wife, that orgasm ideally was to occur for both during penetrative sex. This point was further emphasized by some manuals claiming that healthy sex meant simultaneous orgasm, thus reinforcing the concept of sex as vaginal-penile intercourse or, as described by one marital manual, the act that "concludes with the ejaculation—or emission—of the semen into the vagina, at the nearly simultaneous culmination of sensation—or orgasm—of both partners."[51] During the 1920s and 1930s, marriage manuals placed great emphasis on simultaneous orgasm, something sociologist Michael Gordon referred to in his examination of marital advice literature as a mutual orgasm cult.[52]

But though the manuals stressed that normal, healthy sex meant penetrative sex, they remained mindful of the clitoris and the need for the organ to receive stimulation. Marriage manuals provided detailed descriptions of sexual positions and techniques to assist couples in achieving mutual orgasm.[53] These positions called attention to the importance of the clitoris in female sex arousal, for, as Hannah and Abraham Stone noted in their 1935 *A Marriage Manual,* "in many women the sexual response can only be evoked by direct stimulation of the clitoris."[54] Marriage manuals expected women to orgasm during sexual intercourse, so marriage guide authors discussed numerous positions to educate readers. The two most commonly discussed positions were the husband on top and the wife on top. When the husband was on top, Theodore Arden in his 1939 book, *Handbook for Husbands and Wives,* suggested that wives place their heels "in the cavity back of the man's knees or circles her legs about his waist" in order to "bring more direct pressure to bear upon the clitoris."[55] Oliver Butterfield, in his 1940 guide, suggested placing a "firm pillow under the woman's hips" to change the "slope of the pelvis so that this contact may be more easily maintained."[56] The female on top position was seen as more advantageous and an easier position for women "to control the degree of stimulation she receives," according to Millard Everett.[57] J. Rutgers told married couples to allow for the "traditional position" to be "reversed, and the husband to lie underneath, so that the undersurface of his penis glides along in her vulva" allowing her clitoris to be rubbed during the act.[58] Couples were encouraged to think of positions beyond missionary as healthy; as Evelyn Millis Duvall and Reuben Hill stated in their textbook, "Any activity or position in coitus is normal and acceptable if it brings satisfaction to the couple."[59]

But the marriage manuals also acknowledged that some women failed to have an orgasm at all during penetrative sex. If women did not receive their own "satisfaction," marriage commentator Frederick Harris sympathized, they could come to view sex with "fear and loathing" and refuse to participate in the act that was the "supreme sensuous expression of the sense of unity and partnership."[60] Millard Everett, professor of philosophy at Roosevelt College in Chicago, told husbands in his 1939 *Hygiene of Marriage* that it was "essential that he sees to it that her orgasm is brought about, even though it has to be done artificially by stimulation of the vulva and particularly the clitoris" with his fingers.[61]

Physician H. W. Long advised husbands who arrived at orgasm before their wives that it was *"perfectly right for him to substitute his fingers, and satisfy her in this way."* He warned husbands against making this a regular practice though, for it was not as satisfying for the wife, "but it is *far better than for her not to be entirely gratified."*[62] In similar fashion, a 1935 marriage manual told men should they reach orgasm before their wives, they had to stimulate her clitoris till she reached orgasm too, no matter how tired they may be.[63] At least one marriage manual signified that such "artificial means of stimulation" was not uncommon among couples. As M. J. Exner wrote, "clitoris friction" was quite frequently "resorted to" in "preliminaries to coitus, as variety in lover's technique, and especially to 'finish' the wife when coitus has terminated without her having reached orgasm." When stimulating the clitoris was "employed as a supplement," Exner continued, "and carried out as a love act, it has helped many a couple to a well-adjusted sexual regime."[64]

Married couples apparently did not object either. According to one study conducted in the 1920s, married couples had intercourse in a variety of sexual positions and engaged in stimulating the clitoris. Though his study was small and not representative of the American population, G. V. Hamilton found that, of the two hundred spouses he interviewed to uncover "problems of sex in the marital relation," at least some seemed to incorporate attention to the clitoris to enable female orgasm. Of the one hundred men interviewed, four told Hamilton they performed cunnilingus in answer to the question "What, if anything, do you do to make it possible for your wife to have an orgasm?" Twenty-eight (including, perhaps, the four men who stated they performed cunnilingus) told him they "handled their wife's genitals." Interestingly, when the question was asked, "What, if anything, does your husband do, either before or during the sex act, to increase your pleasure?" of the one hundred women, eight told Hamilton their husbands performed cunnilingus and twenty-five said they manipulated their genitals. Moreover, both men (twenty-two) and women (thirteen) provided "cunnilingus" as the answer to Hamilton's question "Does your husband ever vary his method of performing the sex act with you," implying perhaps that men and women saw oral sex as a sexual position and not just a method of foreplay.[65] Additionally, both men and women noted trying a variety of positions, possibly with the intention of increasing female orgasm (they could provide Hamilton with more than one answer to a question): twenty-seven women told Hamilton sometimes they engaged in intercourse on top of their husbands; twenty-two told him they had sex in a variety of unspecified positions; twenty indicated they had had sex with their husbands entering them vaginally from behind; six noted they had had intercourse in a "sidewise" position; and five that they had sex sitting up. Three women said they had had sex with their husbands in "all known positions." Men, in contrast, were a bit less detail minded: seventy-four simply told Hamilton they engaged in sex with their wives in various positions.[66]

Medical Tensions over Sex

Not every physician regarded sex as healthy outside the narrow parameters of missionary and penetrative. In 1937, a New York physician anonymously wrote to the query section of *JAMA* asking about the "treatment" of a woman, a "graduate nurse," who masturbated. In response, the *JAMA* contributor noted—in addition to saying that "operations on the genitals are of no value unless some distinct condition aside from the habit is present"—the treatment depended on her marital status. Setting aside the concern about the genital treatment for a single woman who masturbated, I am going to here concentrate on the response given as applied to married women whose husbands' practiced withdrawal before she reached orgasm. As a result, the woman or her husband "titillates her clitoris to bring on the orgasm." According to the person writing the response for *JAMA*, "This practice must be absolutely interdicted," and both the husband and the wife "should be instructed in the art of normal coitus."[67]

The *JAMA* response illustrates a central tension regarding prescriptive sexual literature during this time. On the one hand, some physicians and marriage manual authors believed only a strict adherence to orgasm during coitus should be regarded as healthy and normal. Couples were instructed in the variety of sexual positions to enable mutual orgasm, often with the assumption that the male orgasm was a given but that women often needed alternative positions. On the other hand, some physicians and marriage manual authors encouraged stimulation and even orgasm outside the parameters of normal coitus, believing that although an orgasm outside of intercourse may not be ideal, it was better than the woman not having an orgasm at all. The man who failed to give his wife satisfaction "ultimately defeats his own," stated *The Hygiene of Marriage* author Millard Everett. Referring to two studies, one with 310 women, two-fifths of whom "experienced orgasm, one-fifth had it sometimes, and two-fifths never experienced it," and another study with one hundred women, half of whom did not experience orgasm, Everett blamed the husbands who were "ignorant of the importance of his wife's having an orgasm." Everett noted that, when women did not experience orgasm, they ceased to enjoy the marital embrace and became "an unwilling sex partner."[68]

As the studies above indicate, despite the variety of positions encouraged by the marriage manuals, not all women experienced orgasm during intercourse with their husbands. Robert Latou Dickinson, the gynecologist keenly interested in women's ability to experience pleasurable (heterosexual) sex, saw more than one thousand married women during his years of practice from the late nineteenth through the early twentieth centuries. In the copious records he kept regarding these women, he noted that the usual reason for their first visit to him was related to childbirth, a pelvic disorder, or for marital advice regarding their sexual lives.[69] Of the more than one thousand women he maintained records on, Dickinson separated out the fifty newlyweds he saw, the majority married for only four months when he first saw them. Of these new brides, he recorded the reason for the first visit of forty-nine. Twenty-seven expressed a problem with adjustment to sex, and only half of the forty-nine were "having satisfactory coital relationships."

Of the entire group of married women, 442 told him about their marital orgasms, with 40 percent saying they had experienced an orgasm at least once, but only 2 percent said they usually did, 15 percent said sometimes, 10 percent told Dickinson they rarely did, and 26 percent said they never experienced one with their spouse. When asked whether they considered their relations "normal," most answered yes, meaning that the husband was able to enter and have an orgasm. Dickinson noted that most of his patients had sex in the missionary position and that they told him of their orgasms "afterwards by clitoris friction." One sexually frustrated woman showed Dickinson a book that told of fifty-nine ways to engage in sex and remarked "that she had tried most of them."[70] Breaking down his figures, Dickinson estimated that for every five women, two had had an orgasm during intercourse, two had not, and one did sometimes.[71]

Part of the motivation of many of those writing marriage manuals, as well as those reading them, was to avoid unhappy marriages and prevent divorce.[72] But, despite the resources of marriage manuals describing sex positions and encouraging attention to the clitoris, the marriage education courses that informed students about sexual physiology, and the marital clinics, many couples found intercourse lacking. In her study of marriage and divorce from the 1880s to the 1920s, historian Elaine Tyler May found that conflicts around marital sex changed little: women argued that their husbands sexually abused them by desiring too much sex and men accused their wives of denying them reasonable amounts of intercourse.[73] As part of the depiction of companionate marriage, men came to expect their wives' sexual participation, a participation that culminated in an orgasm. Not doing so indicated a resistance to the companionate marriage ideal emphasizing love and comfort, part of which was provided through sex, and men often cited this as a complaint in their divorce.[74]

Divorce rates reveal that sex was often a source of contention for couples. Dickinson noted that the husband of one of his patients told her he "could divorce any woman who didn't" have an orgasm and that he would seek out other women "if she was cold."[75] In his 1920s study of one hundred married couples, C. V. Hamilton perceived the suggestion of a correlation between the lack of female orgasm and divorce, as eleven of the fifteen women who divorced during the time of his study did not have an orgasm during their first year of marriage.[76] A women's lack of orgasm during penetrative sex with her husband was sometimes labeled frigidity, which was considered grounds for divorce. Physician William Robinson in 1929 stated that frigidity was "legally considered a sufficient cause for divorce or for the annulment of the marriage."[77] Indeed, one of the reasons for the increasing numbers of marital sex manuals in the 1920s and 1930s was the common belief that marriage as an institution was failing; the manuals were presented as a means to cope with this perceived crisis while not challenging gender norms—norms which were being challenged during these decades as more women attended college and worked outside the home.[78]

Clitoral Surgery for Sexual Pleasure

With the importance of orgasm to marital relations becoming more expected and accepted by happily wed couples, the question necessarily arose of why some women were orgasmic and others were not. Though gynecologist Robert Latou Dickinson believed it took "two persons to make one frigid woman," some women looked for the answer on their own bodies.[79] By the early twentieth century, Americans largely saw medicine as a legitimate authority, and increasing numbers sought medical attention and expected to be treated through medical intervention.[80] This expectation extended to sex-related problems. And to keep their marriages intact, some women who struggled with experiencing orgasm turned their attention to a fault of their own bodies, and thus to physicians for assistance. And, once again, the culpable character was the clitoris, and the correction was surgery.

In 1937, Frank Iiams, a gynecologist in Houston, noted that he, like many other gynecologists, was "confronted with the sex problems of the woman, many who relate their incompatibility with their mate." These women had husbands who achieved "sexual satisfaction but the woman does not," and, while in most cases Iiams believed the problem could be remedied by "education of the mate," there were times when physical intervention on the wife was necessary. These cases occurred when the woman was "passionate" and "eager for intercourse and there is no fault with the mate but, near the beginning of the act the woman becomes frigid and is left somewhat nervous." Iiams suggested that when presented with such a case, the doctor should examine the woman to see whether she had adhesions on her clitoris or whether the organ was elongated. "Simple removal of the adhesions will make the woman sexually normal" but, should the adhesions reform, "she has a definite indication for circumcision and will surely be benefited." The operation, he noted, could be "done either in the office, under local anesthesia, or in the hospital."[81]

In cases when women failed to experience orgasm, some gynecologists examined the clitoris and recommended removing any adhesions should they be found.[82] Adhesions were a problem, for, as more than one doctor wrote, adhesions between the hood and the clitoris prevented "the development of the glans clitoridis and lead to aneroticism."[83] An adherent hood could so bind down the clitoris that during intercourse the penis failed to stimulate the organ, "and as a result the woman has no orgasm."[84] Clitoral adhesions keep the clitoris from being properly stimulated, some physicians claimed, but with the removal of the adhesions, these women would experience the pleasure of intercourse. C. S. Bacon, in a paper he presented to the Chicago Gynecological Society on January 21, 1898, noted that "adhesions of the prepuce in the female" could lead to "aneroticism."[85] Theodore Arden stated that adhesions to the clitoris "may delay orgasm" and that a "physician can remedy this by loosening these delicate adhesions and drawing the hood back over the head of the clitoris."[86]

After seeking a medical consultation, "some unresponsive wives find that the clitoris is at fault" when they failed to orgasm during sex with their husbands because it was bound down by adhesions, according to Robert Morris.[87] Recall from chapter 3 how this noted New York gynecologist believed that nearly 80 percent of women he described as "Aryan-American" had adhesions binding the glans of the clitoris to its hood. In quoting Morris, Eugene Bernardy, the physician with whom I opened this chapter, stressed to his peers the need to examine the clitoris specifically for such adhesions, particularly when married female patients noted their lack of orgasm. Bernardy was "firmly convinced" that it was "absolutely essential" for the clitoris to be in a "healthy condition or the orgasm will be a failure." Presenting before the Philadelphia Medical Society, Bernardy stated that "the orgasm in women is of such a complex nature" and "so evenly balanced, that the slightest deviation renders it inert."[88]

Doctors believed the reason adhesions could prevent a woman from reaching orgasm with her husband was that they trapped the organ, preventing it from being stimulated by the penis during sex. When clitoral adhesions were not present, during sex "the erection of the clitoris is followed by a pushing forward of the sensitive glans," which then "rests on the dorsal surface of the male organ, and orgasm occurs," according to Bernardy. But if adhesions were present, "no such act occurs" because the "sensitive glans is held down and a thick layer of tissue lies before it." Thus trapped, the "act on the part of the woman proves a failure." Bernardy told members of the medical society that he had examined many married women "suffering with preputial adhesions," all of whom, prior to his intervention, complained of a lack of orgasm. Bernardy described breaking up clitoral adhesions as a simple operation, though "very painful" and so "demands the use of cocaine." The procedure, however, did not take long to perform.[89]

Though Bernardy spoke to the medical society in the late nineteenth century, concerns about the role clitoral adhesions played in preventing female orgasm continued into the twentieth century. In his 1937 book, Arkansas physician LeMon Clark maintained that an adherent hood prevented the stimulation of the organ. In *Emotional Adjustment in Marriage*, Clark told married couples that though the couple may try a variety of positions to increase pressure upon the clitoris during intercourse, in some cases "because of various structural differences—a small clitoris, or one which is unusually well hooded—it will be quite impossible to secure adequate stimulation in face-to-face intercourse." An adherent hood on the clitoris could, he noted, "inhibit normal sensation to a considerable degree."[90]

During his lectures to students at Indiana University about sexuality, Alfred Kinsey suggested the possibility of loosening an adherent hood to assist with women's orgasms. After describing the clitoris as the primary sexual organ for women in a lecture he gave in the spring semester of 1940, Kinsey told his students that normally the clitoris should have "a hood-like structure above" it, extending "from there on down to the inner lips of the female genitalia." But, Kinsey stressed, "in cases where the foreskin has become adherent, it will completely cover the clitoris and will produce pain." Treatment, however, was "very simple, for with a tool the physician can strip the clitoris, allowing the foreskin to roll back and may make a distinct difference in the response of the female."[91]

Breaking up clitoral adhesions may have formed part of the premarital medical checkup for women. In their textbook for marriage courses, Duvall and Hill noted that physicians were "often able to speed up a woman's response by preparing her more fully for marriage, by helping her dilate her hymen, and by freeing the clitoris from the folds that may cover it." By freeing the clitoris, they contended, it better enabled the husband to "make full use of the excitability" of his wife's erogenous zones, "especially the clitoris."[92]

Sometimes physicians did not leave quite as clear of an indication of how they enabled the husband, and the woman, to "make full use of the excitability" of a woman's erogenous zones. For example, in 1904, a young woman calling on Wallace Abbott, a physician in Chicago, told the doctor that she "had failed, during two years of marital life, to respond to the marital embrace, though her desire was ardent." She further informed Abbott that she always waited "for something to happen but it never did." Abbott examined the young woman and found a "well-formed clitoris" entirely hooded. "A very slight [but unspecified] operation under cocaine anesthesia remedied the [unspecified] abnormality, and the woman waited no more for the 'something to happen.'"[93]

While Abbott perhaps removed the adhesions between the hood and the clitoris of this woman, he may instead have removed the prepuce for her to reach orgasm with her husband. Other physicians did this, as the following cases illustrate. In 1900, A. S. Waiss, a Chicago gynecologist, removed the clitoral hood of Mrs. R., a twenty-seven-year-old woman who had been married for seven years and who was "absolutely passionless," something that greatly upset her. She apparently loved her healthy, passionate, and "kind and good-hearted" husband, a man who had "borne up patiently" his wife's disinterest in, and unresponsiveness during, sex. Mrs. R., Waiss wrote, submitted to intercourse "out of love for the man alone." Her unresponsiveness, however, troubled her, or her husband, enough for her to seek a medical remedy. Waiss found Mrs. R.'s clitoris "entirely covered" by its hood. He circumcised the clitoris and the patient "became a different woman"— she was, the doctor wrote, "lively, contented," and "happy," and sex now brought her satisfaction.[94] In 1912, Douglas H. Stewart in New York City saw a "fairly robust woman" who, though desirous for sexual intercourse, when the act was attempted found "there 'was nothing in it.'" Upon examination, Stewart found the clitoris of the patient to be "buried" and then, with the assistance of fellow physician Clement Young, preceded to circumcise the woman to reveal the organ.[95] Charles Lane, a physician in Poughkeepsie, New York, believed the clitoris "a very important organ to the health and happiness of the female" and performed circumcision on women who were unable to reach orgasm. In a 1940 article concerning his use of circumcision on a patient—Mrs. W., a twenty-two-year-old woman who had recently married but had yet to experience an orgasm—Lane noted "that little trick did it all right."[96]

Physicians, both in print and at medical society meetings, had discussed that "little trick" for decades. In a paper he gave before the fiftieth annual meeting of the AMA in 1899, Chicago gynecologist Denslow Lewis presented evidence for the benefits of female circumcision when a woman was anerotic. "In a large percentage" of women who failed to find marital passion, Lewis stated, "there is a preputial adhesion, and a judicious circumcision, together with consistent advice, will often be successful." Lewis had treated thirty-eight women with circumcision and had "reasonably satisfactory results in each instance."[97]

In addition to describing the benefits of female circumcision, Lewis also described the sexual act between (married) men and women as being an event both parties should enjoy. And to do so, he stressed the need for men to pay attention to the clitoris, for the "titillation of the most sensitive regions" was responsible for the "repeated orgasms on the part of the woman, very much to her satisfaction." For many women, this came about when "the penis is in direct contact with the clitoris and introis vaginae."[98] Circumcision was meant to better facilitate such direct contact during penetrative intercourse. This surgery, like the removal of adhesions, was seen as better exposing the clitoris to stimulation during penetrative sex, a therapy that reinforced both penetrative sex and the role of the clitoris in female sexual pleasure as normative.

JAMA did not accept Lewis's paper, though it was customary for the journal to accept all papers presented at the annual meeting of the AMA; the editors did not care for his graphic description of sex at the beginning of the article and told him that if he cut that part, they would publish it.[99] Lewis heard similar sentiments after he delivered the paper as well; Howard Kelly, a physician from Baltimore, stated he was "sorry" it had been read and that he was "opposed to dwelling on these elementary physiologic facts in a public audience." Charles Chamberlin, a physician from Ohio, agreed with Kelly and further opposed Lewis's idea to steer young people from sexual ignorance. But B. Sherwood-Dunn, a physician from Boston, endorsed Lewis's paper, calling it courageous and reminding his peers that there was "not a gynecologist in this room" who had not been called upon by women who "have not told him" about their ignorance and confusion regarding sex. Underlying these disagreements was the question of where the discussion about sex should take place. For Kelly, the discussion about "elementary physiologic facts" was a private one, "guided by our common sense and experience."[100] For Lewis and Chamberlin, however, the "physiologic facts" of sex were not "elementary" to lay people, and more information needed to be made public.

While knowledge of the clitoris as a sexual organ appears to have been medically common, not all physicians who knew of female circumcision as a therapy for an inability to have an orgasm recommended it. Arthur Hale Curtis, for example, in his 1938 *Textbook of Gynecology*, wrote that a "hooded clitoris" was "a common occurrence" in women, with irritation "from accumulated smegma" frequently a result. Curtis stressed that breaking up the adhesions with "a simple dorsal slit of the prepuce" would relieve "this difficulty." But he also noted "circumcision, formerly resorted to for relief of frigidity, is rarely indicated."[101] Curtis's referral to the procedure as one formerly used could be taken to suggest female circumcision as a treatment for orgasm difficulties went away in the late 1930s. Indeed, Curtis did not include this information in his 1942 or 1946 editions.[102]

But it also can be read as a reflection of an increasing tension regarding ideas about the role of the clitoris in healthy female sexual expression and how (or whether) physicians intervened to treat the organ. Physician M. J. Exner's advice to couples in his 1932 marriage manual illustrates this. Exner told couples that there was no "physiological or psychological" objection to "clitoris friction" to enable a wife to have an orgasm; indeed, wrote Exner, the "reactions do not differ essentially from those in normal intercourse except that there may be less of the finer, vivid psychic context and that there is less likelihood of full vaginal climax along with clitoral climax."[103] Though Exner believed normal intercourse meant penetrative intercourse, he also saw nothing wrong with stimulating the clitoris before, during, or after "normal" sex. But his description of the clitoral orgasm as slightly less "full" than the vaginal orgasm points to a newly emphatic discussion about female sexuality: the assertion that there was not only one normative sort of healthy sex but that that there was also only one kind of normal and healthy female orgasm, and it was vaginal.

Chapter Five

Female Circumcision as Sexual Enhancement Therapy during the Era of the Vaginal Orgasm, 1940–66

In a paper given before the third annual meeting of the Academy of Psychosomatic Medicine in October 1956, Chicago obstetrician and gynecologist William S. Kroger stated that "even though the American woman looks and acts as though she is capable of sexual gratification, many do not have orgasm during intercourse." Kroger declared these women frigid and described several types of frigid women. According to Kroger, some women were frigid because they thought they were not supposed to feel sexual pleasure because sex was "indecent" and others who perhaps become aroused but failed to achieve orgasm. But the label of frigidity also applied to women for "whom sexual response occurs only after clitoral stimulation." Women were truly frigid who had a "total incapacity for vaginal orgasm." Because he defined true frigidity as a lack of vaginal orgasm, Kroger told his audience that "circumcision of the clitoris is valueless" as therapy.[1]

Kroger explained the importance of differentiating between the clitoral and vaginal orgasm, noting that the "vaginal and clitoral theories for evaluating frigidity and orgasm differ so much that discussion cannot be attempted without defining them." The majority of the followers of Sigmund Freud, Kroger stated, "adhere to the vaginal theory of orgasm and label 75 per cent of American women frigid" because they cannot reach orgasm vaginally without clitoral stimulation. Many followers of Freud advocated this theory, in opposition to, Kroger wrote, what "a disciple of Kinsey or a proponent of the clitoral theory" believed. Those who maintained women had clitoral orgasms thought "less than 25 per cent of these same women are frigid." Kroger went on to note that this "difference of opinion" confused physicians and was "disturbing to millions of American women." This confusion had only been "compounded" by the "barrage of lay articles, medical treatises, and public and private discussions" about whether a healthy, mature female orgasm was clitoral or vaginal.[2]

Freud, Kroger noted, originated the idea of distinct and hierarchal female orgasms in the early twentieth century, with the vaginal orgasm promoted by some as not just the "optimum type of sexual response," as Kroger called it, but also as the only one that signified a woman had reached healthy feminine sexual maturity.[3] This theory of the primacy of the vaginal orgasm remained popular from the mid-1940s through the mid-1960s, a period coinciding with the popularity of psychoanalysis in general.[4] The diagnosis of a lack of a vaginal orgasm—a woman's inability to transfer her erotic feeling from her clitoris in order to reach a vaginal orgasm because she was not passive and receptive enough—was a useful therapeutic tool for those who sought to reinforce strict gender divisions between masculine men and feminine women in the Cold War era.[5] As such, it appeared in popular marriage manuals and popular advice articles, and it was used within marital education and counseling.[6] The theory came to be regarded, as Stephen Jay Gould wrote in the late 1980s, "a shibboleth of pop culture during the heydays of persuasive Freudianism."[7]

Feminists in the late 1960s and early 1970s, as well as some later scholars, largely viewed the opinion espoused by Kroger on the primacy of the vaginal orgasm as the dominant narrative in the United States from the 1940s until at least the publication of *Human Sexual Response* by William Masters and Virginia Johnson in 1966.[8] Kroger and others like him posited that a vaginal orgasm was mature and healthy, while a clitoral orgasm was not. Although some who believed in the primacy of the vaginal orgasm did not necessarily disavow the clitoris as a sexual organ, they maintained that sexually healthy adult women had vaginal, not clitoral, orgasms. As suggested in Kroger's 1956 lecture, however, some physicians continued to treat a lack of female orgasm through surgical intervention on the clitoris, implying that these physicians regarded clitoral orgasm as healthy—otherwise, why treat this organ in order to enable orgasm?

Saving my discussion of *Human Sexual Response* for the next chapter, this chapter ends in 1966, the year Masters and Johnson published this book providing "new" evidence of the clitoris as the organ primarily at the center of female sexual sensitivity. By doing so, I extend upon historian Thomas Laqueur's contention that knowledge of the sexual purpose of the clitoris would have been "a commonplace to every seventeenth century midwife and had been anticipated in some detail by nineteenth century investigators" by explaining that it also would have been commonplace knowledge for gynecologists in the 1940s, 1950s, and 1960s. Laqueur wondered about the "great amnesia" that had to have befallen "scientific circles around 1900 so that hoary truths could be hailed as earth-shatteringly new in the second half of the twentieth century."[9] But physicians, perhaps especially gynecologists, and even some psychiatrists and psychoanalysts, did not forget that the sole purpose of the clitoris was sexual. Indeed, some physicians applied this knowledge of the sexual purpose of the clitoris by treating the organ to better enable sexual stimulation.

Sigmund Freud and the
Origins of the Vaginal Orgasm Theory

There can be no doubt that Freud's work regarding sexuality and the unconscious greatly influenced American academics and popular culture in the first half of the twentieth century. As historian Nathan Hale Jr. claimed in his book about Freud's impact in the United States, Freud made conflict about sexuality central to life.[10] I am concerned with just one aspect of his theories regarding sexuality here, however: his contention that healthy and sexually mature adult women experience a vaginal, not a clitoral, orgasm.

As others have noted, Freud can be difficult to study because he said different things at different times.[11] Moreover, his theories and attitudes were often complex, and, regarding female sexuality, he often stated that while he sincerely tried to understand the sexual life of women, this was something of a "dark continent" for him, as Freud biographer Peter Gay wrote. That said, his ideas about the clitoris as an inferior organ and the need for females to abandon it to reach mature sexuality were remarkably stable and seemed to him "well established," according to Gay.[12] Perhaps more importantly, many of his followers advanced these theories on female sexuality.

Freud laid the foundation for his hierarchal female orgasm in his *Three Essays on the Theory of Sexuality*, first published in 1905. Here Freud argued that both boys and girls develop sexually through stages, that they may stop at one stage or even regress, and that how they proceed through this series amounts to a reflection of their personal lives. But even though the path to healthy sexual maturity varied according to the individual, the end point was to be the same: heterosexuality.[13] Though Freud's focus was on sex, it was a traditional notion of sex, what Nathan Hale Jr. called "'civilized' morality," an idea that defined appropriate sexual behavior and provided models of the "manly man and womanly woman."[14] To understand how a girl became a womanly woman, Freud recommended looking to the clitoris, the central erotic area for female children, as evidenced by girls masturbating their clitorises. But when the female child became a female adult engaged in the sexual act, Freud argued that a mature and healthy woman moved her central erotic area away from the external clitoris internally to the vagina. This did not mean the clitoris ceased to be important, however, for according to Freud the clitoris still retained a "function: the task, namely, of transmitting the excitation to the adjacent female parts," namely, the vagina. For Freud, the purpose of the clitoris was similar to that of "pine shavings" which could be "kindled in order to set the log of harder wood on fire."[15] The clitoris could be stimulated during foreplay, but the real orgasm needed to occur in the vagina for the woman to be engaged in mature sex.

Freud's theories prior to World War I hinted at his assumption that males were the superior sex, according to Gay, and that the penis was the superior organ because it was the active organ. This did not mean that he believed women were not sensual beings; indeed, through the first two decades of the twentieth century, Freud described the sexual development of boys and girls as mirrors of each other, with differences created by social pressures. His ideas of boys and girls reflecting each other, Gay contended, was why Freud's original theory on the need for women to transfer the location of their sexual sensitivity went largely unchallenged among other psychoanalysts. By the 1920s, though, Freud began adopting the theory that a little girl was a failed boy; no longer were boys and girls on parallel paths to sexual development. Anatomy, Freud quipped, was destiny, and this destiny was the observable difference between the male and female genitalia. During this decade, he added another concept phase of sexual development, the phallic phase. For girls, this new phase introduced penis envy, the discovery that they did not possess the visible and powerful penis.[16]

Though Freud wrote that "anatomy has recognized the clitoris" as the "organ that is homologous to the penis" in his 1908 "On the Sexual Theories of Children," he also described the clitoris as not equivalent to the penis. Though, according to Freud, the clitoris "behaves in fact during childhood like a real and genuine penis—that it becomes the seat of excitations which lead it to being touched," it was in truth a stunted organ, a "small penis . . . which does not grow any bigger." A woman could not have a real penis—this was the organ of masculinity. Instead, Freud saw the clitoris as an immature sexual organ for women.[17] In her humiliation at not having the mature organ, the girl turned from her mother, the figure of attachment for both boys and girls in infancy and during their toddler years, to her father. In doing so, she also abandoned her infantile sexual organ, the clitoris, in favor of the adult vagina. She then developed a corresponding wish for a baby to replace her missing penis.[18] Girls, then, needed to make two laborious shifts that boys did not: girls needed to transfer their love from mother to father and then repress their masculine organ to embrace the uniquely feminine organ of the vagina for "the woman to emerge."[19] Freud recognized that this emotional and unconscious transfer from the clitoris to the vagina was not an easy one for women to make; indeed, women risked suffering more psychological ailments than men because of their need to make this difficult transfer.[20] Along the way, women, Freud acknowledged, could fail: as a result, they might give up sex altogether, refuse to give up the masculine clitoris, or become overly submissive. For those who managed to make this transition and enjoy any sexual pleasure, this pleasure was principally to be achieved through the vagina—otherwise there would be no need for a man.[21]

Freud, it should be noted, never actually used the phrase "vaginal orgasm." His work did, however, stress that for women to progress along their mature sexual destiny and reach normal femininity, the route was through the vagina, ditching the clitoris along the way. As a medical doctor, Freud knew anatomy well, and instead of ordering the physical removal of the clitoris to fit his theory, he ordered it to simply no longer matter.[22] It is difficult to believe Freud was unaware of normative anatomical ideas about the clitoris as the equivalent to the penis and that the clitoris, not the vagina, was regarded as the location of female sexual pleasure.[23] Physicians recognized the clitoris as the organ comparable to the male penis and similarly the organ of normative erotic sensitivities—beliefs that were maintained both before and after 1905. From a physiological perspective, Thomas Laqueur argued that Freud's reconstruction of the clitoris and the vagina was a "farce," one not supported by "common medical knowledge available in any nineteenth century handbook."[24] Freud's view, then, is not about anatomy but, rather, was "intended as the story" of the sexual destiny of women, how girls stopped being "little men."[25] Rather than being based in a physiological assessment of the two organs, Freud's vaginal orgasm was "a narrative of culture in anatomical disguise," according to Laqueur.[26]

The Dissemination of the Vaginal Orgasm Theory

Though Alfred Kinsey in the early 1950s labeled Freud's idea of vaginal transfer a "biological impossibility," those who believed in the vaginal orgasm theory began to disseminate it within the medical community as well as popularly in the United States in the decades prior to World War II.[27] Like psychoanalysis in general, the vaginal orgasm theory, first proposed (though not named as such) in 1905, did not immediately ignite either the popular or the medical imagination. While Freud's international reputation began to grow in the late nineteenth century, it was not until 1909, when he visited the United States for the first and only time, when his influence began to be felt in America. Within two years, psychoanalysis went from "merely one of a number of competing medical psychologies" to a professionally organized movement in America, according to Hall.[28] By the onset of World War I, the majority of Freud's work had been translated and was available in the United States, and a small but important group of analysts worked throughout the country to make psychoanalysis a subspecialty within medicine. Physicians outside of this subspecialty learned about psychoanalysis through publications, and some medical colleges began teaching the theory in the decade leading up to World War I.[29]

The advancement of the vaginal orgasm theory began in the United States to a limited degree in the 1920s and 1930s.[30] For example, according to physician W. F. Robie in his 1921 book, *The Art of Love*, while a woman "may have an orgasm or sexual climax from manipulation of the clitoris alone," he called such an orgasm incomplete and not as "natural as when the sensations begin in the external and are gradually carried over to the internal organs and have their culmination there."[31] Similarly, in a 1927 article, psychoanalyst Wilhelm Reich outlined how a woman, upon "the emission of the penis" into the vagina should move her feeling from the clitoris to the vagina "without any kind of rivalry" between them.[32] And in the early 1930s, Karl Menninger, a Kansas psychiatrist, began publishing an advice column in *Ladies Home Journal* answering readers' letters regarding questions of mental health. Many of these letters expressed women's frustration with their lack of orgasm during (presumably penetrative) sex with their husbands. Menninger responded, saying the problem was always "psychological in origin," calling lack of orgasm during intercourse frigidity—a "kind of disease" women needed to recover from. He insisted "the only way that you can get rid of this with any degree of certainty is by psychoanalysis."[33]

But while these men advanced the theory of vaginal orgasm, historian Jane Gerhard, in her work examining the history of feminism and American sexual thought, stated that "few doctors worked harder to define frigidity and the pathology of the clitoris" than Edward Hitschmann and Edmund Bergler did in the 1930s and 1940s.[34] Indeed, they are credited with the introduction of "vaginal orgasm" as a household term.[35] In 1936, they published *Frigidity in Women*, the first book on the psychoanalytic basis of frigidity.[36] In it, Hitschmann and Bergler wrote that a woman's transfer from clitoral to vaginal orgasm did not normally occur "until she has been deflowered." In their influential tome, Hitschmann and Bergler stated that the "sole criterion of frigidity is the absence of the vaginal orgasm."[37] Unlike Freud, Hitschmann and Bergler did not believe the clitoris could still be used to ignite passion in healthy adult women; rather, clitoral sexuality for them was a cause of neurosis and ill health. But a woman's ill health was not limited to her physiology: a woman who refused to make the transfer to the vagina was refusing her feminine social role. The vaginal orgasm transfer, then, was not just about sex; as Gerhard described, "Vaginal orgasm encapsulated the idea of feminine woman who knew her place in bed and in the family."[38] This idea resonated during the Cold War era.

Though Menninger and others did much to popularize psychoanalysis in the 1930s, it was not until after World War II that psychoanalysis truly "exploded" in the United States as part of the rise in wider acceptance of psychology in general.[39] Before the war, psychotherapy had been a marginal treatment, but the needs of returning soldiers and their families provided the impetus for the rise in the application of psychoanalysis.[40] Psychiatry, which had been largely confined to an institutional setting, moved to a clinical one: by 1947, half of the members of the American Psychiatric

Association worked in private practice. Many psychoanalysts found employment in teaching positions within medical schools and in clinics, thus
enhancing the professional standing of those who practiced psychoanalysis
as well as shaping others practicing medicine.[41] Freud's influence, and the
influence of psychoanalysis in general, extended far beyond the discipline.[42]
Coinciding with America's retreat into a more culturally and politically conservative attitude, psychoanalysis flourished within the medical and psychological professions, as the theory placed a stronger emphasis on internal
controls over individual's sexual behavior. Popular support grew, and both
the number of people waiting to see psychoanalysts and those seeking to
become psychoanalysts increased.[43]

While not all psychiatrists and sexual theorists agreed with him, Freudian
concepts greatly influenced American ideas about sex and about how to treat
sexual problems during this time, according to historian Vern Bullough.[44]
During the "heyday of analysis" in the 1950s, historian John C. Burnham
contended, psychoanalysis grew as a result of a larger cultural rise in the
prestige of science and the belief it could not only cure illness but also provide a route to happiness.[45] The growth of psychoanalysis between the mid-
1940s and the mid-1960s is what Hale called the "golden age" of the practice
and popularization of psychoanalysis.[46]

Psychoanalysis both reflected and reinforced narrow definitions regarding gender roles and expectations in American culture. As historian
Eli Zaretsky wrote, "Postwar psychoanalysis became a veritable fount of
homophobia, misogyny, and conservatism, central to the post war project of
normalization" with its resanctification of heterosexual love and marriage
as being central to healthy womanhood.[47] Psychoanalysts, argued Mary Jo
Buhle in her history of psychoanalysis and feminism, eschewed their former
avant-garde status in favor of aligning with mainstream ideas in the United
States, a mainstream increasingly misogynistic.[48] Women, or at least healthy
and mature women, were to be passive in their social and sexual roles. In
postwar culture, many white families idealized the home in an effort to find
security during the Cold War, an idealization that domesticated and subor-
dinated women.[49] Since the 1920s, white women had increasingly joined the
paid workforce, but during the 1950s their proper role became more stridently defined as housewife and mother, with her world to be centered on
children, consumption, and housework.[50] The stereotype of the Cold War
era shows a suburban world of white, female homemakers. But, as other historians have pointed out, while many women did indeed fit this stereotype,
others did not. Postwar culture was complex; acknowledging the diversity
of women's actual lives, nevertheless, there existed a cultural narrowing of
gender roles in postwar America.[51]

These beliefs supported the idea of the mature orgasm located in the
vagina, as it both implicitly and explicitly reinforced childbearing by

requiring healthy sex to be potentially procreative as well. As one psycho-analytically inclined obstetrician gynecologist wrote in 1961, a career would no longer matter to a woman and, during intercourse, "her unconscious phantasy" was that her husband "might make her with child."[52] The vaginal orgasm became, historian Carolyn Herbst Lewis argued, "the epicenter" of heterosexuality for women because it "served both as the site of the success-ful performance of heterosexual intercourse and as the only healthy outlet for female orgasms."[53] Many psychoanalysts, psychiatrists, and psychoanalyti-cally inclined physicians worked hard to depict use of the clitoris as patho-logical, arguing that aggressive and neurotic women experienced clitoral orgasm while mature and healthy women experienced passive and healthy vaginal orgasms. The vaginal orgasm combined the sexual with the repro-ductive and conflated sexuality with gender. This conflation made "psycho-analysis useful for social commentators and antifeminists in the post–World War II period who insisted that healthy, normal women were sexually pas-sive, essentially maternal, and happily devoted to home and hearth," accord-ing to historian Jane Gerhard.[54]

In 1951, Chicago gynecologist William Kroger and San Francisco phy-sician S. Charles Freed, prominent advocates of the vaginal orgasm the-ory, declared that the role of the woman "during the sex act" was "one of passivity and receptivity," whereby a "woman's passive acceptance of the penis" was a necessary sign of a sexually mature woman.[55] J. P. Greenhill, a Chicago gynecologist, restated this position, writing in 1952 that the "transference of sexual satisfaction and excitement from the clitoris to the vagina" occurred as part of a woman's "emotional maturation."[56] In their 1947 book written largely for a popular audience, *Modern Woman: The Lost Sex*, psychiatrist Marynia Farnham and journalist Ferdinand Lundberg likewise noted that though it was quite common for women to "obtain sexual gratification only with the manipulation of the clitoris," a woman's ability to transfer her orgasm internally was an "essential part of the sexual maturation."[57] During their sex education classes in New York City in the 1940s and 1950s, doctors and marital sex guide authors Lena Levine and Abraham Stone noted the importance of the clitoris to pleasurable sex for women but stressed the vaginal orgasm as the superior and mature orgasm. While telling those attending their classes that the clitoral orgasm was bet-ter than no orgasm at all, they urged the women to work toward achieving a mature vaginal one.[58] And physician Marie Robinson, in her 1959 book, *The Power of Sexual Surrender*, echoed this line, noting that the clitoris was "extremely sensitive to stimulation" but that in the "fully mature woman this sensitivity often diminishes, giving way to the vagina as the primary source of the greatest sexual pleasure."[59]

Bergler, one of the loudest advocates of the vaginal orgasm as the only normal orgasm for healthy adult women, believed women were unable to fake a vaginal orgasm. A husband, Bergler wrote, "can be deceived by a clever woman in many things," but a woman could not voluntarily contract her "pelvic and perineal muscles at the end of the sex act." This, Bergler believed, was the "only sure criterion that a man can use to determine whether a woman is frigid." Women who did not transfer their orgasms from their clitorises to their vaginas, who were unable to, or who were found to be attempting to fake their vaginal orgasms were regarded as unhealthy. The "consequences of frigidity," Bergler believed, were "tragic for the woman" and included "depression" and "hysterical symptoms" including a "denial by the woman that she is ill."[60] Marie Robinson told her readers that having a clitoral, not a vaginal, orgasm was a form of frigidity and, "psychologically speaking, pathological."[61] These women, argued Eugene Hamilton, an obstetrician gynecologist in St. Louis in 1961, were "childish and false" because they rejected their femininity when they rejected the vaginal orgasm. In contrast, a woman who obtained orgasm vaginally was the definition of appropriate self-effacing femininity, including that though she may "fail to reach an orgasm once in a hundred times," she would take pleasure "in the very obvious pleasure that she is able to give her husband."[62]

Espoused as such, the vaginal orgasm theory reinforced and promoted female sexual passivity as an extension of the female's subservient role in the family and in society. The vaginal orgasm was, asserted Carolyn Herbst Lewis, the "prerequisite for marital stability."[63] Regarded as such, women who failed to make the transfer risked more than just their health: they also risked the well-being of their families. Edmund Bergler maintained that 90 percent of "all cases of infidelity on the part of the woman are traceable to frigidity."[64] Eugene Hamilton stressed that the "importance of the problem [of frigidity] can be appreciated by all," for frigidity in women was often one of the "common factors leading to divorce, separations and marital infidelity."[65] Hitschmann and Bergler noted that men could easily become unfaithful to their frigid wives, seeking satisfaction "with aware and potent women." A frigid woman could lose her husband and then "only too easily becomes lonely, neglected, betrayed, neurotic, dejected—and ill."[66]

In a paper they presented at the Sixth Annual Meeting of the Academy of Psychosomatic Medicine held in Cleveland before it was published in the spring of 1960, physicians R. N. Rutherford, A. L. Banks, S. H. Davidson, W. A. Coburn, J. Williams, and F. H. Zaffiro noted that many a frigid woman was neither aware of nor disturbed by her frigidity and sought medical help only "because her marriage is imperiled unless she becomes an 'adequate' partner (usually adequate according to her husband's definition)."[67] Similarly, but with less sympathy to women, in their popular 1947 *Modern Woman*, Farnham and Lundberg wrote that a large number of women were sexually "disordered" and that "their disorder is having terrible social and personal effects" on men. Farnham and Lundberg saw a woman stepping outside her social role as wife and mother as detrimental to "her home, husband, and children." According to the authors, "the more educated the woman is, the greater chance there is of sexual disorder," including frigidity.[68] Edward Podolsky, a psychiatrist in Brooklyn, agreed, stating that frigidity was "the cause of the break up of a great many marriages."[69]

According to Podolsky, frigidity was "more common than is popularly supposed."[70] Like Podolsky, psychoanalysts, psychiatrists, and physicians worried over the extent of what they regarded as the common problem of an absence of vaginal orgasm. Though Farnham and Lundberg, for example, stated they had "no way of determining accurately how widespread the condition is," they believed its prevalence to be "enormously high."[71] Writing in 1950, Kroger and Freed estimated that nearly three-quarters of women "derive little or no pleasure from the sexual act."[72] In a paper with Bergler three years later, Kroger estimated the rate to be even higher, with 70–90 percent of women failing to reach a vaginal orgasm.[73] The reason for such high numbers, Bergler believed, was that "the majority of women are incapable of shifting the excitement to the passive receptivity of the vagina."[74] Chicago gynecologist J. P. Greenhill wrote that, based on his clinical experience, "surely more than one-third of all women fail to enjoy the pleasures of sexual intercourse."[75] A decade later, Eugene Hamilton estimated that 40 percent of women "suffer frigidity in some degree," referring back to the various forms of frigidity outlined by Bergler.[76] In 1966, one article gave the proportion, while "having in all probability diminished," as still "high" at between 30 and 50 percent of women.[77]

In 1954, Bergler and Kroger argued that frigidity was "so widespread in our culture that it is the emotional plague."[78] But, for those who argued about the necessity of the vaginal orgasm, it was an emotional plague based on woman's bodily construction. As Kroger and Freed pointed out, Freud's contention that anatomy was destiny indicated "his belief that the clitoris does not often come into contact with the male organ during intercourse." This, they said, provided the anatomical proof of the necessity for healthy adult women to transfer their orgasm from the clitoris to the vagina, an organ the penis did contact during penetrative intercourse.[79] Those who advocated for the transition to the vaginal orgasm, then, worked to make the clitoral orgasm seem not just unhealthy to both the woman and her family but also anatomically impossible without "artificial clitoris-penis contact," according to Bergler.[80] As Bergler further described, women who tried to attain orgasm from clitoral stimulation during penetrative sex resorted to "substitute acts" to establish "artificial contact between the penis and the clitoris" such as using "acrobatic movements only to achieve the aim of penis-clitoris contact" or by holding their "thighs closely together."[81] Because there was "no mechanical intensification of arousal of the clitoris through friction during coitus," without such behavior, Bergler argued, women's anatomy decided the necessity of vaginal orgasm to her healthy heterosexuality.[82]

What Counted as Frigidity?

Los Angeles psychiatrist Judd Marmor wrote in 1953, "The conclusion that clitoral sensitivity must ultimately give way to vaginal sensitivity in the normal female seems never to have been seriously questioned in the psychoanalytical literature."[83] Yet his contention does not hold true, either within the psychoanalytical literature or the wider medical literature. In fact, some of those who followed Freud, like Ernest Jones, "sturdily disagreed" with Freud on the nature of female sexuality as moving from clitoral to vaginal.[84] As part of this disagreement, many writing on the subject of female sexuality and frigidity noted that there were two theories regarding female orgasm, clitoral and vaginal, with some suggesting that the two orgasms should be seen as normal companions to each other rather than as distinct and hierarchal. Additionally, those writing about women's sexual response or lack thereof noted the absence of a uniform definition of frigidity, with definitions ranging from a lack of desire to a lack of any orgasm to a lack of a specific sort of orgasm. Finally, many writing about the vaginal orgasm observed that it was a controversial theory within medical discourse.

Some scholars have noted the debate between advocates and detractors of the vaginal orgasm theory, and some have suggested that medical voices of dissent challenged those in the dominant position—those who believed in the vaginal orgasm as superior.[85] Loud and well placed, advocates of the vaginal orgasm theory dominated the discussion. But this discussion was never uniform in its presentation of the vaginal orgasm or in its attending complaint, frigidity. Nor was it, perhaps, the dominant position within medicine. Looking closely at relevant texts from this period suggests that the reason for their volume could be that proponents of the vaginal orgasm theory were arguing outside established medical ideas regarding the organ of female sexual response.

Those enmeshed in the debate recognized that there were two theories regarding healthy female orgasm at this time. Recall that, in the discussion that began this chapter, Kroger acknowledged both. Writing in 1953 with Bergler in a challenge to Alfred Kinsey's work regarding the female orgasm as clitoral (discussed below), they noted there was a "problem" in "defining, scientifically, female orgasm" because there was "no unanimity of opinion," with "one school of thought" claiming "that vaginal orgasm does exist" while the "other school of thought . . . denies this claim, putting clitoris orgasm in the center."[86] Discussion in the literature about female orgasm noted, as a mid-1960s article in *Minnesota Medicine* did, that "two distinct types of orgasm have been postulated: clitoral and vaginal."[87] In their July 1959 article adapted from a paper they gave at the Fourth Annual Meeting of the Academy of Psychosomatic Medicine in Chicago, physicians R. N. Rutherford, A. L. Banks, S. H. Davidson, W. A. Coburn, and J. Williams noted that some "authors maintain that the vagina has virtually no sensory nerves and that the orgasm, therefore, is largely clitoral in nature," while others "maintain that true orgasm is vaginal in nature, not clitoral, which is really dual masturbation."[88]

While some believed the vaginal and clitoral orgasms were distinct and hierarchal, others saw no reason to separate them. Analysts like Melanie Klein had in the 1920s written about the clitoris and the vagina together rather than about the subordination of one for the other.[89] Four decades later, Terence McGuire and Richard Steinhilber, psychiatrists at the Mayo Clinic in Minnesota, tried to bridge the two. They argued that women whose clitoris had been removed still experienced orgasm, while also noting "worldwide preferential sexual positioning favors those positions that predispose to the greatest clitoral stimulation during intercourse." Moreover, anatomical studies indicated "that the clitoris is proportionately more richly supplied with sensory nerve endings than the larger male homologue, the penis." This "indirect corroboration," McGuire and Steinhilber stated, made them believe that "both clitoral and vaginal orgasm exist with doubtless degrees of admixture of the two in normal heterosexual activities."[90]

Four years before this article, psychoanalyst Helene Deutsch chaired a panel on frigidity in women at the December 1960 meeting of the American Psychoanalytic Association.[91] Though in her 1945 book Deutsch had called the clitoral orgasm "infantile sexuality" because it was "useless for reproduction," she was now reconsidering her position.[92] In her introduction of the panel discussion, she chose to "take a stand based on her many years of work in female psychology" about "so-called frigidity." "Shocked by the high incidence" of, and psychoanalytic treatments for, frigidity, she came to question "whether the vagina was really created by nature for the sexual function we assume and demand for it."[93] Her clinical experience showed to her that many healthy feminine women did not have vaginal orgasms, even after analysis, while many women she described as masculine (and unhealthy) did experience such orgasms.[94] Based on her own professional experience, Deutsch returned to the "conviction that the female sexual apparatus consists of two parts with a definite division of function." The clitoris was the sexual organ, and the vagina "primarily the organ of reproduction." The clitoris held a central role, communicating sexual desire to the vagina.[95] Though Deutsch still accepted the vaginal orgasm, she also saw room for the clitoris as a healthy and normal sexual organ that worked with the vagina in effecting sexual gratification.[96] Taken literally, historian Reuben Fine noted, Deutsch's revision was a "complete about-face" from the vaginal orgasm theory.[97]

On that same panel, psychoanalyst Burness Moore reported that, based on his review of the literature, perhaps too much focus had been placed on the importance of the vaginal orgasm as better than the clitoral orgasm.[98] He further stated that, possibly as a result of so much attention to the vagina as the appropriate location of female sexual sensation, frigidity had not been "sufficiently clarified."[99] Perhaps this lack of a definite definition for frigidity could be attributed to the debate regarding the two theories of female orgasm. Though historian Carolyn Herbst Lewis maintained that, although frigidity in the mid-twentieth century was at times regarded as the absence of any sexual desire or sensation, "physicians and psychiatrists primarily stressed the importance and pervasiveness of frigidity as *inappropriate*, not absent, sexual outlet." As such, frigidity manifested "itself in the failure to achieve a vaginal orgasm—or, worse yet, a consistent reliance on the clitoris for pleasure," according to Lewis.[100]

But though Bergler and Hitschmann defined frigidity as a lack of a vaginal orgasm, others defined it more broadly, including an inability to reach any orgasm.[101] Some defined frigidity as a lack of sexual response. In a 1966 seminar at the Mayo Clinic, those attending noted that since the "presence of vaginal orgasm is doubted by some and the presence of orgasm—whether vaginal or clitoral—is often hard to determine, it would seem more reasonable to define frigidity as the total or relative absence of pleasurable response to erotic stimuli."[102] Others defined frigidity as the absence of sexual desire and of pleasurable sensation during intercourse. Josef Novak, an obstetrician gynecologist at Columbia University, described frigidly as "both absence of sexual desire *and* lack of pleasurable sensation in coition with a man of normal sexual potency."[103] And still others considered the label frigid to describe a woman who did not have sex.[104]

These diverse definitions were noted in the literature—indeed, even Bergler acknowledged that there was "by no means complete agreement" over the "definitional and terminological demarcation of this malady."[105] At the 1966 seminar on frigidity in women at the Mayo Clinic, those assembled noted that there was "no generalized agreement regarding the exact definition of frigidity in women."[106] Two years earlier, psychiatrists at this clinic noticed the diverse definitions of frigidity as consisting of not just the "conscious revulsion or disinterest in sexual intercourse" or the "absence of the sexual aspect of love in the female" but as also applying to women who desire but experience no pleasure in sex. Thus, attendees Terrence McGuire and Richard Steinhilber observed, "We have a spectrum running the gamut from vaginismus and dyspareunia through vaginal anesthesia and ultimately up to only an occasional failure to achieve orgasm, all being represented by divergent authors as varying degrees of frigidity."[107]

Writing in *General Practitioner* in 1966, William A. Layman, Gerald H. Rozan, and Morton L. Kurland noted that among the "many patients with sexual problems encountered by the modern doctor, the most frequent, and perhaps the least understood, is the 'frigid woman.'" As they further noted, the label of frigidity was "used so loosely" it was "without real scientific meaning." When a woman was labeled as frigid within popular culture, it was not clear, they argued, "whether the woman's sexual functioning is being considered or whether she is simply being denigrated." This was true even "within the medical community," because frigidity "has come to cover a broad spectrum."[108] Part of this confusion about frigidity was that there were different levels and different sorts of frigidity; Bergler and Hitschmann, for example, originally enumerated eighteen forms of frigidity, and in a 1947 article Bergler wrote that he could now "add a few other forms."[109] Others held there was a difference between "true frigidity" and "pseudo-frigidity," with different causes and treatments. In 1946, LeRoy Ritmiller and Roy Nicodemus, gynecologists in Danville, Pennsylvania, wrote that frigidity was either classified as constitutional (individuals having a "physical imperfection and/or organic disease"), pseudo-frigidity ("due to ignorance of coital technic on the part of either partner or both, or they are clinging to some false sexual theories"), or true frigidity.[110] Layman, Rozan, and Kurland believed the term "total frigidity" should be reserved for those women who never attain orgasm—a condition they believed was relatively rare. "The more common forms would be better classified as *relative frigidity*," they argued, and included "women who can achieve orgasm only by manual manipulation of the genitalia, those who can only infrequently achieve orgasm during coitus and those whose drive is so limited that they desire sex only on rare occasions."[111] The Chicago obstetrician gynecologist Greenhill made a demarcation between true frigidity and pseudo-frigidity as well, noting that pseudo-frigidity was the result of impotent husbands or husbands who ejaculated prematurely, as well as "clumsiness, ignorance of the proper technic on the part of the husband, misunderstandings, quarreling and ill health."[112]

This lack of agreement on what frigidity meant clinically translated into a variety of treatment options. If, as Ritmiller and Nicodemus believed, true frigidity comprised the majority of cases, because it was based in "an abnormality or disturbance in the psychosexual development," the necessary treatment consisted of psychoanalysis.[113] Others, such as John Paul Brady, a psychiatrist at the University of Pennsylvania, argued for a more direct, less time-consuming route than psychoanalysis: relaxation of the woman through the use of drugs.[114] But if frigidity was due to "ignorance of coital technic," education regarding sexual anatomy and positions was the therapy for both partners—though some physicians thought the male partner perhaps needed it more, like Milwaukee obstetrician and gynecologist F. Jackson Stoddard, who wrote, an "inept, immature husband is often the cause" of female frigidity.[115]

Some practitioners, like Robert Rutherford, who believed most cases of frigidity were psychological in origin, still stressed the need to conduct a physical examination "to exclude a bona fide organic cause."[116] Such structural causes that could result in frigidity included a tight hymen or a small vagina, thus prohibiting penetration.[117] Greenhill also noted the importance of a physical examination—of both the husband and the wife—to reveal any "structural reasons for frigidity."[118] Though gynecologist Josef Novak believed frigidity often had its origin in unconscious inhibitions, he also listed several potential physical reasons for frigidity, including malnutrition, diabetes, or a disease of the thyroid or ovaries, all of which "may cause loss of sexual desire and satisfaction."[119] If frigidity was a result of a "physical imperfection," however, treatment such as hormone therapy was seen as possibly capable of correcting this imperfection.[120] In their 1950 gynecology text, Arthur Hale Curtis and John William Huffman noted that while they found estrogen therapy to have been "disappointing," a prescription of oral testosterone had "been helpful to many frigid patients."[121]

Treatment was also sometimes applied to a specific part of the body when women failed to reach orgasm during intercourse.[122] The West Virginian obstetrician gynecologist Archibald Perrin Hudgins wrote about a local ointment that was "available for application to the external genital organ." This "frigidity ointment" could be prescribed to women, "when deemed necessary by the physician," and was to be applied "gently for five minutes" upon the "sensitive area (clitoris) every night."[123] This treatment reflects a recognition of the clitoris as an impaired sexual organ resulting in frigidity and an assumption that organ could be treated. Edward Podolsky, a Brooklyn psychiatrist who defined frigidity as "the incapacity of the woman to experience a vaginal orgasm" also suggested that sometimes frigidity could be caused by "malposition of the clitoris" and, when this was the case, a recommendation for "a new coital position" to bring the clitoris "in closer contact with the penis is of value."[124] In a way, this conflation makes no sense—if frigidity is the lack of vaginal orgasm, why apply an ointment to the clitoris or recommend a change in sexual positions to better stimulate the clitoris? Possibly these recommendations were made to help the woman transfer her orgasm from the clitoris to the vagina once the clitoris has been stimulated. But this seeming contradiction—made even by one who believed frigidity was the absence of a vaginal orgasm—can also be seen as an understanding of the vaginal orgasm as an ideal that did not supplant the normative belief in the clitoris as the principal sexual organ for women.

The Controversial Vaginal Orgasm Theory

The vaginal orgasm theory was controversial during its heyday—a controversy explicitly noted by many at the time.[125] In their 1959 article, R. N. Rutherford, A. L. Banks, S. H. Davidson, W. A. Coburn, and J. Williams noted that though "Freud originally believed that transfer of sensation took place from the clitoris to the vagina," the "discussion still rages, based on certain anatomic truisms."[126] Others, including Bergler and Kroger, indicated that the vaginal orgasm theory was contentious: there was "considerable difference of opinion" regarding "whether orgasm in the female" was from "vaginal or clitoric stimulation" and "controversy rages in the psychiatric literature" on the issue.[127]

Though Bergler, Hitschmann, Kroger, and others maintained the centrality of vaginal orgasm to female health, the vaginal orgasm was possibly not considered a necessary component of mental health by psychoanalysis overall. As psychoanalyst Jules Glenn and psychiatrist Eugene Kaplan noted in their 1968 critical review of the definition of orgasm in women, though Hitschmann and Bergler both believed it was necessary for female mental health, the vaginal orgasm was not listed as one of the requirements for completion of therapy at the Symposium on Termination of Analysis in 1950.[128] Glenn and Kaplan further noted that the vaginal orgasm theory was not listed in major texts on the techniques of psychoanalysis published in the 1940s or 1950s.[129] For example, in his 1949 *Basic Principles of Psychoanalysis*, A. A. Brill, one of the most noted advocates of psychoanalysis in the United States, listed nothing in the index of his book for the clitoris, clitoral orgasm, vagina, vaginal orgasm, or for frigidity.[130] Nor were either the vaginal orgasm theory or frigidity listed within the 1950 *Freud: Dictionary of Psychoanalysis*. Instead, the concept that girls should transfer their "dominant erotogenic zone" prior to becoming a mature female from the clitoris to the vagina "wholly or in part" was found under the definition of "phallic phase in girls"—not under its own listing as vaginal orgasm.[131] As a final example of the nonuniform acceptance of the vaginal orgasm theory, in the 1958 *Comprehensive Dictionary of Psychological and Psychoanalytical Terms: A Guide to Usage*, there not only was no listing for vaginal orgasm, the clitoris was defined as "a small organ of erectile tissue, part of the external female genitals, stimulation of which is an important source of sex pleasure."[132]

Even Bergler and Kroger noted in 1953 that the acceptance of the vaginal orgasm theory was still in its growth state, writing "from discussion and recent publications, the theory of vaginal orgasm is receiving increasing recognition."[133] Bergler, this time with Hitschmann, had also highlighted the theory's nondominant status in an earlier attack on Alfred Kinsey. In a late 1940s article restating their definition of frigidity as a lack of a vaginal orgasm, they noted that their definition recently "got a boost from an unexpected quarter." Kinsey, they wrote, "in his *Report*, not only denies the existence of vaginal orgasm, but denounces the mere possibility of existence of 'such a thing' like vaginal orgasm." They further objected to Kinsey's stance that the vaginal orgasm was an "allegedly unfounded opinion" and denigrated Kinsey's "claims that the opinion is widespread among psychiatrists and other clinicians." Either overly modest, or possibly flattered, Bergler and Hitschmann further wrote that "we hope that Kinsey has statistical proof for at least that statement: we are unaware of the fact that the Hitschmann-Bergler theory is so widespread."[134]

This lack of widespread, uniform, and perhaps even official acceptance of the vaginal orgasm theory within psychoanalytical discourse, let alone medical discourse, is perhaps why Bergler and Hitschmann wrote so harshly in condemnation of proponents of the clitoral orgasm, most notably, but not solely, Alfred Kinsey. I will turn to Kinsey and his followers after I examine the attacks made upon the clitoral orgasm theory. Looking at the denouncements of the clitoral orgasm in the context of established medical understandings of the clitoris as a sexual organ provides a different way to view critiques against the clitoral orgasm: as responses not to an alternative and marginalized theory but to the accepted theory that the clitoris was the principal sexual organ of women—and that healthy women could have a clitoral orgasm.

Those who were most vocal in their attacks on the clitoral orgasm theory were, not surprisingly, those most vocal in their advancement of the vaginal orgasm theory, Bergler being in the fore. Bergler worried about the "group of scientific investigators" who were of the "opinion that a woman is sexually normal if capable of achieving a *clitoridian* orgasm." Clitoral orgasm proponents, Bergler argued, believed that orgasm "*after* coitus, in the clitoris, through masturbation with the help of the man" was an acceptable form of "emotional satisfaction" for women.[135] Such beliefs, Bergler contended, meant that the practice of a woman who demanded her husband "massage her clitoris for about half an hour" though she remained "cold" during intercourse or a woman who "detested" "vaginal intercourse" and who after would masturbate "with her own hand" or a woman who "attained orgasm through cunnilingus alone" were all "normal." According to Bergler, these practices were not normal, and the "opinion that there are no rules in sexual life but that each must seek for happiness in his own way is wrong."[136]

In addition to condemning the theory of the clitoral orgasm (and the "not normal" means of achieving a clitoral orgasm), Bergler and others also attacked its proponents. In 1949, Bergler and Hitschmann restated their views on the primacy of the vaginal orgasm and how frigidity was the "incapacity of a woman to have a *vaginal orgasm*." But more importantly, in this paper not only did they restate this view; they attacked those who denied the "existence of vaginal orgasm."[137] One such person was G. Lombard Kelly, an anatomy professor at the Medical College of Georgia.[138] Hitschmann and Bergler quoted Kelly describing them as "two Austrian physicians" who laid "great stress upon what they call the vaginal orgasm" and who claimed "that any woman, no matter how passionate she is, who cannot attain orgasm in normal intercourse, [and who] requires massage of the clitoris, is frigid."

These two psychoanalysts, they quoted Kelly as arguing, "have invented what they call the vaginal orgasm and call frigid the hottest woman in the world who cannot have one (whatever it is)."[139]

Hitschmann and Bergler criticized Kelly for suggesting men bore some of the responsibility to ensure women received stimulation during penetrative intercourse. Kelly's suggestion that couples try different positions, or even more problematic for Hitschmann and Bergler, viewing "clitoris-masturbation during intercourse" as being "normal prerequisites," seemed to them to be "an extreme concession to frigidity making out of woman's neurotic habit a virtue, blaming the victimized man to boot." Attacking the idea that "there are no frigid women, only inexperienced men," as Kelly had said, Hitschmann and Bergler labeled this a "misconception" that denied the "existence of frigidity and places all the blame on the man." Moreover, they argued "even if the husband proposes prolonged masturbation, he gets tired of obligatory and prolonged clitoric masturbation," calling this "more work than pleasure."[140]

But though Bergler and Hitschmann were critical of Kelly, the person of greater concern to them, because of his popular influence, was Alfred Kinsey. "Many dynamically oriented psychiatrists are protagonists of the theory of the vaginal orgasm, and are sharply critical of Kinsey's statistical and nonmedical approach," Bergler and Kroger wrote in 1953.[141] Advocates like Bergler and Kroger were most distressed by Kinsey's denial of the vaginal orgasm as having a physiological basis. Bergler and Kroger charged that Kinsey "denies the existence of vaginal orgasm" and were critical that Kinsey instead argued that "most of the physical stimulation which the female receives from actual coitus comes from contact of the external areas of the vulva, of the areas immediately inside the outer edges of the labia, and of the clitoris, with the pubic area of the male during genital union."[142]

The next year, Bergler and Kroger again challenged Kinsey in a January 1954 letter to the editor subsequent to *JAMA*'s review of *Sexual Behavior in the Human Female*.[143] Beginning by claiming Kinsey "merely 'dusts off' many abandoned theories" regarding female sexual sensitivity, they then launched into a vicious attack, one they felt was justified because "millions of persons" were "uncritically accepting" the report. Physicians, Bergler and Kroger believed, were being "bombarded with questions concerning the Kinsey report; therefore, prompt correction of Kinsey's faulty inferences is mandatory to prevent their perpetuation as dogma." Bergler and Kroger spent a large amount of time in their letter criticizing the report's denial of the vagina as sexually sensitive. Noting that Kinsey tested the insensitivity of the vagina "by gently stroking the walls with a glass, metal, or cotton-tipped probe in a gynecologist's office," Bergler and Kroger maintained that an "erect penis certainly cannot be compared with a wisp of cotton on an applicator." But where they really condemned Kinsey was for the implications of an insensitive vagina: the denial of the vaginal orgasm. And here one sees Bergler and Kroger, who had in the past stressed physiological evidence in support of the vaginal orgasm—the location of the clitoris—stress social and authoritative reasons instead. The vaginal orgasm, they wrote, was considered by "most authorities" to be "more desirable than the clitoral one." Unlike Kinsey and other proponents of the clitoral orgasm, Bergler and Kroger continued to regard as abnormal women who required "perverse acts to achieve orgasm" from clitoral stimulation. According to Bergler and Kroger, "quality rather than quantity" mattered when it came to a "healthy sexual response."[144] And they deemed the vaginal orgasm of more quality.

Proponents of the Clitoral Orgasm Theory

Quality over quantity may have mattered to advocates of the vaginal orgasm like Bergler, but not all women agreed with what that quality entailed or that it included the necessity of transferring their orgasms internally. Eugene Hamilton, an obstetrician gynecologist in St. Louis, noted that women who had clitoral orgasms were "often difficult to treat because they often deny the existence of frigidity."[145] According to Marie Robinson, physician and author of *The Power of Sexual Surrender*, many women defended their clitoral orgasm as "perfectly normal and adequate," though she assured them "it is not." She recommended therapy to help these women experience the "profound pleasure of true orgasm," vaginal orgasm. Robinson noted that many of her patients who had clitoral orgasms brought in the results of Alfred Kinsey to defend their form of orgasm as normal. "Somehow or other," Robinson complained, "women with this difficulty do get hold of the Kinsey 'results.'" She called it a "sad thing" that "the Kinsey report is often used to bolster the neurotically defensive attitude of women who are able to achieve only clitoral orgasm." Robinson noted that many of her colleagues also reported "similar experiences," something she labeled as "unfortunate."[146]

Alfred Kinsey received his PhD in entomology from Harvard and accepted a position at Indiana University, spending the first two decades of his academic career studying gall-forming wasps. Asked in 1938 to help with a student-demanded course on sex, he began researching the topic but found little on human sexual response. So he began gathering the information, first by interviewing students and then branching out and traveling on weekends to interview people outside the university and the state. With the university's backing, he formed the Institute for Sex Research, securing Rockefeller Foundation money and reluctantly giving up his wasp studies. In his sex research, Kinsey followed his taxonomic perspective: he gathered a large and varied range of samples and he passed no judgments on them.[147] Most of the current theories about sex, Kinsey wrote, were "developed without any adequate appreciation of the anatomy which is involved whenever there is sexual response."[148] This is what Kinsey sought to remedy through interviews with thousands of women, testing parts of the body, and direct observations of intercourse of both human and nonhuman mammals.

In 1953, Kinsey and his staff at the Institute for Sex Research published *Sexual Behavior in the Human Female*, a book based on 5,940 interviews with white women collected over fifteen years. Calling it the second progress report (the first being on male sexuality published five years earlier) to discover "what people do sexually," Kinsey and his fellow researchers hoped to show through this large accumulation of data the way humans actually behaved.[149] The interviewers used orgasm as a measure of pleasurable sex in their study. Though believing that orgasm was "not the final test of the effectiveness of a sexual relationship," noting that sex could still be a powerful connection even when it did not lead to orgasm, "the female's failure to respond to orgasm" was, they found, "one of the most frequent sources of dissatisfaction in marriage, and it is not infrequently the source of other types of conflict which may lead to the dissolution of a marriage." Kinsey's data indicated as many as two-thirds of marriages at some point experienced "serious disagreement over sexual relationships," and in a "considerable number, there is constant disagreement." Moreover, Kinsey estimated that in nearly "three-quarters of the divorces recorded in our case histories, sexual factors were among those which had led to divorce."[150]

Women in the study who reached orgasm (they did not specify vaginal or clitoral) did so during around three-quarters of the time during sex acts with their husbands. The percentage varied considerably depending on the woman's age and length of her marriage; younger newly married women reached orgasm on average only 63 percent of the time, while women married for twenty years or longer reached orgasm around 85 percent of the time. The interviewers found that in 95 percent of the married women interviewed, their husbands manually stimulated their wives' genitals before intercourse, and a little over half did orally. Nearly all couples reported the most common position to be the female supine underneath, facing the male, though half of the younger generation reported engaging in intercourse frequently with the woman on top. In addition, Kinsey and his associates found a correlation between premarital sex with orgasm during sex once married and that most women had reached orgasm through masturbation or premarital heterosexual or homosexual petting, activities which favored the stimulation of the clitoris.[151]

What Kinsey and his team learned from these thousands of interviews was that women did not report sexual feeling in their vaginas but in their clitorises. As biographer James Jones noted, Kinsey could have simply used this information from interviews as evidence that the vaginal orgasm theory had no physiological merit, but this "would have been contrary to his nature."

Always the gatherer of data, Kinsey sought to supplement his case histories by also engaging with physicians investigating sexual response, carrying on "lengthy and highly technical correspondence" with those conducting histological studies of vaginal tissues as well as of the role of hormones and the quantity and distribution of nerves in the external genitalia, vagina, and cervix.[152] Five gynecologists (three men and two women) also worked with Kinsey to test the sensitivity of the clitorises and the vaginas of nearly nine hundred women. The gynecologists lightly stroked or applied soft pressure to both areas. Of this group, less than 14 percent were aware that their vaginas were being touched, confirming for Kinsey that the "vaginal walls are quite insensitive in the great majority of females." In sharp contrast, 98 percent were aware that their clitorises were being stimulated. Though Kinsey noted "awareness of tactile stimulation or of pressure does not demonstrate the capacity to be aroused erotically by similar stimuli," it seemed to him "probable that any area which is not responsive to tactile stimulation or pressure cannot be involved in erotic response." Kinsey called this evidence a "precise and important body of data on a matter which has heretofore been poorly understood and vigorously debated."[153]

Based on the information gleaned from the interviews and from the laboratory tests, Kinsey and his associates declared the clitoris important to female sexual arousal and orgasm. "There are many females who are incapable of maximum arousal unless the clitoris is sufficiently stimulated," he wrote. In light of this finding, as well as what the women he interviewed told him and his colleagues, Kinsey rejected the psychoanalytic idea of the vaginal orgasm. "Some of the psychoanalysts," he wrote, "ignoring the anatomic data, minimize the importance of the clitoris while insisting in the importance of the vagina in female sexual response." He further noted that some "psychoanalysts and some other clinicians insist that only vaginal stimulation and a 'vaginal orgasm' can provide a psychologically satisfactory culmination to the activity of a 'sexually mature' female." Examining his findings, Kinsey found it difficult in "light of our present understanding of the anatomy and physiology of sexual response, to understand what can be meant by a 'vaginal orgasm,'" since sensory stimulation of the vagina was "a physical and physiologic impossibility for nearly all females."[154]

Taking Freud directly to task, Kinsey noted that Freud knew the clitoris to be highly sensitive, "but he contended that psychosexual maturation involved a subordination of clitoral reactions and a development of sensitivity within the vagina itself," something that had never been indicated as possible. The question of vaginal versus clitoral orgasm, Kinsey argued, was not purely theoretical. Indeed, the question "is of considerable importance" because some clinicians, psychoanalysts, psychologists, and marriage counselors "have expended considerable effort trying to teach their patients to transfer 'clitoral responses' to 'vaginal responses.'" Women in his study, like "many thousands" of others who saw "certain clinicians," have "been much disturbed by their failure to accomplish this biologic impossibility," Kinsey wrote. Kinsey stressed that Freud failed to conduct any research on sex, and he was amazed at the small empirical base upon which Freud's entire theory rested.[155] Finally, Kinsey believed that while Freud spoke of distancing himself from nineteenth-century condemnations of sexuality, he merely changed the labels from sinful to clinical ones.[156] As one historian of psychoanalysis noted, Kinsey "was no friend to psychoanalysis."[157]

Scientific and popular reaction to *Sexual Behavior in the Human Female* was at first muted, then fierce.[158] With his rejection of the vaginal orgasm, among other aspects of psychoanalysis Kinsey regarded with skepticism if not outright dismissal and hostility, psychoanalysts' reaction to his findings were strong and went beyond just a critique of his gathering of case histories from volunteers.[159] Kinsey was in some ways an easy target. He received a lot of popular attention when he published *Sexual Behavior in the Human Female*, and his negation of the vaginal orgasm was easy to attack by those in support of this theory, and they did so with the same kinds of criticism as those lodged by other Kinsey critics: his statistics were wrong, he did not have a diverse population base, his volunteers were lying to him.

Alfred Kinsey has been portrayed as a solitary voice in opposition to the vaginal orgasm theory during these decades, with his stand largely drowned out by the negative response to other aspects of his study on female sexuality.[160] Kinsey was actually one of many voices who were not so much challenging the vaginal orgasm as arguing for accepted beliefs about the clitoris as an organ of sexual response in the female. For example, Havelock Ellis, writing in the 1930s, called the clitoris the "chief focus of sexual sensation in women." Though noting it was "sometimes said by psycho-analysts that this is only true for an early age, and that with adolescence sexual sensation is normally, if not constantly, transferred from the clitoris to the vagina," Ellis found it "difficult to account for the origin of this notion." Such an idea, Ellis wrote, "might have easily been dispelled by a little knowledge of women." According to Ellis, although it was "natural" an adult woman would find pleasure in vaginal intercourse, it was "incorrect to speak of any 'transfer'" of orgasm.[161] Or, as pediatrician turned marriage counselor Rebecca Liswood put it bluntly in 1961, there was "no such thing" as a vaginal orgasm.[162]

Albert Ellis, a New York marriage counselor, also took the vaginal orgasm theory to task in 1953 with his essay "Is the Vaginal Orgasm a Myth?"[163] Written when he was still a practicing psychoanalyst, Ellis concluded that, first, the "so-called vaginal orgasm seems to be misnamed" and should be referred to as "orgasm obtained through intercourse," as the vagina was largely insensitive to sexual stimulation, and, second, that, as a result of "falsely teaching that women who do not have orgasms through intravaginal stimulation are missing something essential in their lives, or that they are immature, we may easily *make* such women emotionally or sexually disturbed"; and, third, that "orgasm is orgasm, however experienced."[164]

Like Albert Ellis, others worried about the effects of false teachings regarding female orgasm. During a symposium on female sexuality hosted by the Society for the Scientific Study of Sex in the late 1950s, New York University obstetrics and gynecology professor Sophia Kleegman noted that while Freud and "modern psychiatry have been powerful forces to help us evolve" from ideas that considered women as happily sexless creatures, she blamed a "small group of psychoanalysts" who held "a theory of frigidity in women that is in my opinion antiphysiologic and has caused much confusion."[165]

Sandor Rado, a psychiatrist in New York City and dean of the New York School of Psychiatry, stated at the same symposium that the transferring of the orgasm from the clitoris to the vagina now sounded like Victorian folklore.[166] But it was folklore some women believed they needed to play out. Albert Ellis, also speaking at the symposium, stressed that the shame many women felt about not having a vaginal orgasm during penetrative intercourse was unwarranted. "Literally millions of American women," he said, "are employing noncoital sex methods only as preliminary or love play techniques and are not using them, when necessary, up to and including the achievement of orgasm." They restricted themselves, he believed, out of shame: "that is, they feel that they should not require digital manipulation of the clitoris, oral-genital relations, or other techniques of coming to climax." This, Ellis maintained, "is perfectly illogical and is almost entirely a consequence of their arbitrary notions of what is 'shameful.'" There may be many reasons for frigidity in American women, Ellis contended, "but chief of these, today, is not a deep-seated or unconscious feeling of guilt, anxiety, or hostility, as many orthodox psychoanalysts would still unfortunately mislead us into believing." Rather, it was the "socially acquired feelings of shame, inadequacy, and the horror of making a mistake or being incompetent" that were the main "culprits" for frigidity in women. These were the "ideas and attitudes that should be forthrightly attacked, questioned, challenged, and uprooted by the psychologist, psychiatrist, marriage counselor, or physician who specializes in sex problems," Ellis concluded.[167]

Ellis continued with his forthright challenge to the vaginal orgasm in his book *The American Sexual Tragedy*, published in 1962. According to Ellis, popular sex manuals contributed to the "folklore of married sex relations, particularly in their consideration of such things as female orgasm." Too many such manuals, he wrote, "follow the mistaken lead of Freud in differentiating between so-called clitoral and so-called vaginal orgasm when, in point of fact, no such thing as vaginal orgasm appears to exist." Ellis noted he both read the literature and interviewed "scores" of women he labeled as either "sexually normal" or "disturbed," a process that "forced" him to conclude, "the so-called vaginal orgasm is largely a myth." But it was a myth, he worried, that was "exceptionally widespread in contemporary America, and is causing immense needless anguish" to "innumerable women who are having perfectly satisfying and legitimate orgasms" but are convincing themselves, or having themselves convinced, "that they are missing something unique, and are making themselves and their husbands miserable." Normal women, Ellis wrote, "may no more experience vaginal orgasm than the normal male experience his climax in his scrotum." As way of an example, Ellis related the story of a woman physician who came to him wanting to know what was wrong with her because, though she experienced clitoral orgasms regularly, she could not reach a vaginal orgasm. Ellis explained that "many women were quite incapable of having a regular orgasm from intercourse alone, but that most of these women could fairly easily obtain regular orgasm by clitoral manipulations." She was, Ellis assured her, perfectly "adequate" and normal and she had been "mislead by the books she read which ecstatically described the virtues of vaginal orgasm."[168]

Others echoed the assertion that women had been misled. Physician Sophia Kleegman, who had been a student of Robert Latou Dickinson (whom she called "one of our greatest teachers in the sex problems of women"), said most of the women she had seen who were unable to reach a vaginal orgasm were not "neurotics" but rather "victims of our unfavorable cultural patterns" that regarded sex as "repressive." According to Kleegman, "a woman whose main source of stimulation had been the clitoris, and who with marriage receives little or no stimulation before entrance, and no clitoral contact after entrance, finds it physiologically impossible to achieve orgasm." For these women, "bells don't ring, and birds don't sing," and they, who had thought sex would be a wonderful thing, are disappointed and nervously "upset with a feeling of inadequacy and often with a feeling of guilt," as if only a "pervert" enjoyed sex when her clitoris was stimulated.[169] Los Angeles psychiatrist Judd Marmor, in a paper he read before the Society for Psychosomatic Medicine of Southern California in the fall of 1952, stated that women were often fearful or resentful or objected to "any form of clitoral manipulation for a variety of unconscious reasons," including "masturbatory guilt, shame about her genitals," and "anxiety that such manipulations" amounted to "'perverse,' 'unnatural,' or neurotic'" practices.[170]

Occasionally it was not the woman who worried that her need to have her clitoris stimulated was perverse or abnormal but her husband. Physician Rebecca Liswood noted, "Sometimes a husband is disturbed because his wife will achieve orgasm very quickly under manual stimulation but be unable to come to a climax during actual intercourse." This was because some men believed the penis "produces the orgasm in a woman—or should." Too often men thought the "objective during a sexual relationship is to penetrate the woman's vagina and achieve orgasm for both of them through an ejaculation," but this, Liswood counseled, was "not absolutely necessary." Liswood told worried men and women who were "convinced that the wife should be aroused only if the penis has entered the vagina" that there were "no nerve endings for sex stimulation inside the vagina." Liswood advised women to "make the most of what nature gave" them and provided instructions on ways to engage in coitus that stimulated the clitoris.[171]

Like Rebecca Liswood and Albert Ellis, Sophia Kleegman based her rejection of the vaginal orgasm on her "knowledge of anatomy and physiology of coitus," as well as her "vast clinical experience."[172] Others also based their support for the clitoral orgasm as healthy and normal on their own clinical experience. E. W. Hardenbergh, a professor in Pennsylvania, wrote four years before Kinsey's study was published about his own study regarding women and location of orgasm. Hardenbergh developed a questionnaire and asked sixty-two married college women to tell him where they experienced an orgasm. Thirty-nine answered the question, with the majority indicating the clitoris.[173]

Reflecting the information found in anatomy and gynecology texts, New York psychiatrist Sandor Rado wrote in the late 1950s that it was "generally known, the sexually most responsive areas of the female organ are the clitoris, the minor labia, and the entrance to the vagina."[174] In their 1951 book, *Patterns of Sexual Behavior*, Yale University professors Clellan Ford, an anthropologist, and Frank Beach, a psychologist, noted it was "well known that at least the majority of women derive sexual excitement from clitoral stimulation." Ford and Beach also stressed the normality of the clitoral orgasm through their cross-cultural study of sexual behavior, especially their finding that the woman on top position provided the best method of stimulating the organ during intercourse. Additionally, they observed that when the man was on top, moving "backward and forward" while thrusting "likely" enabled his penis to rub against the clitoris. They further noted that these were the most common positions Americans engaged in during sexual intercourse, citing Kinsey, and that these positions were also common among other cultures.[175]

By pointing to the cross-cultural attention to clitoral stimulation, Ford and Beach emphasized the ubiquity and normality of the clitoris as a sexual organ, as did other proponents of the clitoral orgasm. Havelock Ellis quoted "so authoritative a gynecologist as Dickinson" as "truly" stating that "'a large proportion of women have orgasm only from pressure in the clitoris region, and this is perfectly normal.'"[176] These proponents, even when writing in the professional literature, reassured women and men that though a vaginal orgasm was regarded by some as perhaps the more full orgasm to experience with a spouse, many women had difficulty experiencing one, and a clitoral orgasm was also healthy and normal. In her book, Rebecca Liswood reiterated a story fellow physician Sophia Kleegman told at a meeting of the American Association of Marriage Counselors. In the story, Kleegman talked about a woman who told her she was worried "because the only sexual activity we have is when my husband manipulated my clitoris." Kleegman asked the woman what was wrong with this, to which the woman replied, "But I didn't marry a finger." To which Kleegman replied, she "didn't marry a penis either."[177]

G. Lombard Kelly, the anatomy professor at the Medical College of Georgia with whom Bergler stridently disagreed, took "definite exception" to the idea that women who had a clitoral orgasm were not normal.[178] In a letter to *JAMA* in response to an editor's assertion that female circumcision was "not justified" since the vagina "in the normal adult woman" was the "principal sexual organ," Kelly argued that "thousands of women who are normal in every way sexually and have one or more orgasms spontaneously in each act of intercourse will testify that the clitoris is the principal erogenous zone."[179] Kelly further stated that in his "opinion there is no such thing as a 'vaginal orgasm,' for there are no genital corpuscles in that organ." In both men and women, Kelly noted, the nerves were found "only in the head of the phallic organ" and only by stimulating this area of the body "can the orgasm be initiated and felt."[180] In a letter published a month later, Maurice J. Small, a physician in West Virginia, agreed with Kelly and also took exception with the *JAMA* editor. Small noted that he too had seen "many normal, well balanced, adult married women whose complaints of lack of sexual pleasure were remedied by showing them or their husbands the position of the clitoris." Their "apparent frigidity," he wrote, was "cured by a change of intercourse positions so that the clitoris was stimulated, or by manual stimulation." But he also argued, like Kelly, that the idea of a vaginal orgasm made no sense since the clitoris was "morphologically similar to the glans penis and possess the neurogenic mechanism for orgasm by friction" and as such was the chief area of orgasm arousal in women.[181]

Like Small, others suggested sexual positions and techniques for the stimulation of the female organ that corresponded to the male sexual organ. Liswood, deeply concerned about the lack of information concerning sex available to married couples, founded in the 1950s the Marriage Counseling Service of Greater New York. Initially a pediatrician, Liswood in the 1930s returned to school for psychiatric training. Though she was a proponent of the Freudian theory of penis envy for girls, she did not accept that mature women needed to transfer their orgasms to their vaginas. She stressed the need for men and women to understand their own and each other's anatomy, in particular the clitoris, describing it as "the most important female organ for sex stimulation."[182] Both the nerve endings at the entrance of the vagina and the "contact with the clitoris, as well as the friction of the penis against the sensitive vaginal opening, will create excitement for the woman," she stated.[183] Liswood told couples it did not matter which position a couple chose so long as the clitoris was stimulated. "Don't worry if an orgasm is clitoral or vaginal or anything else someone has told you about."[184] Sophia Kleegman similarly recommended that women, and their husbands, look to sex guides for new techniques to stimulate the clitoris—and then that they throw away the book and write their own. "Rigidity of attitude as well as frigidity ruins sex pleasure," she said. For Kleegman, the theory of vaginal orgasm represented "rigidity about sex that is most destructive."[185]

But Kleegman further noted that orgasm depended upon more than just the stimulation of even the clitoris. Orgasm, she noted, involved a woman's whole body, as well as her personality. "Perhaps there would be less disparity between our two points of view if we could learn to communicate," she suggested.[186] Kleegman was not alone in her contention that the division and hierarchy of orgasm location were both unnecessary and anatomically untrue. During the discussion following a presentation on the sexual response cycles of men and women given by Masters and Johnson in the early 1960s at the University of California, Berkeley, on sex and behavior, the questions soon turned to the difference and division between vaginal and clitoral orgasms.[187] Charles Rogers, of the Yerkes Laboratories of Primate Biology in Orange Park, Florida, asked whether "some females show maximal arousal with clitoral stimulation, while others do so in response to vaginal stimulation." In response, Masters noted that this was based on the individual woman, with some women responding more to one over the other. "However," he added, "from an anatomic point of view there is absolutely no difference between an orgasm stimulated by pure vaginal stimulation or pure clitoral stimulation." Benson Ginsburg from the University of Chicago asked for clarification: "When you speak of vaginal orgasm and of the stimulation being controlled, am I correct in assuming the clitoris is not stimulated?"[188] In response, Masters replied that this was "incorrect" since, even when sex was penetrative, the clitoris received stimulation from the "penile thrust" along the "labial hood of the clitoris."[189]

Proponents of the clitoral orgasm theory did not rule out that many women enjoyed penetrative sex. Rebecca Liswood reassured women they could feel enjoyment from the sense of fullness in their vaginas when their husbands were inside; a woman "may call this sense of fullness a vaginal orgasm, and that is all right too."[190] Positing a similar position, Sandor Rado called the clitoris woman's "most precious biological equipment." Rado noted that his "observations corroborate Dickinson's findings that in the healthy female clitoral and vaginal stimulation complement each other in the production of sexual arousal and orgasmic satisfaction." But by suppressing "her clitoral sensations," Rado continued, "the female cannot possibly augment her vaginal responses; she can only reduce her capacity for sexual performance, health, and happiness."[191] And, though Albert Ellis labeled the vaginal orgasm a myth, he did not disavow the pleasure of penetrative heterosexual sex. But he qualified this statement, noting that while penile-vaginal intercourse was "*one* of the most satisfying of human sex experiences, it is not necessarily *the* most satisfying experience for all men and women." While Ellis saw no harm in a couple trying to "adjust themselves sexually so that they each achieve an orgasm during intercourse, and often achieve it simultaneously," he also stressed that "orgasm is orgasm, however and whenever achieved, and may be thoroughly enjoyable on a non-simultaneous basis."[192]

Statements by proponents of the clitoral orgasm, however, should not necessarily be read as empowering women's sexual autonomy. Some, like Albert Ellis, definitely noted and encouraged as healthy the capabilities of women outside penetrative sex. Others, however, like Sandor Rado, while stating that women feel "obliged" to satisfy the desires of men for penetrative intercourse, also noted that women desired it from "maternal feeling."[193] As historian Carolyn Herbst Lewis noted, for many sex meant the penetrative sort in a loving, married relationship.[194] What I want to stress, however, is that the clitoris was seen as important even within the context of beliefs that vaginal sex was the only normal and healthy form of sex for women: the clitoris was incorporated into this vision of normal and healthy sex. The recommendations, then, of a change in sexual positions or of the application of an ointment to enable the clitoris better stimulation were both therapies for lack of orgasm that necessitated such an understanding. Like both of these therapies, the use of female circumcision to treat lack of feminine orgasm further illustrates an understanding of the clitoris as the principal sexual organ in women and of clitoral orgasm as healthy.

Female Circumcision during the Heyday of the Vaginal Orgasm

Recall that in the 1956 speech with which I began this chapter, Kroger told his audience that "circumcision of the clitoris is valueless" to treat frigidity.[195] This was not a random comment by Kroger. Along with San Francisco psychoanalyst S. Charles Freed, Kroger had warned against circumcision in an article they published in *JAMA* in 1950, calling it a "valueless treatment."[196] The pair did so as well in a book published in 1951 and again in 1962: since there were an "enormous number of cases of frigidity being seen by an all too meager number of competent psychotherapists," Kroger and Freed noted that many women sought a "more rapid form of therapy," including female circumcision. They stressed, however, that the "surgical procedures [such] as circumcision of the clitoris are valueless."[197]

Kroger's short ruminations against female circumcision as treatment during this time for lack of orgasm were not isolated. Many of the references to the therapeutic use of female circumcision to treat a lack of orgasm were not case reports but rather recommendations *against* using the surgery. In the 1964 *Case Studies in Obstetrics and Gynecology*, a book written in a question and answer format, one question asked when female circumcision should be performed. Milwaukee obstetrician and gynecologist F. Jackson Stoddard's answer was "circumcision of the female to expose the clitoris has never been of proved value."[198] Gynecologists Arthur Hale Curtis and John William Huffman, in their 1950 gynecology textbook, wrote that they found "little foundation" for the belief that circumcision of an adherent clitoris would enable orgasm. "Circumcision seldom increases libido," they wrote. But though Curtis and Huffman said there "appears to be little foundation" for circumcision as therapy for frigidity, they did find that freeing the clitoris from a tight prepuce "by a simple dorsal slit ordinarily accomplishes all that can be achieved with circumcision." Circumcision, however, they believed "cannot be recommended except in rare instances."[199]

Discussion within *JAMA* about the use of female circumcision as a sexual surgery similarly highlights awareness of the practice. In 1940, M. F. Smith, a physician from New Mexico, wrote to the journal asking about female circumcision. In response, the *JAMA* commentator noted that the procedure was "not often required" and that there appeared to be "little foundation for the belief that an adherent clitoris is often responsible for frigidity." Circumcision, the commentator went on to add, "seldom increases libido."[200] Six years later, in the late winter and early spring of 1946, in the Queries and Minor Notes section of *JAMA*, a small and brief interchange of ideas again took place concerning the value of this procedure. A letter from Frank Hyde, a physician from North Carolina, initiated the discussion when he asked, "What is the general opinion among gynecologists as to the value of operations on the clitoris for frigidity or reduced libido?" In response, the *JAMA* commentator stated that such operations "have practically no effect on frigidity or reduced libido" because "gynecologists, psychiatrists, and psychoanalysts" all "agree that in all cases of frigidity there is a large psychic element." Because of this "psychic factor in frigidity, operation on the clitoris are [*sic*] not justified," the commentator argued. But the commentator further noted that women have "two sexual organs," the clitoris and the vagina, and that while the clitoris is important for the child before puberty, the vagina "in the normal adult woman" is the "principal sexual organ."[201] Though editorializing against female circumcision as therapy, like Kroger, this commentator's reaction to the surgery suggests it was being used as a therapy to enhance female sexual sensation.

Positive references to female circumcision (and other clitoral interventions) were similarly often quite short. C. F. McDonald, a physician in Milwaukee, wrote in a 1958 article about the benefits of female circumcision to some of his patients. Noting that the women who complained to him of difficult or painful intercourse often had borne three or four children, he examined them and found that the prepuce hid their clitoris. To reveal the organ, he removed the prepuce, with "very thankful patients" as the reward. "For the first time in their lives, sex ambition became normally satisfied," he wrote, presumably meaning these women reached orgasm during coitus by having their clitoris stimulated.[202] Another physician, Leo Wollman, a New York gynecologist, simply noted that he had removed the clitoral hood of more than one hundred women from 1953 to 1973.[203] Gynecologist Le Mon Clark described two cases of married women for whom orgasm occurred after he removed the smegma and peeled back an adherent hood.[204] And sometimes lay publications also offered up this therapy for women having orgasm difficulties. For example, in his 1940 *Sex Satisfaction and Happy Marriage*, Alfred Henry Tyrer noted that for some women "intercourse terminates" in a "partial orgasm." Women experienced this, Tyrer believed, because of "a hooded clitoris," which he noted could be "corrected by a trifling operation in a few minutes by a surgeon."[205]

One physician published a longer article discussing the merits of female circumcision as a sexual enhancement surgery. California physician W. G. Rathmann published "Female Circumcision: Indications and a New Technique" in 1959. In it he argued that the clitoral prepuce could hamper sexual relations for women. The prepuce existed "for the protection of the clitoris," Rathmann wrote, and in its normal state was "useful," but if it was excessive "it can prevent contact and is harmful." Rathmann believed that the main indications for need of circumcision were functional—a "lack of ability to have a climax or ability to have one only with considerable difficulty"—or anatomical. He believed there were three sorts of patients for whom circumcision was of benefit: first, an overweight woman, because the surgery could help remove tissue blocking the clitoris; second, a woman whose husband was "unusually awkward or difficult to educate," because circumcision would "sometimes make the clitoris easier to find"; and third, a woman with a clitoris that was "quite small" and "difficult to contact," because "circumcision might help by making it more accessible." Rathmann advised against using the operation when frigidity occurred "from psychologic causes, such as fear of pregnancy, early adverse training and experiences," or problems between the husband and wife, such as "abnormal jealousy."[206]

Rathmann believed certain women benefited from circumcision, and he provided Mrs. R.B., age thirty-four and married five times before seeing Rathmann, as an example. She had a rather large amount of coverage over her clitoris and "had never experienced climax." After seeing many doctors for assistance with her inability to orgasm, she visited Rathmann, who circumcised her. Mrs. R.B. subsequently remarried the last man she had divorced, experienced "no more sexual problems," indeed, telling Rathmann she had "wasted four perfectly good husbands."[207]

Curious to see how many other women experienced orgasm following the procedure, Rathmann sent a questionnaire to all the women he circumcised over the past fifteen years, and 112 were completed and returned (Rathmann did not say how many questionnaires he sent out). Of these women, seventy-three had never experienced an orgasm before surgery but sixty-four did so following, while, of the thirty-nine who had experienced orgasm only with difficultly prior to the operation, thirty-four said their ability had improved postsurgery. This led Rathmann to advise that so long as the cases were selected based on the criteria he outlined, doctors could expect "85 to 90 percent to show satisfactory improvement" following female circumcision.[208]

Rathmann devised a simple vice-grip set of pliers to circumcise women, with "specially designed jaws for this procedure." The pliers had a screw on the handle that allowed the doctor to adjust for the "various thickness of the prepuce before the pliers are clamped." After grasping and holding the prepuce for five minutes, Rathmann then used a scalpel to "excise the prepuce within the upper jaw" of the pliers, being "careful to stay close to the inner wall of the clamp." He called the technique "extremely simple, accurate, and bloodless," one that produced "excellent results because of the reduced healing time and absence of scar tissue." Rathmann advised codeine or Percodan for "postoperative discomfort," and if the surgery were done on a Friday, the patient could return to work that following Monday, though he noted that complete recovery took about ten to fourteen days.[209]

While published accounts of the use of female circumcision are not plentiful, this can be explained partly as a reflection of the procedure itself: it was a quick outpatient procedure easily performed in a physician's office. The operation may well have been performed in a physician's office more often than the published records show, as two accounts published in the 1970s indicate. The first, *The Consumer's Guide to Successful Surgery*, published in 1976 by doctors L. M. Elting and Seymour Isenberg, recounted the positive sexual effects of female circumcision for making orgasms easier and noted that the surgery had been "quite popular in the 1950s and a clamp was even devised to free the clitoris from overriding tissues," perhaps referring to the clamp Rathmann devised.[210] In the second reference to the procedure's popularity, published in 1973, James Semmens, an associate professor of obstetrics and gynecology at the Medical University of South Carolina, also noted that during the 1950s female circumcision was popular "and a clamp was even devised to accomplish this particular feat," again possibly referring to Rathmann.[211]

What should be made of the possibility that clitoral circumcision was popular during a period when some physicians and nonphysicians told women to ignore this organ? One way to make sense of this is to consider that physicians saw the vaginal orgasm as an ideal, while in reality women still had (and were perhaps even encouraged to have) clitoral orgasms. Many practitioners do not seem to have altered their ideas about the clitoris as the principal female sexual organ, and common medical knowledge as reflected by anatomy and gynecology texts also continued to consider the clitoris as such. But perhaps, too, even those who accepted the vaginal orgasm theory may have regarded the vaginal orgasm as an archetype rather than the norm, and on an individual patient level perhaps recommended different sexual positions, prescribed clitoral ointment, or removed clitoral foreskins to enable their patients to more easily have an orgasm during penetrative sex. Theory, then, was one thing; clinical application was another. The doctors who recommended and even removed the hood of a clitoris did so with the belief that it would make the organ more sexually sensitive and enable a woman to reach orgasm during penetrative sex. Female circumcision as a therapy for lack of orgasm, then, relied on the idea that women could have a clitoral orgasm and be healthy. The therapeutic use of female circumcision to enable female orgasm in 1950 again illustrates, just as the use of physiological interventions on the clitoris to treat masturbation in 1900, an understanding of the clitoris as a sexual organ, though an organ in need of medical intervention to function appropriately.

Chapter Six

Female Circumcision and the Divisive Issue of Female Clitoral Sexual Pleasure Go Public, 1966–81

Catherine Kellison first heard about female circumcision from a friend, who told her she had undergone the procedure and now experienced "greater sexual sensations" and "higher levels of orgasm" than she had prior to the operation. Writing in *Playgirl* magazine in 1973, Kellison, who admitted being ignorant about her genitalia, raced to the library to look up information on her body after learning about the operation. She discovered that the clitoris "exists for the sole purpose of giving pleasure" and that women are "multi-orgasmic." After reading about the clitoris, Kellison noted she was "more than mildly distressed." If, she wrote, women "are so potentially erotic, seething on the inside with great bursts of passion flames, what happened to it all?"[1]

In search of an answer, and encouraged by the fact that a second friend had "treated herself to the circumcision," Kellison made an appointment with Stanley Daniels, a gynecologist in southern California, who had removed the clitoral hood of her two friends.[2] Daniels, Kellison wrote, "was great" and very "enthusiastic." He informed Kellison that although the "clitoris responds well to both direct and indirect pressures," an "awesome 75 percent of women are hindered from feeling the full extent of the sensations due to a condition most commonly known as a 'hooded clitoris.'" The clitoral hood on these women was "too long or too thick (or sometimes both) and the clitoris lies buried, forgotten, but by no means gone." Circumcision, done "strictly for pleasure," was the surgical solution to this condition, he informed her.[3] This was enough information for Kellison, who elected to undergo the operation to find out for herself.

When Kellison was writing for *Playgirl* in the 1970s, information about the proposed benefits of female circumcision was being touted directly to women through stories in popular magazines and books about cosmetic surgery. No longer was this information mostly limited to medical texts and articles, and Kellison was not the only woman to learn about, seek out, and undergo female circumcision as a sexual enhancement surgery from the late 1960s through the early 1980s. Edward Wallerstein, in his history of male circumcision, noted that though there was no accurate data regarding how often women chose to undergo circumcision, he estimated that of the "approximately 5,000 operations performed annually on the external female genitalia" for the years 1968, 1973, and 1977, "possibly two to three thousand were circumcision." These numbers, however, were for operations performed in a hospital; according to another study, "the ratio of this operation performed in doctor's offices to hospitals is about 50:1," a figure Wallerstein noted was "not projectable" but, if true, meant that more adult women elected for circumcision than adult men in the 1970s.[4]

While estimating how many women underwent circumcision for sexual enhancement during this time is not possible, evidence of its reach can be found indirectly. Several physicians in southern California reported circumcising hundreds of women, and the operation was not geographically limited, as a doctor in Fayetteville, Arkansas, and another in Dayton, Ohio, also claimed to have circumcised hundreds of women.[5] In addition to the popular and medical articles in which these particular physicians described their use of clitoral circumcision, that a national health insurance company refused to continue paying for the surgery further hints at the extent female circumcision was performed in the United States during this time. In May 1977, Blue Shield Association recommended that its individual plans stop routine payments for twenty-eight surgical and diagnostic procedures considered outmoded or unnecessary by groups such as the American College of Surgeons and the American Hospital Association. Of the twenty-eight, one of the procedures deemed not medically necessary was "the removal of the clitoral hood."[6] Apparently enough women in the 1970s were requesting Blue Shield pay for a surgery on their clitoris that it warranted a national discontinuation.

While none of this information is translatable into an actual estimate of how many women elected to have their clitorises circumcised, it suggests the procedure was a modestly popular elective surgery. And this was perhaps because, as one doctor who performed the surgery said in 1976, it would "uncover the clitoris and make it more subject to direct stimulation" thus increasing "sensitivity and pleasure of contact."[7] This doctor, like many of the physicians who performed female circumcision in the late 1960s through the 1970s, as well as the many women who underwent the procedure during this time, regarded this as a liberating decision meant to enhance or even enable female sexual response during penetrative sex.

The Simple Operation for Supreme Sexual Pleasure

The clitoris, as described by sex therapists Benjamin Graber and Georgia Miller Graber in a 1974 *Playgirl* article, "is located at the upper junction of the two inner lips of the vagina." The convergence of the lips created a fore-skin covering the clitoris—"just like the foreskin of the uncircumcised penis." When the foreskin of the clitoris was pulled back, "the clitoris is revealed as a small pea-size structure." However, in some women, this foreskin was so "attached to the head of the clitoris" it could not be retracted. This "not uncommon" condition resulted for some women in reduced feeling during sex. Removing the adhesions was a "simple office procedure done under local anesthetic with very little pain involved," according to the Grabers.[8] Removal of the adhesions involved moving a blunt probe between the clito-ris and the foreskin, thus loosening their connection without removing the clitoral hood.[9] The purpose was to enable the clitoral hood to retract, thus allowing for more stimulation during sex.

Some sex therapists believed that the loosening of the clitoris from adhesions enabled a woman previously unable to reach orgasm to do so.[10] Breaking up the adhesions that bound the foreskin to the clitoris sufficed for certain women. But for other women an "excess amount of foreskin"—a clitoral hood that was "too large or too thick"—indicated the skin needed to be removed, not just broken, according to the Grabers.[11] Indeed, "an exces-sive amount of tissue covering the clitoris," said Stanley Daniels, a physician who performed female circumcision, could result in "creating an actual mechanical problem," an inability to orgasm during penetrative sex.[12] For these women, circumcision was indicated.

Doctors who performed female circumcision routinely called it an easy operation. Two doctors writing in the 1970s in *Cosmopolitan* described the surgery as incising the hood, "'trimmed' as the operative notes say."[13] North Carolina gynecologist Takey Crist described female circumcision as "retracting and excising the foreskin around the clitoris." The fore-skin, according to Crist, was "pulled forward, an outline made of the tissue to be removed, the tissue excised, and loose edges sutured with cat-gut."[14] Nonphysician David Haldane, writing for *Penthouse Forum* in 1978, described it as removing "that small triangular piece of flesh which covers the clitoris." Imagine, he instructed his readers, the "foreskin of the clitoris to be a triangle with the clitoris under it somewhere near the center." To circumcise the clitoris, a doctor cut "from the center of the triangle's base to its tip," removed the two now-loose flaps on either side, and sutured the cut.[15] While before the operation the clitoris was covered, following cir-cumcision the organ was exposed.

The procedure was done under local anesthesia and physicians consid-ered it much easier to perform than male circumcision.[16] Patients in Crist's clinic rested for around fifteen minutes after the surgery before being dis-charged, were told to take a sitz bath following the surgery twice a day for three days, to apply a topical ointment following the bath, and to return six weeks later for a postoperative exam. Women were discouraged from having sex for a week to ten days following circumcision.[17] Most often the surgery was performed in the doctor's office. One doctor said only two of the one hundred circumcisions he had performed were done at the hospital—and this was only because of the women's request.[18]

Prices varied from fifty to two hundred dollars for the surgery during the 1970s.[19] For their money, women were told their clitoris would be free, "making it more accessible to direct stimulation by the penis" during intercourse, according to Haldane.[20] Leo Wollman, a New York gynecologist, stated in 1973 that, "based on clinical experience," the "sensuality of the clitoris is greater when there is no tissue covering the clitoral head." Wollman believed that the "ideal result of female circumcision, where it is indicated, is an increase in quality of the orgasm, as well as increased rapidity in achieving this sensual result in love-making." Wollman noted that though the patient had the final say in whether to have the operation, it was the "duty of the gynecology surgeon, who is in fact the expert, to explain fully the reasons for surgery and the possible benefits that accrue from surgical intervention." He based his assessment of the success of the operation on one hundred cases in which he removed the hood of a woman's clitoris. Ninety-two women told him their orgasms had improved, seven said there was no difference, and one said her orgasms were worse.[21] In 1975, William Walden, another New York physician, stated that probably 15 percent of women would benefit sexually from circumcision and that he had performed the operation on fifty of his own patients.[22] Physicians like Wollman and Walden performed female circumcision on women whose anatomies they believed held them back from experiencing full sexual pleasure.

The Clitoris and *Human Sexual Response*

Though Leo Wollman noted that it was not seen as "stylish nowadays to ascribe sexual problems to physical causes," he was certain a "small percentage of women are anatomically unable to have clitoral climaxes," a problem circumcision was supposed to treat.[23] Wollman's sentiments regarding women having clitoral climaxes stemmed from William Masters and Virginia Johnson's physiological evidence about the clitoris as a sexual organ published in *Human Sexual Response* in 1966. Though the pair's findings about the clitoris as a sexually sensitive organ were standard medical knowledge, their work provided greater physiological support for the concept of the organ as sexual, evidence that was then picked up by the nonmedical community.

Masters, an obstetrician and gynecologist clinician and researcher at Washington University in St. Louis, was forty in the mid-1950s when he proposed his study of the physiology of human sexual response; his initial research of the obstetrics and gynecologic literature convinced him that his field had an aversion to the topic. But, unlike Kinsey, he wanted to directly observe the body's functioning during sex, thus focusing on clinical observation instead of patient recollections.[24] Masters began his studies by interviewing male and female prostitutes but, because he wanted his research to be regarded as normal, decided against using his original subjects in anything he published. He also decided around this time to add a woman to his research team, and hired the non–medically trained Virginia Johnson.[25] Masters later said he would have preferred a female physician, but such a person was hard to find and he knew a woman physician would demand a more equal footing with him as well as be hesitant to take a controversial position.[26] Regardless, Johnson proved to be "particularly important," according to historian Vern Bullough, especially for the work that resulted in *Human Sexual Response*. With Johnson, Masters gave greater emphasis to female sexuality than to male and because of this saw great value in having women play an important part of the research process.[27] Johnson was central to recruiting educated women in their twenties and thirties around Washington University in the 1950s and 1960s willing to have sex for a nominal fee and the promise of anonymity.[28]

Working from the belief that their research would benefit people directly and be useful in sex therapy, Masters and Johnson wrote that the "widespread problems of human sexual inadequacy will not be attacked effectively by either medical or behavioral personnel until more definitive information is accumulated" on how humans engaged in sex. As part of their research on how bodies reacted during sex, Masters and Johnson measured their volunteers' physical reactions to determine the sexual response cycle. Masters and Johnson directly observed individuals engaging in masturbation and heterosexual couples engaging in intercourse. They created a research environment that enabled them, as they wrote, to "observe, to record, and to evaluate the patterns of physiologic and psychological response to effective sexual stimulation" in a way and a degree "never possible previously in a medical or behavioral environment."[29]

Though they believed in the positive importance of masturbation in the development of sexual identity, sex for Masters and Johnson remained of the heterosexual variety, preferably married. Heterosexuality, they argued, was natural, and the natural sexual activity was penetration. They described all other forms of sexual activity as foreplay. This can be at least partly explained by their biological model of sex as a reproductive function.[30] Their view can be explained further because, first and foremost, Masters and Johnson were sex therapists who hoped their work would help people with sexual problems, and the majority of people seen by sex therapists were married heterosexuals. Unlike Kinsey, as Paul Robinson wrote in his 1976 critique of Masters and Johnson, "the therapist tends to accept the established order and seeks to adjust the patient to it," while the scientist "is free to imagine a better order." Masters and Johnson did not see beyond this frame; their entire conceptual framework, Robinson argued, "appears to have been devised to highlight a single phenomenon, the orgiastic platform." Moreover, Robinson maintained that while Masters and Johnson took strong positions on the sexual status of women, they for the most part conceived of sex as existing within lasting, heterosexual relationships and so did not challenge the idea that a healthy sexual life was a married one.[31] Following Robinson years later, psychologist Jane Ussher added to this critique, noting that Masters and Johnson considered female sexuality in relation to male sexuality, with the expectation women would "experience sexual pleasure and orgasm during heterosexual intercourse, and . . . be aroused by a man (or by anticipation of penetration from the penis)."[32] Indeed, in their research sample, Masters and Johnson accepted only women who said they achieved orgasm during penetrative sex and who took part in prolonged foreplay with their partner before sex, something that Robinson suggested led the duo to a prejudice in favor of the clitoris in their research sample.[33] This also gave an obvious bias to women who were orgasmic during penetrative intercourse, a bias Masters and Johnson then extended to the entire female population.

To best measure these women's sexual responses and to measure the sensitivity of the vagina and the clitoris specifically, radiologists created artificial penises made of plastic containing optics allowing for observation, enabling Masters and Johnson to see the vagina's response during intercourse. Because they were able to literally watch the physical reactions of women during sex, they discounted the idea that the clitoris was a small penis, noting that it reacted to sex differently, becoming smaller, not larger, as orgasm approaches.[34] Much of their evidence on the orgasmic response of the clitoris was gathered through watching women masturbate. No two women masturbated in the same fashion, though nearly all did so without directly stimulating the organ. Observing women while they were using "mechanical and manual masturbatory techniques" answered the question of how and how much the clitoris needed to be stimulated.[35] Masters and Johnson found that the clitoris responded best not to direct stimulation like the penis but to stimulation of the general area.[36] They labeled the clitoris a "unique organ in the total of human anatomy" with its only purpose a sexual one. No such organ, they stressed, existed for men. Based on their findings, they rejected the idea that there were two separate sorts of orgasms, the clitoral and vaginal. Noting that the "literature abounds with descriptions and discussions of vaginal as opposed to clitoral orgasms," from the anatomic view, Masters and Johnson found no difference.[37]

Devoting a whole chapter to the organ, Masters and Johnson described and lamented the lack of cultural acceptance for the role the clitoris played in sexual response. "Why has female orgasmic expression not been considered to be a reinforcement of woman's role as sexual partner and reproductive necessity?" they wondered. Masters and Johnson could find "neither totem, taboo, nor religious assignment" to account "for the force with which female orgasmic experience often is neglected as a naturally occurring psycho-physiological response."[38] Noting the influence of Freud, Masters and Johnson held that whatever his analytical merits may have been on the couch, he was wrong about what happened in the bed.[39] From their research, Masters and Johnson believed that orgasmic physiology had been established, and "the human female now has an undeniable opportunity to develop realistically her own sexual response levels."[40]

Prior to the publication of *Human Sexual Response* in 1966, Masters and Johnson tried to get medical journals to publish their findings without much luck; their first published results appeared in the non-peer-reviewed *Western Journal of Surgery, Obstetrics and Gynecology*, in 1962.[41] In this article, they presented the findings of their direct observation of more than two hundred women, ages twenty to sixty-one, and relayed how these women stimulated their own clitoris to reach sexual satisfaction and the physiological reactions of the organ during orgasm.[42] The popular press, however, did not pick up this article. Indeed, their book deal, signed in the fall of 1964, was originally for a text aimed for doctors and residents. *Human Sexual Response*, however, soon saw a much larger market, receiving seven hundred reviews and notices in popular and peer-reviewed journals, including a favorable review in *JAMA*, a journal that, like other major peer-reviewed medical journals, had once rejected their work for publication. And while receiving a lot of "drop dead" mail, they were also featured on the cover of *Time* magazine on May 25, 1970.[43]

Later histories of this time often credit Masters and Johnson's work as fundamental to discrediting the myth of the vaginal orgasm.[44] But, as outlined in previous chapters, their research should not have surprised most gynecologists, or even most physicians. What Masters and Johnson's work did do, however, as historian Carol Groneman noted, was push the controversy of the vaginal versus the clitoral orgasm to the larger public's attention.[45]

Masters and Johnson's research on human sexuality was an aspect of, and helped support, the sexual revolution of the 1960s and early 1970s. During these decades, sexual matters became a visible part of the public sphere. The sexual revolution was not just about anonymous sex or open relationships; it was also about unmarried heterosexual people in monogamous relationships being able to obtain birth control and openly live together and about gay men and lesbians having their desires not classified as a mental disease. By the end of the 1960s the idea that sex was a source of personal meaning became widespread in the United States and was no longer limited to marriage.[46] The revolution, however, was not an instant one nor was it the

same for everyone everywhere in the United States. As historian Beth Bailey
outlined in her book on the history of the sexual revolution in the Midwest,
the agenda "was not created by a set of radicals on the fringe of American
society and then imposed on the rest of the nation." The national events
that occurred and were publicized through the mass media affected people
on a local level, and their responses were very much intertwined with their
local situations.[47]

The very physiological basis of *Human Sexual Response* made it more easily acceptable to many Americans. Moreover, the book appeared when science was still revered, and both its physiological approach and the medical
credentials of one of its authors helped make it a palatable and popular
text.[48] But *Human Sexual Response* was also acceptable to a large number of
Americans because of its focus on heterosexual, married couples—in other
words, those regarded as socially normal.

During the late 1960s and early 1970s, the number of sex therapists in the
United States increased, many of them trained by Masters and Johnson.[49] In
their 1970 *Human Sexual Inadequacy*, Masters and Johnson claimed successful
treatment of sexual dysfunction, further increasing the number of sex therapy clinics across the United States.[50] Before Masters and Johnson's work
in advancing the field of sex therapy, most often those who had received
counseling for sexual problems had gone through psychoanalysis; now some
men and women turned to sex therapists instead.[51] This change reflected
both the dominance of Masters and Johnson's therapeutic style and a parallel decline in the authority and attention given to psychoanalysis.[52]

Psychoanalysis and the Challenge
to the Vaginal Orgasm Theory

A few months before *Human Sexual Response* was published, physician Mary
Jane Sherfey published "The Evolution and Nature of Female Sexuality in
Relation to Psychoanalytic Theory" in the *Journal of the American Psychoanalytic
Association*.[53] In the early 1960s, Sherfey discovered that endocrinologists
had been theorizing for a decade that the mammalian male was derived
from the female, not, as had been previously thought, the reverse. Though
the theory had been discussed a little in the literature, "nobody," Sherfey
wrote, "save the few endocrinologists who developed the theory, had ever
heard of it." But to Sherfey the conclusion was "breath-taking" and historic
and one, she reasoned, that had been "ignored unconsciously because both
the men who made the discovery and those who read the duly recorded data
did not *want* this fact to be true." She decided she had to bring this theory
to the fore, especially to the attention of psychoanalysts, since this biological
reality "would strike a body blow at the Freudian concepts of female sexual

development," including the theory that to be a healthy, mature female women had to transfer their orgasm from the clitoris to the vagina.[54]

To present this concept to psychoanalysts, Sherfey decided to examine other evolutionary theories, but she could not find any evidence of the vaginal orgasm in them. According to Sherfey:

> The evolution of the clitoral mechanism was clear and unquestionable; yet I could find no more physical reason for how a vaginal orgasm came about in the most primitive monkeys, or any other animals, than in women. This was a crucial point, I thought, for if the inductor theory was right, then one had to explain why, if the vagina developed first, it then acted like a new structure, or an old one with a new function imposed upon it, so new that only women had it or so new that it could only operate after a long and proper psychological conditioning during childhood. All organs are subject to psychic influences, but none like this, none that requires psychic influences in childhood in order to operate at all. The inductor theory and Freud's vaginal orgasm seemed to confront each other like diametrically opposed mutually exclusive ideas. One or the other was wrong.[55]

Sherfey examined "masses of embryological, genetic, and endocrinological data" trying to answer her question, but, after a year of looking, she found what she wanted purely by chance. On a Saturday afternoon in 1962, sitting in the New York Academy of Medicine, she came across the 1960 issue of the *Western Journal of Obstetrics, Gynecology, and Surgery* and the article by Masters and Johnson on the anatomic response of the vagina during sexual response. After reading this article as quickly as she could, she then "ripped through all subsequent journals to see if more articles had appeared," finally reading their third study on the clitoris. It was, she recalled, "a Eureka-moment for me." This Eureka-moment led her to conclude "Freud was wrong. Men were wrong. Women were wrong. Common sense was wrong. There was no such thing as the vaginal orgasm as heretofore conceived."[56]

According to Sherfey, with the way now "wide open," she went home that night and started writing. Six months later, she submitted her piece to the *Journal of the American Psychoanalytic Association*, seeking to reach the largest number of those in the field with her challenge to the vaginal orgasm theory. Because of a backlog of articles to be published, according to Sherfey, her article did not appear until 1966—three months before *Human Sexual Response* appeared. It was, she later noted, "nice timing."[57] Drawing on the research published by Masters and Johnson in the early 1960s, as well as works in embryology and endocrinology, Sherfey strongly argued for the end of the vaginal orgasm theory as not based in biological reality. There was, she argued, "no such thing as an orgasm of the vagina."[58]

She saw the vaginal orgasm as a cultural reality that resulted in frustration for many women and men. The work of Masters and Johnson seemed to Sherfey to clarify that seeing the vaginal orgasm as normal was not physiologically accurate, though "almost all psychiatrists and physicians (excepting gynecologists and endocrinologists) are still committed to the belief in the existence of the vaginal orgasm as distinct from the infantile clitoral orgasm and consider the vaginal orgasm to be a vital sign of feminine development." Sherfey posited that perhaps the endemic sexual neuroses of many women were a result of this belief and thus were iatrogenic; the eradication of the vaginal orgasm theory would be, she believed, "formidable" because a "large block of professional and public opinion . . . want the vaginal orgasm to exist."[59]

Though Ludwig Eidelberg, in his 1968 *Encyclopedia of Psychoanalysis*, wrote that "most psychoanalysts specifically define frigidity as the incapacity to have a vaginal orgasm," many psychoanalysts came to accept the evidence presented by Masters and Johnson and Sherfy by the late 1960s and early 1970s that a purely vaginal orgasm was not physiologically possible.[60] The research of Masters and Johnson, and the larger changes regarding sex and sexuality within society, were "the facts that we have to face," as one British psychoanalyst noted in 1968.[61] Moreover, as I showed in the previous chapter, the profession had already been discussing the validity of the vaginal orgasm theory prior to the published results in *Human Sexual Response*. Though movement toward a rethinking of the vaginal orgasm had begun prior to 1966, with the publication of Sherfey's article, "this equivocation came to an abrupt end," historian Mari Jo Buhle noted. The discussion regarding female sexuality now, however, occurred during what one analyst called an "identity crisis" in psychoanalysis. As Buhle argued, though the number of trained analysts had risen dramatically since the end of World War II, the profession had begun to fall from its position of esteem, as attacks on the validity of its therapeutic claims, begun in earnest in the 1950s, peaked in the late 1960s as part of a larger revolt against psychiatry. One of the major assaults would come from feminists, whose challenge to Freud, and in particular here to the vaginal orgasm theory, came at what Buhle called a "portentous moment."[62]

The Organ of Liberation

The transformation in the 1960s of attitudes regarding sex occurred alongside and often overlapped other cultural revolutions, most importantly here the women's movement. During the late 1960s and early 1970s, this movement can be viewed in a simplistic manner as having two parts, one led by women we could call liberal feminists, the other led by women we could call radical feminists.[63] Though members of the two groups were often intertwined with the New Left and civil rights movements, these feminists saw gender as a core component of their oppression, something many men within the other movements failed to understand.[64] Liberal feminists were largely (but not entirely) made up of white, middle-class, professional women seeking the same social and political opportunities men traditionally enjoyed. They sought changes by working within the existing political structure. By contrast, radical feminists were largely (but not entirely) younger women dissatisfied with the sexism in the civil rights and New Left movements. Though their movement was far from unified, these women for the most part had a more radical approach to the advancement of women's rights; instead of working within the established structures, they wanted to destroy them. For radical feminists, the sexual revolution revealed much about sex roles and men's power and less about women's pleasure.[65]

Gender oppression, many radical feminists argued, played out in a myriad of ways, from familial to cultural, but was often seen as an individual lacking control of her own body. In response, many women began demanding a right to control their bodies and pressed for a variety of reforms, such as in rape laws and in the legalization of abortion. But they also fought for knowledge about their bodies, with the idea that women themselves should be the authorities on the subject; the personal was political, as the slogan declared. The process of consciousness raising became fundamental to radical feminism, an intimate protest enacted dramatically differently from the mass actions of those engaged in the anti-Vietnam movement.[66]

Beginning in the late 1960s, one aspect of women's lives that consciousness raising brought to the fore was the treatment of women by physicians. Women collectively began challenging the authoritative role that physicians, most often male, held over their bodies, in particular in areas related to reproductive and sexual health. During the early 1970s, women gathered in their kitchens, in the basements of churches, and in community centers to discuss health matters as a key feminist issue and launch the local, independent, yet unified women's health movement. Women within the movement expressed frustration that male doctors were condescending and that routine passages of women's lives—birth control, pregnancy, childbirth, menstruation, menopause—were overmedicalized.[67]

The feminist critique of the health-care system in general, and of doctors in particular, charged that men dominated medical care and knowledge, thus exercising control over women's bodies. In 1969, a group of women in Boston at a health conference formed the Boston Women's Health Book Collective, and published what became the defining text of the movement, *Our Bodies, Ourselves*.[68] The women who formed the collective wrote that they "had all experienced similar feelings of frustration and anger toward specific doctors and the medical gaze in general." By writing the book, they attempted to "do something about those doctors who were condescending, paternalistic, judgmental and non-informative."[69] As the feminist journal *off our backs* noted in 1971, women were "crippled by our ignorance about our bodies," and this ignorance about how "our bodies are put together and how they work means we have no control over ourselves."[70]

Those in the women's health movement, historian Wendy Kline noted, privileged individual experience over scientific evaluation, thus allowing "for a more democratic, less hierarchal approach to learning about female biology—something potentially quite revolutionary."[71] In addition to popular texts such as *Our Bodies, Ourselves* and the establishment of feminist health centers, women also gathered to learn about their bodies at gynecological self-help meetings, by going to self-help clinics, and by reading self-help pamphlets and publications.[72]

Feminists' demand to understand and control their own bodies extended to a right to sexual pleasure and freedom on their own terms.[73] Many of these women turned to the new research on the clitoris, seeing in it the opportunity to embrace their own sexual pleasure independent of men. Masters and Johnson were neither the first nor the only to challenge the idea of the supremacy of the vaginal orgasm, but their research provided physiological evidence at a time when women were questioning medical and therapeutic knowledge about the female body. So while Masters and Johnson were accepted popularly because of their scientific grounding and their focus on improving heterosexual sex, radical feminists embraced their work regarding the clitoris as evidence that women were capable of erotic independence from men.

Though the vaginal orgasm theory was not ubiquitously held within medicine, other historians have noted the theory's widespread acceptance and dissemination within popular culture in, for example, advice columns in women's magazines well into the 1960s. This shaped the expectations and frustrations of many women.[74] As expressed in a memoir about three women's experiences during the 1960s, Susie Berman recalled never having had an orgasm, that her husband had never touched her clitoris, and that she had not even been sure where her clitoris was on her body. "Freud and [her husband's] father informed him that mature women have vaginal orgasms." Susie faked all her orgasms with her husband to meet this expectation. It was not until 1968, when she discovered the research of Masters and Johnson by attending a meeting with other women speaking about being treated poorly by the men in their lives, that she learned about her body's sexual potential.[75]

Berman's discovery occurred at a time when many radical feminist polemics were leveling what historian Mari Jo Buhle called "potshots" at Freud and psychoanalysis. Between 1970 and 1971 alone, four major feminist texts appeared charging Freud with misogyny: Kate Millett's *Sexual Politics*, Shulamith Firestone's *The Dialectic of Sex*, Eva Figes's *Patriarchal Attitudes*, and Germaine Greer's *The Female Eunuch*. According to Buhle, of all the theorists,

Freud received the most criticism from feminists.[76] And though Freudian psychoanalysis as a whole was challenged (and not just by radical feminists), providing in hindsight what psychiatrist Ethel Spector Person called a "wake-up call" for the discipline, specific to this story was the radical feminist attack on the vaginal orgasm theory.[77] Using Master and Johnson's research, feminists were hardly, as Buhle stressed, "cutting-edge and added nothing to the well-publicized evidence" from Masters and Johnson. Nevertheless, Buhle argued, "they compensated for their lack of originality by mercilessly targeting Freud."[78]

Writing in 1971, Alix Shulman called their research a clinical confirmation of "what women know to be true from their own experience."[79] Anne Koedt, in her classic challenge to the vaginal orgasm theory made in 1968, used Masters and Johnson's research in her critique, "The Myth of the Vaginal Orgasm." Originally printed by the New England Free Press, it sold for a dime as a yellow tabloid sheet folded in half.[80] "The Myth" was, historian Christine Stansell noted, "an underground sensation, distributed through feminist newspapers and women's centers."[81] Koedt, historian Buhle argued, created the political frame for the feminist discussion about the vaginal orgasm.[82]

Koedt tied sexual expression not to heterosexuality or homosexuality but to a sort of feminine sexuality, one not bound to social designations. In her article, Koedt debunked the idea of sex "in terms of what pleases men" and challenged women to "redefine our sexuality" to "discard the 'normal' concepts of sex and create new guidelines that take into account mutual sexual enjoyment." She denied the Freudian analysis of the vaginal orgasm and insisted that women need to "demand that if certain sexual positions now defined as 'standard' are not mutually conducive to orgasm, they must no longer be defined as standard." Koedt argued that the "establishment of the clitoral orgasm as fact would threaten the heterosexual *institution*" as a clitoral orgasm allowed for women to obtain pleasure "from either men *or* women, thus making heterosexuality not an absolute, but an option."[83] Koedt challenged the entire cultural conception of sex and encouraged women to see the sexual not within the parameters of heterosexuality or homosexuality but rather of pleasure.[84]

Like Koedt, Susan Lydon, in her 1969 essay in *Ramparts*, also challenged the vaginal orgasm myth, "codified by Freud," as responsible for women's conception of their sexuality as "repressed and channeled, denied and abused." The theory, she argued, was useful because it "provided a convenient basis for categorization" of women as either clitoral—and thus "neurotic, bitchy, and masculine"—or as vaginal and thus "maternal, feminine, mature, and normal." For Lydon, the Freudian theory was almost "demoniac" in its repression of female sexuality. In comparison, the work of Masters and Johnson enabled women to see that there was "infinite variety in female sexual response," and that one sort of orgasm was not superior, just different. Though noting that the "sexual problems of our society will never be solved until there is real and unfeigned equality between men and women," Lydon ended her essay with the hope that "if the Masters and Johnson material is allowed to filter into the public consciousness, hopefully to replace the enshrined Freudian myths, then woman at long last will be allowed to take the first step toward her emancipation: to define and enjoy the forms of her own sexuality."[85]

Arguing along similar lines in her 1968 essay, "Vaginal Orgasm as a Mass Hysterical Survival Response," Ti-Grace Atkinson charged men with oppressing women with the vaginal orgasm hegemony. Women, she wrote, learned to orgasm vaginally because that was what men wanted, and women acquiesced in order to survive.[86] Similarly, Cathy, a member of the Chicago Women's Liberation Union, in an article for *Womankind* in 1972, noted that while previously the expectation had been that men enjoyed sex and women endured it, the "new slant" for this was that "men are trained to enjoy sex and women are trained to enjoy men enjoying sex."[87]

Feminists like Koedt and Atkinson believed men feared the clitoris because it allowed women to experience orgasm without them.[88] And indeed sexual pleasure and sexual self-determination came to be seen by some women as not just sexually important but also politically important for their liberating potential. For these women in the 1970s, the clitoris became a feminist organ, existing purely for female pleasure, unlike the vagina, which bound women to the confines of both motherhood and heterosexuality.[89] Some women, most famously perhaps Betty Dodson, regarded self-exploration and masturbation as liberating sexually and mentally, and as a political statement of independence.[90] Other women saw lesbianism as the only truly feminist sexual expression, though, as historian Christine Stansell noted, some women who regarded lesbianism as the best political choice failed to support women who loved women for reasons other than political conviction.[91]

As historian Jane Gerhard stated, sex mattered in a whole new way to these women; it was "perhaps short-lived, perhaps misguided, most certainly selective, but for a moment, sex was at the center of women's impending liberation." Women envisioned sexual pleasure as "empowering, as helping men become more human, and as a route out of patriarchal repression of the body." And while pleasure may not have meant the same thing for every woman, it nonetheless became momentarily equal with liberation. Sexual freedom for this new generation of feminists meant determining what happened to their bodies, empowering women's sexual desires, and changing the perceptions of male experts and partners. For these women, the clitoris was the organ of liberation.[92]

Finding the Clitoris

As part of the critique of (male) medicine's dominance over information about female bodies, as well as part of the idea within the women's health movement that individual experience mattered as much as other, more traditional forms of evidence, some feminists advocated women examining their own—and each other's—genitals to better understand their own bodies and the differences among women's bodies.[93] The popularity of the vaginal self-exam in the early 1970s among some feminists was based in its novelty, its rejection of conventional middle-class respectability, and the "enthusiasm for experimentation," historian Michelle Murphy argued. Carol Downer, one of the originators of vaginal self-exams and the gynecological self-help movement, remembered it as a "mind-blowing" experience.[94]

Self-exams did not just involve looking at the internal vagina and cervix, however, but also the external genitalia, including the clitoris. In her 1972 book, *Vaginal Politics*, Ellen Frankfort documented how many women did not understand the diversity of female genitals. One woman, while attending a gynecological self-help course, recalled her gynecologist telling her she had a "meaty" clitoris. As she told Frankfort, after seeing other women's clitorises at the self-help course, she realized that clitorises differed "enormously" from one another, with one "meaty," another concealed, and another protruding. Frankfort further noted in her book that, once women learned about not just the diversity of the shape and size of their clitorises but also their erotic capabilities, they no longer felt "hesitation about stimulating themselves and bringing themselves to climax."[95]

Feminist health texts highlighted the importance of the clitoris to female sexual arousal and satisfaction and provided drawings to help women find their own clitorises. The second printing of *Our Bodies, Ourselves*, published in 1971, included a drawing of a woman's external genitals, labeling the clitoris and clitoral hood. In the text below the drawing, the authors noted the importance Freud placed on the vaginal orgasm as being the orgasm of maturity but said that "fortunately for women," Masters and Johnson "finally proved Freud wrong" by showing that "all orgasms happen in the same way—in the clitoris."[96] A year earlier, in Carol Horos's book *Vaginal Health*, a drawing of the female external genitals noted the clitoris as having a glans and a prepuce, and the text noted the internal "hidden" portion of the organ, the crura. Horos further called the clitoris "the most sexually sensitive organ in the female reproductive system," an organ "similar to the male penis in both form and function," having "erectile tissue" and "an abundance of nerve endings." Like *Our Bodies, Ourselves*, Horos noted that "all orgasms are related directly or indirectly to clitoral stimulation or arousal," citing the work of Masters and Johnson as debunking the earlier Freudian myth of the "purely" vaginal orgasm.[97] In *The Ms. Guide to a Women's Health*, first published in 1979 and then in 1981, the clitoris was described as consisting of "erectile tissue" and as the "most sensitive of all the female genital organs."[98] The 1981 *Woman's Body: An Owner's Manual*, described the clitoris as "the center of orgasm." According to the book, the clitoris corresponded exactly to the penis and was similarly "made up of erectile tissue."[99] And in the 1980 *Self Help*, published by the National Women's Health Network as part of their series on women's health, the clitoris was described as "covered with sensitive nerve endings" and as "the center of orgasmic pleasure for most women." The only purpose for the clitoris, the text noted, was "sexual sensation and pleasure."[100]

But it was the 1981 book *A New View of a Woman's Body*, published by the Federation of Feminist Women's Health Centers, that took the embrace of the clitoris to a new level by envisioning the clitoris as not just important to female sexuality but as the *center* of female genitalia. As the authors noted in the first chapter, illustrator "Suzann Gage's well-researched illustrations are designed to lift the veil of medical mystery from women's bodies and reveals the truths that, though simple, have been hidden up to now." In the chapter "The Clitoris: A Feminist Perspective," the authors stressed their intention of challenging "deeply entrenched myths" about female sexuality and the clitoris in particular, including the myth of the vaginal orgasm and the myth of there being a "correct" way to have an orgasm. Through the use of "self-examination, personal observation and meticulous analysis," the authors "arrived at *a new view of the clitoris*." The authors noted their pleasure in learning "that the clitoris has many distinct parts in addition to its visible structures, such as bodies of erectile tissue, muscle, nerves and blood vessels." In essence, the authors relabeled all the external genitals in reference to the clitoris: the vagina became the "clitoral opening to the vagina," the hymen the "hymen of the clitoris," the fourchette the "fourchette of the clitoris," and the labia the "inner lip of the clitoris."[101]

Adriane Fugh-Berman, in her review of *A New View of a Woman's Body* for the feminist journal *off our backs*, noted that the authors saw "the redefinition of the clitoris" as "broadening of the concept of women's sexuality to deemphasize orgasm reached by penis-in-vagina intercourse." The "detailed research," Fugh-Berman wrote, done by a "small group of women," encouraged other women to learn from their own bodies. But she also questioned the extension of the clitoris to encompass all the external genitals, calling it "self-indulgent." Noting that by labeling the perineum as "part of our sex organ" made an episiotomy "a mutilation of the clitoris," Fugh-Berman argued that one could similarly "define the brain as composing the central nervous system along with the spinal cord, but that doesn't make a spinal tap a lobotomy."[102]

The authors of these medical guides for women, from *Our Bodies, Ourselves* to *A New View*, regarded the clitoris as not just important for women to know about, but also an organ neglected or misrepresented within standard medical texts. But, as I discussed in the introduction to this book, though only a few anatomy and gynecology texts explicitly noted the sexual purpose of the organ, many implicitly regarded the clitoris as sexually important.[103] Were anatomy and gynecology texts embracing the clitoris in the same manner as *A New View* or as critics like Koedt who regarded the clitoris as the potential organ of liberation for women? Hardly. But this does not mean that medicine—represented here by anatomy and gynecology texts—neglected information about the clitoris as a sexual organ prior to the findings by Masters and Johnson. Indeed, physicians had been acting upon such an understanding of the organ by removing the clitoral hood to enable the clitoris to better receive stimulation for decades.

Surgery to Liberate the Liberating Organ

The women's health and the self-help movements were critical of medicine during a time others were also critical of medicine and medicalization. Beginning in the 1970s, some social scientists began questioning the expansion of medicine into many aspects of life that had previously not been under medical purview.[104] Though the medicalization critique began with a focus on the more general idea of medical imperialism and used "case studies" on subjects like mental illness, it quickly expanded to other areas.[105] These theorists viewed the medical model as assuming a moral neutrality medicine did not actually have. Medical designations were a form of social judgments, these theorists argued.[106]

Though people historically have actively pursued their desired medical treatment, for a variety of reasons patients became consumers in the late twentieth century, and elective physical enhancement surgery was at the fore of consumer-driven medicalization.[107] Cosmetic surgery was part of this trend, and it began to move from the margins to the mainstream in the 1970s, with elective female circumcision part of that movement. Whereas in the early twentieth century "beauty surgery" was considered the practice of quacks and charlatans, by the 1950s it was regularly featured in women's magazines; by the 1970s, cosmetic surgery was well established and thriving. The development of cosmetic surgery, historian Elizabeth Haiken argued, was driven by consumer desire and changes in perception. As Haiken observed, with the economic gains American women made in the decades after World War II, by the 1970s "more women than ever before could afford to buy the things they wanted, and among other goods they bought were smoother faces, bigger breasts, and thinner thighs."[108] As surgery of all kinds became both more widely available and acceptable in the 1960s and 1970s, more people sought surgical procedures, and increasingly the surgeries were elective.[109] Some of these elective surgeries were promoted as a means of achieving self-determination and empowerment; cosmetic surgeons advertised procedures like breast enhancements as a feminist decision where women took control of their bodies.[110]

Perhaps inevitably, some physicians pointedly connected the removal of the clitoral hood as a surgical method for women to take control of their bodies. Female circumcision was promoted as a surgical means toward women's sexual empowerment, a message sent directly to women in articles published in magazines such as *Cosmopolitan*. By removing the hood of the clitoris, these physicians argued, the organ would be better able to receive stimulation and thus women could better control their orgasms. Physicians Seymour Isenberg and L. M. Elting wrote in *Cosmopolitan* that "sometimes" to "revive sexual pleasure, or bring it within reach for the first time" surgery of the body's "most private parts" was necessary. Clitoral circumcision was one such operation they advocated. Isenberg and Elting wrote that, for about 10 percent of the female population, circumcision uncovered the organ and made stimulation easier. In a direct appeal—or perhaps challenge—to women to surgically take control of their sexual lives, Isenberg and Elting noted that if a man "walked in for circumcision strictly on an elective basis he would be swiftly booked for surgery," while many women feared their doctor would "think the reason for the surgery improper."[111] In a similar manner, Richard Scotti, a gynecologist in Santa Cruz, California, labeled those who opposed the surgery as "people with sex hang-ups" who viewed sex as meant only for procreation.[112]

Though Catherine Kellison, whose *Playgirl* story began this chapter, did not see Isenberg, Elting, or Scotti for her circumcision, she agreed with their assessment that the surgery was meant purely to enhance female sexual response.[113] Kellison decided to ask the doctor whom her friends had seen for their circumcisions if he believed she was a good candidate for the surgery. To determine the answer, physician Stanley Daniels had her pay close attention to the difference in pressure he applied to the clitoris when covered by the foreskin and when he pulled the foreskin back. "The difference," Kellison wrote, "was quite distinct and favorable." The doctor told Kellison that she would be a candidate for the surgery, though he also said that in her case the operation would not "drastically" change her sensations. Kellison decided to see for herself and scheduled surgery two days later.[114]

Kellison described the prep work for the surgery: the pubic area was cleaned with alcohol, and then the clitoral hood was injected with local anesthetic (she wrote this stung—"not unlike the initial ouch! of a dentist's needle which is there for an instant and gone the next"). After the foreskin was deadened, surgery began. The doctor made an incision that left "loose flaps" he removed and sutured. He then dusted the area with antiseptic powder. The operation was over within twenty minutes. She left with a prescription for painkillers, some salve to apply, and instructions to abstain from sex for at least two weeks. The doctor charged her fifty dollars for the surgery, which Kellison decided was a "bargain" because he had been performing it for thirteen years. What she called the "Moment of Truth" arrived when Kellison again had sex, the orgasm she had known was now "elevated to a new position of glory and lofty power."[115]

Other women Kellison interviewed for her articles spoke equally highly of the operation. One woman, Willy (Kellison did not include the women's last names), who had the procedure in 1972, compared it to having her tonsils out, "except that it was cheaper, a lot less painful and it sure made me feel a hell of a lot better." Another woman, Susan, thought sex was now "far more sensuous, more than anything I've ever experienced, really," for her orgasms now reminded her of "honey, slow and very sensuous."[116]

Kellison and the women she interviewed were not the only ones to sing the praises of the procedure in popular magazines. Twenty-eight-year-old Linda Marx told *Penthouse Forum* that she had been having great difficulty reaching climax during sex. When, during her routine annual exam, her gynecologist suggested circumcision, Marx flinched. At first. "I'd never heard of such a thing and frankly the idea of being sliced down there scared me to death!" But after he explained what the procedure entailed, Marx decided to go ahead. Two months following her circumcision, Marx called the results amazing. Since the circumcision, she was "still climaxing every time my boyfriend and I have sex."[117]

In her article about female circumcision in *Viva*, journalist Terri Schultz interviewed Doris, a legal secretary, who was thirty when she had her clitoral hood removed by Stanley Daniels, the physician who also operated on Kellison. Calling herself a "level-headed woman" who usually didn't go for "fads," Doris (Schultz did not include last names of the women) told Schultz she decided to undergo circumcision because she was "desperate." Doris said that though her husband turned her on, she consistently failed to reach orgasm during intercourse. When Doris informed her doctor about what she called her "frigidity," Daniels suggested circumcision as treatment. Eight weeks after her operation, when Daniels asked Doris whether she noticed any difference in her ability to respond sexually, Doris "smiled quietly and nodded," Daniels recalled for Schultz. "She said she had so much sensation the first time she reached orgasm that she started to scream and cry," he continued. "Her husband thought he was hurting her and tried to pull out, but she grabbed his buttocks and kept him in and had a fantastic orgasm." Doris also told Schultz, in less graphic terms, her happiness with the surgery. "I get incredible feelings of exultation and ecstasy that were never there before." Sex was finally "fun" for her, something she looked forward to and planned her day around to allow for "my husband and me as much time as possible for having sex."[118]

Constance Knowles, interviewed by David Haldane in *Penthouse Forum*, underwent circumcision in 1972. She told Haldane that prior to her surgery she considered herself "lucky to experience even one orgasm during intercourse," but, following the removal of the hood of her clitoris, she often experienced several and "the intensity is greatly increased." Knowles, reportedly working on her master's degree in marriage and family counseling, decided to make her thesis a long-term follow-up on the surgery that so excited her own sexual life. Seventy-five percent of the women who participated in her study reported a "significant and lasting improvement in their sex lives as a result of circumcision." Part of her decision to look at the long-term effects of the surgery was to share information about the procedure. "I found out that very few doctors know about female circumcision," she told Haldane, and she wanted other women to learn. "I think that the information should be available so that they can make their own choices."[119]

During research for her article, Schultz asked a number of women who had their clitoris intact their thoughts about the operation. Some thought the surgery was another example of a right hidden from them, while others doubted the efficacy of the procedure. Was clitoral circumcision, Schultz pondered, a "new male myth, a frivolous cosmetic surgery created to exploit women's growing interest in their own sexual response, or is it an advance for female sexuality?" Regardless of their views about the procedure, however, every woman Schultz spoke with "savored" the possibilities of a surgery to enhance female sexual response during intercourse. But though Schultz concluded her article by calling female circumcision a waste of money, she refused to dismiss it entirely. "Why not circumcision, after all, instead of a new dress, a diet, or pierced ears?" It was, she wrote, "cheaper than sex therapy, and for some it does seem to work."[120]

"One of the Most Controversial Procedures in America Today"

Of course, not everyone was pleased with the availability of such a purchase. Though some physicians, as noted at the beginning of this chapter, believed the operation was effective for those women with a large or thick clitoral hood, according to David Haldane the vast majority of gynecologists had either never heard of the operation or refused to perform it. "The fact is," he wrote in *Penthouse Forum*, "this simple operation is one of the most controversial medical procedures in America today."[121] While taking into consideration Haldane was purposefully adding drama to his story, he was not alone in calling it controversial. Physicians Seymour Isenberg and L. Melvin Elting, in their *Cosmopolitan* article singing the praises of female circumcision, had also noted that there was "considerable debate" over the necessity of the operation.[122]

Many doctors doubted the purported effectiveness of surgically interfering with the clitoris to promote female orgasm. David Kentsmith and Merrill Eaton, professors of psychiatry at the University of Nebraska College of Medicine, said in 1979 that the only evidence of female circumcision working was anecdotal, with "little objective evidence to demonstrate that the removal of the clitoral hood which keeps the sensitive clitoris exposed during plateau or orgasm enhances sexual responsiveness in women."[123] Physician Donald Sloan, head of the Sexual Therapy Clinic in New York City, noted that while some women claimed the surgery helped them, others said it did not. "It's hard to get any concrete evidence," he told journalist Terri Schulz for her article about the surgery.[124]

Still other physicians and sexual therapists openly questioned the efficacy of clitoral circumcision, and one gynecologist worried that the popularization of the operation "may open up a whole new field for medical charlatans."[125] Leon Zussman, a gynecologist and a sex therapist in New York, believed female circumcision was rarely, if ever, needed.[126] John Money, professor of medical psychology at Johns Hopkins University, called clitoral circumcision "faddist," saying that "some people will tell you they've had better sex after a nose-job operation."[127] Physician A. Stark Wolkoff called the operation "overrated."[128] John Huffman, a retired gynecology professor from Northwestern University Medical School, said in 1976 that based on the several women he had seen who had undergone the procedure, "the operation did not change their sexual reactions or lack of reactions."[129] In the 1977 book *It's Your Body: A Woman's Guide to Gynecology*, physician Niels Lauersen wrote that many women with orgasm troubles decide to have their clitoral hoods removed, though for most "the problem of difficult orgasm remains." These women, Lauersen argued, "probably need more stimulation" and "circumcision will *not* usually help."[130] Indeed, James P. Semmens, an associate professor of obstetrics and gynecology at the Medical University of South Carolina, wrote that because circumcision exposed the clitoris, the "direct contact and lack of protection for it might prove more detrimental than helpful" to women seeking orgasm.[131] And in their 1979 textbook on sexual medicine, Robert Kolodny, William Masters, and Virginia Johnson noted that although there was no evidence to support clitoral circumcision, "because some women's magazines have described clitoral circumcision as a magical way of transforming female sexuality, there are many patients requesting such operations with the expectation that they will experience a new set of sexual feelings and responses."[132]

In addition to the critiques from academics and sexologists, feminists interested in women's health also weighed in on the practice of female circumcision as a surgery for purported sexual enhancement. The June 1977 issue of the Denver, Colorado, feminist newsletter *Big Mama Rag* carried a story from another feminist newspaper, *HerSay*, on Brooklyn physician Leo Wollman's practice of performing female circumcision to "help in situations where the hood-like foreskin which covers a woman's clitoris somehow prevents her from getting enough sexual stimulus to reach orgasm." Though there is no editorial in this short blurb other than the "somehow" in the previous sentence and in the article's title "Better Orgasms?," the implication seems to be that the authors found this to be a questionable surgery.[133]

Though most feminist critiques were wielded against just one practitioner, the obstetrician gynecologist James Burt, whom I will discuss in the next chapter, sometimes the practice of female circumcision was more generally challenged. In both the 1979 and 1981 editions of *The Ms. Guide to a Woman's Health*, physician Cynthia Cooke and activist Susan Dworkin noted that "in most cases, sexual dysfunction is *not* caused by anatomical problems in the genital area," and they cautioned that the suggestion "to somehow alter the genitals" was "very dangerous." Women, they stressed, should "*watch out* for any doctor who suggests the fad therapy, now catching on in popular magazines, which suggests that the skin over the clitoris be surgically loosened so that the clitoris will be more stimulated during intercourse." This, they stressed, was a "nonsense operation" that would not work any better than "additional manual or oral stimulation of the clitoris during lovemaking." Do not, they wrote, "have it."[134]

Americans in the Bedroom

Articles within popular magazines and medical journals both attesting to and questioning clitoral circumcision appeared at the same time as popular sex manuals in the 1970s drew attention to the importance of the clitoris to women for sexual arousal, often including sexual positions for clitoral stimulation.[135] However, while noting the significant role played by the clitoris to female orgasm, many of these texts regarded sex principally as consisting of heterosexual and penetrative intercourse. In the era of sexual freedom, historian Jane Gerhard argued, "vaginal sexuality continued to bear the symbolic freight of proper womanhood." Though women and their partners were now informed about new techniques and positions—even surgery—to stimulate the clitoris, popular sex writers and counselors told women and men that orgasm was still expected to occur for both during penetrative intercourse.[136]

But few women—only 30 percent, according to Shere Hite's 1970s survey—regularly reached orgasm from heterosexual and penetrative sex without additional direct clitoral stimulation.[137] While many Americans continued to see normal sex as missionary position heterosexual intercourse without additional touching of the clitoris, few women reported satisfaction from it. So although some books noted the importance of the clitoris and radical feminists embraced the clitoris as an organ of sexual liberation, the idea of penetrative sex leading to orgasm as normal remained strong in popular culture. In her 1974 book, *The New Sex Therapy*, Helen Singer Kaplan, a sex therapist and professor of psychiatry at Cornell Medical College, wrote that, based on her clinical observations, less than half of women "regularly reach a climax during coitus without additional clitoral stimulation." This, she wrote, was in "sharp contrast to the view held by many experts, and shared by the general public, that coital orgasm is the only normal form of female sexual expression and that orgasm attained primarily by direct clitoral stimulation is somehow pathological."[138] Writing eight years after the publication of Masters and Johnson's work on the clitoris, Kaplan felt the need to challenge what was apparently still the sexual status quo: penetrative sex leading to vaginal orgasm. Feminists had tried to end the validity of the vaginal orgasm in the late 1960s and early 1970s. But a decade later, Lonnie Barbach, an assistant clinical professor in psychiatry at the University of California, San Francisco, Medical School called the vaginal orgasm a "slowly dying theory" in a 1981 article for *Mademoiselle*, "Five Myths about the Big O."[139]

Kaplan's and Barbach's observations reflected the resurgence of conservative notions regarding sex and relations between the sexes in the 1970s.[140] For those who wished to reinforce these notions, the sexual revolution and feminist challenges to conventional ideas about sexual relations and pleasures were wrong. Joseph Oliven, writing to fellow physicians in 1974, said, "radical feminists misinterpreting the Masters' laboratory observations have held that the clitoris is the 'key' to female orgasm" and that through it woman can, in his words, "escape reproductive enslavement and dependence on the phallus." He concluded his short discussion on the "great clitoral controversy" by saying that many women preferred the "fused sex act (i.e., coital thrusting by an organ with a human male attached)."[141]

But while perhaps many women may have preferred the "fused sex act," they may not have derived orgasm from it alone and their partners may not have cared that they did not reach orgasm. A 1978 article by Mary Jane Gray, a professor of obstetrics and gynecology at the University of North Carolina School of Medicine, stated that some women "complain that their sexual partners engage in foreplay grudgingly as payment for coitus" and that men, for a variety of reasons, including "sexual over-eagerness, anxiety about female genitalia, a feeling that 'touching is wrong,' or unfamiliarity with the anatomy of the vulva," omitted foreplay or engaged in it only briefly.[142]

So what were heterosexual Americans actually doing in bed? Surveys concerning Americans sexual habits were far from new, but in the 1970s a great number of them occurred. Surveys about sex not only reported on what people were doing sexually, they also created beliefs about what people should be doing sexually. As Julia Erickson has said in her history of American sex surveys, these surveys provided suggestions for how readers should behave and also provided lessons to the readers on certain types of behavior.[143]

Women who took part in sex surveys revealed how the continued dominance of sex as penetrative affected their sex lives. In 1972, Shere Hite found through her survey that women felt pressured to have an orgasm during intercourse to make their male partners feel good. One woman wrote that she "sometimes felt that reaching orgasm was more a matter of satisfying my partner's desire to satisfy me than my own need for orgasm." Only 30 percent of the women who answered Hite's survey said they regularly had an orgasm from coitus without additional direct clitoral stimulation.[144] Similarly, in its 1975 survey of married women, *Redbook* magazine also found that many women did not have an orgasm during penetrative sex. One woman wrote that she conducted a survey of her friends and found that none of them had ever had a "'real' orgasm through intercourse—only through clitoral stimulation." She reported that men found this hard to believe: "Try convincing a *man* you don't have orgasms his way. He won't believe you." Another woman said that she thought that many women "are faking orgasm during intercourse because they are too embarrassed to tell their husbands or lovers that no matter how long they keep their erection, they just can't make her have an orgasm." This responder begged *Redbook* to print her response to "ease a lot of tensions and make sex a lot better for thousands of women like me."[145]

In her early 1970s article embracing the potential of the clitoris for women, Alix Shulman complained that men treated "the clitoris as simply one more erogenous zone," using it to "arouse a woman sexually so she will permit intercourse." They remembered the clitoris, she wrote, in foreplay, "but for real sex, back to the vagina!"[146] Shere Hite found similar sentiments. In 1981, Hite followed up her sex study on women by publishing one on men. She noted that in the 1970s, clitoral stimulation became a "public issue" and described the diverse ways men reacted. Some men referred to the clitoris with positive remarks, calling it "beautiful and mysterious" or a "little love button." Other men, however, told Hite that they did not know where the clitoris was on their wives or girlfriends. While some men knew it was located in the upper vulva area, others were even more vague, and some were just confused, believing the clitoris to be located in the vagina. Many men who responded to the survey expressed pride in their ability to stimulate their female partners manually though some also felt such behavior was "abnormal" and a juvenile sort of activity. Most men, however, saw it only as part of foreplay, and two-thirds of men similarly thought of cunnilingus as foreplay.[147]

So while feminists in the 1970s recognized the clitoris and with it a woman's ability to orgasm outside of the parameters of heterosexual penetrative sex, for many men and women, sex still meant intercourse. It should not be surprising, then, that ideas regarding what was considered healthy and normal sex were contentious during the 1970s or that because of this clitoral orgasm was often complicated for women during this time. Attention to the clitoris to the point of orgasm often meant having an orgasm before or after coitus with one's male partner, something that bothered some women and often their male partners as well. As in similar sex surveys, a 1981 survey conducted by *Cosmopolitan* magazine discovered that only 34 percent of women usually had orgasms during coitus, while 71 percent usually reached orgasm during manual or oral sex. One twenty-nine-year-old woman from North Dakota wrote that while she liked penetrative intercourse, "I have my orgasms from having my lover touch my clitoris with his fingers."[148]

Though women like the one from North Dakota had orgasms when their lovers touched their clitorises, many women also, like her, expressed enjoying penetrative intercourse. One study by a Pennsylvania State University psychologist found the majority of heterosexual women both believed that the joining of the penis and the vagina was an important part of sex and that sex had not happened until this occurred.[149] But since few women reached orgasm this way, some women went to therapists frustrated because they wanted to experience orgasm during penetrative sex.[150]

Sex therapists Georgia Kline-Graber and Benjamin Graber noted that many women came to their clinic for this reason and that many of the male partners reacted "judgmentally" to the fact that their female partners needed clitoral stimulation during sex.[151] Indeed, one husband who wrote to a popular magazine wanting to know whether his wife was correct when she told him "during marital relations, proper clitoral contact is not felt." Was she correct, this man wanted to know, that his wife needed to "massage her own clitoris (during intercourse) in order to bring about her own climax." The husband felt it "improper" and a "slap at the husband's ability to satisfy his wife."[152]

Women often felt cultural, therapeutic, and relationship pressure to have an orgasm during penetrative intercourse. Following her own circumcision, Catherine Kellison found that during penetrative sex the "usual tension, that responsibility of reaching an orgasm; the *strain* had been taken away." A friend who had the operation agreed, telling Kellison that there was no more "Oh thank God, I did it!" This woman's partner, who apparently overheard the conversation, leaned over, smiled, and nodded "knowingly" to Kellison.[153]

As this man "knowingly" indicated, clitoral circumcision was, of course, not just about the woman's ability to reach orgasm but also about the male ego. For, as the man who questioned whether his wife was correct about the need for him (or her) to manually stimulate her clitoris during sex, many believed a man was responsible for giving a woman her orgasm. In an interview with *Playboy* magazine in 1977, when Shere Hite was asked why women "still have so much trouble having orgasms during intercourse," Hite responded that the assumption was faulty "because intercourse per se does not provide enough clitoral stimulation for most women to orgasm." Women can orgasm during intercourse if their clitoris was stimulated manually at the same time, "but the problem here has always been the idea that men should be able to *give* women orgasms—that women must be provided for here as everywhere else." Because the "definition of sex is intercourse," the definition failed, as Hite said, to "leave a lot of room for creativity, or experimentation, or alternative forms of sexual satisfaction." So while men and women continue to "see intercourse as the only *real* sex, it means that no matter how satisfying anything else they do together is, it's all foreplay without intercourse," Hite responded.[154]

Doctors, then, who advised female circumcisions were not concerned simply with assisting a woman achieve orgasm. It was inability to orgasm during penetrative sex that was regarded as a medical problem, one that some doctors believed surgery could treat. Takey Crist, gynecologist and director of the Crist Clinic for Women in North Carolina, believed a woman would benefit from female circumcision if they reached orgasm only during "masturbation and/or oral sex."[155] While advocating the procedure as a means for women to embrace the sexual pleasures they were entitled to, that pleasure was still supposed to occur during penetrative sex.

Chapter Seven

James Burt and the Surgery of Love, 1966–89

In the late 1970s, journalist Barbara Demick interviewed gynecologist and obstetrician James Burt for a small Boston-area magazine, the *Real Paper*. The Dayton, Ohio, doctor had recently begun generating publicity for a surgery he had designed to improve the sexual capabilities of women. Burt, in an effort to show the positive effects of the surgery, had his secretary arrange for Demick to interview in his office eight women who elected to have the surgery and who were happy with the results. One of these women was Judy (Demick did not use last names). Twenty-seven and married for eight years, Judy told Demick she had not had any problems with sex until after giving birth. In 1977, needing a hysterectomy and bladder repair, she learned about Burt's surgery from a niece and decided to undergo it as well. Her husband, Bruce, went with her to meet Burt, and the doctor showed Bruce, as Judy told Demick, "exactly what he was going to do."[1]

Judy and Bruce were both impressed that Burt took the time to explain the procedure to them, and they were equally happy with the results. Sex was, Judy told Demick, "a whole new thing now." During intercourse "Bruce hits me exactly where he has to." Judy recalled that prior to love surgery she seldom reached a climax during intercourse, but "now I can have as many as I want." The surgery "actually changed my life," Judy said. "Even though I am not the greatest person in the world, to him [Bruce] I am. I feel the pleasure that he does and I feel that I am good for my husband, that I am really extraordinary. I feel more confident in bed, more confident socially." Judy further told Demick that her early sexual experiences were a disappointment—no explosives, no rockets—and she figured that was how it was for all women. But since her surgery she believed differently and was adamant about its benefits: "Women should know they don't have to live the rest of their lives like that. I feel that women just are not made right, seeing how much better I'm made now."[2]

Her words echoed those of James Burt. In the mid-1960s, Burt decided women were made wrong for sex and that he could make them right. Specifically, Burt believed women's internal and external genitals were not aligned in a manner advantageous for heterosexual missionary sex, and he devised a surgery to correct what he saw as this anatomical dysfunction. The surgery, popularly called "love surgery," involved a variation of an episiotomy repair (the sewing up of the cut in the perineum many physicians then made prior to delivery of a baby), cutting the pubococcygeus muscle (located just beneath the vagina), and circumcising the clitoris. In essence, Burt moved the entrance of the vagina closer to the clitoris in an effort to enable women to have both easier and better orgasms by enabling the penis to more easily provide the clitoris with stimulation during penetrative sex.

Though Judy elected to have love surgery in 1977, Burt first practiced his surgery on hundreds of unknowing women after they had given birth beginning in the mid-1960s; it was, he later told them, a modification of episiotomy repair. Between 1966 and the mid-1970s, Burt added and made variations on love surgery. Two years before Judy underwent love surgery, Burt decided he had perfected it to the point where he could promote it as an elective surgery, and both local and national media discussed its benefits. As a result, women from across the country came to Burt's clinic in hopes of a surgically enabled better sex life. Though by the mid-1970s Burt was promoting his surgery as an elective, he continued to perform it on his obstetric patients even when they did not choose to have it. Burt practiced medicine until 1989, when a group of women suing him for malpractice accused him on national television of operating on them without their fully informed consent. After this negative exposure, Burt was pressured to give up his medical license; in early 1989, he voluntarily stopped practicing medicine, though he defiantly maintained he would teach love surgery to any interested physician.

Unlike other practitioners of female circumcision who, it appears, performed the procedure on individual patients either to treat masturbation or to correct a difficulty reaching orgasm during penetrative heterosexual sex for a physiological reason such as a thick hood, Burt seemed to be less patient specific; it was not *a* female body but *the* female body in need of correction. His practice, spanning from the mid-1960s through early 1989, both benefited from an increased acceptance of the sexual in American life and exploited women's concerns about being appropriately sexual for their male partners. And I end this book with Burt because he is perhaps the most famous—some perhaps would say infamous—practitioner of female circumcision in the United States.

The Love Doctor

James Caird Burt Jr. was born on August 29, 1921, in Dayton, Ohio. In 1939, he attended Auburn University and there met his future wife, Lucretia. Burt ultimately received his undergraduate degree from Alabama Polytechnic Institute in 1942 and attended medical school at the University of Rochester in New York, graduating in 1945. He then interned in Houston and spent time in the US Air Force Medical Corps before his residency at the Chicago Lying-in Hospital and the Sloane Hospital for Women. He left Chicago to take a residency at Columbia Presbyterian Medical Center in New York City.[3] On June 21, 1951, Burt received his medical license from the state of Ohio and set up his gynecology and obstetrics practice in Dayton.[4] He obtained surgical privileges at the local hospitals, including St. Elizabeth Medical Center. But soon after, in 1952, the Burts, now with two sons and a daughter, separated, and he filed for divorce. In 1953, with his divorce from his first wife still pending in Ohio, James Burt obtained a divorce in Mexico and shortly thereafter married his second wife, Gerre, in Indiana.[5] After a decade and one child, however, this marriage ended as well. The divorce was not amicable—he countered her claims for alimony, saying the divorce from his first wife was not legal and thus he had never really been married to Gerre Burt. The judge rejected his motion and awarded Gerre Burt alimony and child support, granting her a divorce in July 1966. In 1967, James Burt obtained a stateside divorce from his first wife and married his third wife. His practice now well established and earning him a solid income, Linda and James Burt lived a lavish lifestyle, buying properties in Central America and frequently traveling from Dayton to a condominium in Vail. They hosted grand pool parties, sometimes without swimsuits, and became known around Dayton for their expensive and provocative lifestyle. But by 1973 Linda Burt had left her husband for a ski instructor in Vail and her soon-to-be ex-husband was living with Joan Woodward, a woman twenty-five years younger, who soon became his fourth wife.[6] Joan and James Burt continued an extravagant lifestyle. The doctor often wore gold chains, long fur coats, and sometimes appeared around Dayton clad in a pink safari suit. He was considered flamboyant and eccentric.[7] Burt, a local fellow doctor recalled, cared little for activities like golf—for Burt it "was all indoor games."[8]

It was during this time when Burt was in, out, and between marriages when he was working on, as he saw it, enhancing women's sexual responsiveness surgically. In the mid-1950s, Burt began altering the standard repair of an episiotomy, an incision made from the opening of the vagina toward the anus performed on women during childbirth meant to prevent undue tearing as the baby's head came through.[9] From the 1950s through the 1980s, episiotomies during childbirth were quite common; the standard American obstetrics textbook, *Williams Obstetrics*, noted in its 1956 edition that "except for cutting and tying the umbilical cord, episiotomy is the most common operation in obstetrics."[10] Between 1954 and 1966, Burt made variations on episiotomy repair following a delivery, adding a few more stitches to make the vaginal opening smaller and tighter.[11] But in 1966, Burt discovered two things: the important role played by the clitoris in female sexual response, thanks he said to the recently published research of William Masters and Virginia Johnson, and that the women on whom he had performed his variations of standard episiotomy repair told him their sex lives had improved—even though he had not told them he was performing a surgery meant to do so.[12]

Because of these two discoveries, Burt concluded that women's bodies were not anatomically aligned for heterosexual, penetrative sex. Burt decided the clitoris was too far from the opening of the vagina for women to receive adequate stimulation from the penis during missionary sex and, to correct for this, he began building up the skin tissue between the anal opening and the vaginal opening, thus moving the opening of the vagina closer to the clitoris.[13] In addition, this added tissue also changed the angle of the vagina's opening. During missionary position sex, the changed angle of the vagina forced the penis to hit the clitoris upon penetration.[14] The vagina's redirection, when the woman was on her back, was no longer horizontal but almost vertical.[15] Finally, Burt also circumcised the clitoris in an effort to enable the organ to receive more stimulation. By 1975, Burt claimed to have performed love surgery, in one of its various stages, on more than four thousand women—none of whom had requested it.[16]

It is possible he could have performed this many operations, since Burt was a popular obstetrician gynecologist in Dayton. Working mostly as a solo practitioner and operating mostly at one hospital, St. Elizabeth Medical Center, Burt's medical practice thrived in the 1970s.[17] His office was on the top floor of one of downtown Dayton's tallest buildings.[18] Burt's plush offices illustrated his prosperity as well as his taste for the extravagant and the kitschy: his office included eight examination rooms, a patient waiting room—where one of the couches was shaped like a woman's mouth painted red—a large room for patient files, a consulting room, two bathrooms, a kitchen, and offices for both himself and Joan Burt.[19]

By all accounts James Burt was a genial physician, a stocky man with a short beard who was soft-spoken, listened to his patients, and who possessed a reassuring bedside manner. Former patient Linda Cook recalled Burt having a calm presence, portraying "a peaceful inner self," leaving a patient feeling that he was a "refuge." Burt charged more than other obstetrician gynecologists in Dayton, but he was considered by many to be one of the best in town.[20] His crowded office was a visible testimony to his reputation. Donna Oblinger, whose son Burt delivered in 1970, recalled planning on staying all day at his office when she went in for an appointment "because he'd get called away to deliver babies so often."[21] Part of his popularity with women stemmed from his promise of a pain-free childbirth, achieved by heavily anesthetizing his patients. One former patient, who had three children delivered by Burt, said Burt "guaranteed" no pain and there was none: "If you had one little cramp, you went to the hospital and woke up the next day or perhaps two days later with your baby." Coney Mitchell went to Burt in 1967 pregnant with her third child. Mitchell, who had recently moved to Dayton, recalled Burt listening to her fears concerning childbirth and promising her it would be pain-free.[22]

A core component of Burt's popularity probably was his reassuring personality and his ability to listen to women like Mitchell ask questions and express their concerns and fears. In an era when many physicians, including other obstetrician gynecologists, often did not listen to their female patients, Burt did. And Burt was aware of this, for even he noted it, saying other doctors labeled women as "neurotic and emotionally unstable" when they complained to physicians of their pain upon intercourse, frequent need to urinate, or other problems after childbirth. Burt recalled hearing about other doctors telling these women that they should "get along better with their husbands; get a hobby; see a psychiatrist."[23] Burt sympathized with women who were hesitant to discuss their problems with doctors because of these responses.

Perversely, Burt seems to have benefited from such frustrations, frustrations articulated by the women's health movement of the 1970s, with paternalistic and condescending doctors. But Burt also manipulated and exploited these frustrations. He listened to their worries and complaints but felt it unnecessary to communicate with them that, when he delivered their child or performed a hysterectomy, he surgically altered their bodies to, in his view, alleviate their complaints, all of which—regardless of what the women may have been saying—he felt were based on sex. Indeed, he noted that he performed love surgery on women without their knowledge in a book he published in the mid-1970s.[24]

Burt maintained that love surgery was "conducted with great concern for the welfare of women," to help the many women "with problems involving vaginal intercourse that are either not being adequately addressed or not being addressed at all" by other doctors.[25] He performed the surgery even on women who gave him no indication that they were experiencing problems with sexual intercourse. By the mid-1970s, he claimed he had been performing love surgery, in one of its variations, on nearly all women for whom he delivered a child, "carried out in the delivery room at the time of episiotomy repair," though it was "actually far more extensive than merely closing the episiotomy repair," he wrote. Burt also added the surgery when he performed other pelvic surgeries, including vaginal hysterectomies.[26]

Because of his belief that the female body was pathologically designed for heterosexual penetrative sex, he felt no need to be particular upon whom he operated. In his view, all women needed love surgery. According to Burt, women were structurally inadequate for penetrative sex, in particular missionary intercourse, and his love surgery corrected this "pathological anatomy of the female coital area."[27]

Surgically Created "Monsters"

Though his obstetric practice was thriving, Burt's passion lay in the surgery he invented. And by the mid-1970s, Burt believed that love surgery had evolved to the point where he was ready to share it with others.[28] He tried multiple times to publish in peer-reviewed medical journals; by his own account his folders overflowed with rejections.[29] After repeated refusals, Burt became disgusted with his peers and took his surgery directly to the public, self-publishing his book, *Surgery of Love*, in 1975.[30] Burt gave copies of the book, cowritten with Joan Burt, to patients, sold it through bookstores, and sent complimentary copies to some physicians.[31]

Surgery of Love included chapters with titles like "There Is No 'Foreplay' in Ecstasy of Living and Loving: Only Orgasmic Loving," "Optimal Sexual Functioning Is Sexual Ecstasy beyond the Wildest Imagination of Most People, but within Reach of All!" and "Love as Most People Have Been Living It with Their Mates Will Ultimately Destroy Their Sexual Ecstasy." In the book, Burt outlined his beliefs on marriage and sexuality, as well as the details of love surgery, but, as these chapter titles reveal, the book was largely about Burt's vision of himself as challenging the sexual status quo. In the authors' biography at the beginning of *Surgery of Love*, the Burts wrote that they "manage the children still at home, two small boys, and their homes in Dayton and Vail" and that their "lives are totally dedicated to each other with their hobbies of travel and skiing and writing secondary always to just being together and pleasuring each other."[32] This sentence summarizes what seem to be James Burt's two core philosophies that permeated his surgical practice and his book. The first was that sex should be central and take precedent over everything else in a couple's life. The second, hinted at here and which I will expand upon shortly, was that women should be submissive to their husbands.

Throughout *Surgery of Love*, Burt decried the "current definition of love as defined by the daily living habits of most people." In his view, people needed to restructure their daily living in order to make sex the center if they wished to reach "the ecstasy of living and loving that is potentially possible for all persons." Indeed, Burt repeatedly wrote that people needed to "disregard previous definitions of the word love" and concentrate on his definition if they wanted to attain sexual ecstasy. To do this, Burt advised couples to constantly engage in "innumerable" opportunities for "caressing and intimate manipulation." When the wife was cooking bacon, for example, the husband could approach her from behind and "through her clothing manipulates her clitoris to the point of climax," something that would only take seconds following her surgical reconstruction through love surgery to "optimal sexual functioning." In Burt's view, "love, physical loving and being loved" should be the focus of "every aspect of daily living."[33]

Throughout the book, Burt emphasized the importance of orgasm to women. "The image of the female that has been pounded into the members of our society," Burt wrote, "is that she properly is an erotic receptacle for the discharge of the sexual tensions biologically accumulated in the male." Burt believed women should experience orgasm too and that orgasm ideally occurred through intercourse, and love surgery transformed women's sexual intercourse experience to one of new orgasmic heights. "Other things being equal," Burt wrote, "the more efficient the stimulation of the clitoris would be by the penis during intercourse, the more would the woman's sexual pleasure be." Following love surgery, Burt claimed women could achieve orgasm "almost instantaneously upon manipulation in any manner of the clitoral area." Orgasm postsurgery could be achieved with the slightest of touches—indeed, a husband could bring his wife to orgasm "with his eyelash on the clitoris with a blink or two." Burt described how his operation increased women's orgasmic ability by citing one of his patients, a woman who had experienced only two orgasms during her life, but following the operation her husband told Burt he had "created a monster!" such was the increase in both her orgasmic ability and her desire for sex.[34]

Though espousing the greater ease for women to reach orgasm as the basis for love surgery, Burt very obviously designed the surgery to provide an even greater benefit to men, as the chapter "How Any Man Can Make His Woman into a Seething Mass of Perpetual Passion for Himself: Your Own Private Sex Pot in Your Own Private World!" explicitly attested. While, Burt noted, it took "much more than even the new redesign operation" for couples to achieve new sexual orgasmic heights, love surgery was a definite beginning. Burt maintained that couples who benefited most from love surgery were ones in which the woman had lost all or part of her orgasmic ability following childbirth. This was because, Burt believed, women were too vaginally loose after childbirth, with some women "large enough to drive a truck through sideways." If women were very elastic postbirth, Burt referred to them as "real clappers," meaning that he could put two hands in their vaginas and clap. Burt altered the female body to respond to his perception that men desired small and tight vaginas. Comparing his work with other controversial ideas later accepted by the medical community, Burt described the "reconstructive operation on the female to provide optimal coital area structure" as his effort to alleviate the complaints of husbands postbirth that intercourse with their wives was like "taking it out in a warm room."[35]

Love surgery made the woman "tight enough to offer her husband adequate physical stimulation during intercourse," he wrote, and with his increased satisfaction came her own, for the "knowledge that she is a more adequate partner for her man" increased a woman's sexual satisfaction.[36] Burt was not alone in this belief that women were sexually stimulated by their partners' sexual stimulation; his echoed others in the 1970s like Lois

Bird, who wrote in *How to Be a Happily Married Mistress* that the wife's world should revolve around her husband and that she should fake orgasms so that he will feel like a good lover.[37] For Burt, the man was the active one in sex, the one responsible for his own and his female partner's orgasm, and love surgery helped a man find and show his virility. He sewed one woman so tightly he commented: "if he can't make her come now, he's a real dud." He advised men, "with their superior physical strength" to submit their wives to multiple climaxes. When a man "lovingly physically forces" a woman to have repeated orgasms, "the intensity becomes so great that the woman 'just can't stand it' or screams 'let me breathe, let me breathe,'" he knows he is a truly loving partner. On multiple occasions in *Surgery of Love*, Burt stressed the importance of a man forcing the woman to have repeated orgasms and not taking no for an answer. Burt described the difference between rape and rapture as "salesmanship." Indeed, according to Burt, it was "imperative" that when a woman reached orgasm a man not stop, but, "using physical strength if necessary, force her to submit to more loving caressing," for "further and further and further repeats of climaxing." According to Burt, if a woman was not already lusting for her mate, love surgery would turn her into a "horny little house mouse who couldn't contain her joy and anticipation at the prospect of being loved all over by the greatest Lothario in the world, the only man worthy of her attentions, her husband." After his operation, Burt stated that it was possible for "any man at any age" to "love his woman to exhaustion," because following the operation "every man can be a stud!"[38]

Much of *Surgery of Love* contained such pornographic overtones, with the male as the active, even dominant and forceful, participant in sex. In the chapter "How Any Man Can Make His Woman a Seething Mass of Perpetual Passion for Himself," Burt told of a couple whose loud sex prompted the neighbors to call the police, as they mistook her screams of passion for screams stemming from violence. Though Burt stressed the importance of female orgasm, he quite often seemed to regard it as important more for its effects on the male ego than for the woman undergoing the surgery. Burt suggested that women develop attitudes of "complete eroticism" involving a "total lack of inhibition in deportment, dress, and undress." He offered women ideas such as opening the door naked when their husbands came home from work or hanging mirrors on the bedroom walls, laying a fur bedspread on the bed, or cooking a meal wearing nothing but high-heels and a see-through apron. He also suggested that "as the husband walks into the house" he should be told "by the children doing the dishes that momma wants to see daddy in the bedroom," and when daddy enters the bedroom he sees his "loved and loving wife groomed in some different and erotic manner lying on the bed or the floor," murmuring that she loves him. This would, of course, prompt the man to "throw himself upon her," resulting in sex for "two hours until she has screamed so loudly and longly for so many countless climaxes that both are at the point of exhaustion."[39] One not only wonders what exactly the children were doing while their parents were having loud sex for two hours but also exactly what the woman's role in the sex acts entailed outside of being continually forced to have orgasms.

Men were to force supine women to have repeated orgasms for hours at a time on a regular, maybe even daily, basis: such is the world of imaginary sex. At one point in the book, Burt described his wife Joan Burt as the only one laughing in a theatre where they were watching a pornographic film because she found the film's implication that women only climaxed once laughable.[40] In *Surgery of Love*, Burt conflated real and imaginary sex during a time when many Americans' ideas about sex were being challenged and perhaps changed, in part because of the increased exposure to imaginary sex.

Following World War II, sexuality became more explicit and pornography became more widely available, moving the objectification of women's bodies and of sexuality from the margins to the mainstream.[41] In 1953, the first issue of *Playboy* was printed, with photos of Marilyn Monroe in the nude. By 1967, *Playboy* had a circulation of five million. However, magazines like *Playboy* through the late 1960s still air-brushed over women's genitals, and pornographic movies remained shy of showing explicit sex. That all changed in 1970 when *Penthouse*, the more risqué upstart challenging *Playboy* in mainstream pornography, began showing genitals in the magazine. *Playboy* followed within months.[42] Soon after, sexually explicit movies like *Deep Throat* and *The Devil in Miss Jones* achieved a sort of respectability, attracting large audiences and becoming cult favorites. During the 1970s, newsstands and adult bookstores sold magazines that would have been confiscated by the police a decade earlier. And the invention and popular embrace of videocassette recorders enabled people to rent and view pornographic movies in the privacy of their homes.[43]

Surgery of Love was written and promoted during a time when sexuality was increasingly woven throughout American culture, with the erotic explored in popular literature, film, and television. Changes in the public perception of the role of sex and sexuality in general also produced changes about the place of sex specifically within marriage. The visibility of sex encouraged exploration of the erotic, and though men still typically initiated sex with their wives, other parts of marital sex in the 1970s differed from that only two decades earlier. Married couples in the 1970s reported being twice as likely to have sex in positions other than missionary and oral sex became part of the sexual repertoire. Sexual frequency increased and fewer women described sex as being of no interest to them. The plethora of sex manuals encouraged couples to explore new ways to make love and spice up their sex lives, and both men and women reported enjoying the kind and amount of sex they experienced within marriage. Though many reported they were happy with their married sex lives, this may also have been because unhappy marriages were more likely to end in divorce than a generation earlier.[44] This new focus on sexual pleasures and liberties, then, also brought new stresses and constraints. As Jessica Weiss noted in her work on marriage and the baby boom, for some "the sexual revolution seemed to threaten marriage from the outside while sexual ignorance and dissatisfaction bore away at it from the inside."[45]

Burt sold the idea of love surgery to women (and their husbands) as a surgical route to achieve these higher sexual standards. As Barbara Demick, the journalist who interviewed Burt in 1978, wrote, "Love surgery has frightening commercial potential, especially if it is packaged without Burt's cloying sexual and social biases." Burt promoted love surgery during the climax of the sexual revolution in the 1970s, and an early critic worried that America was "ready, willing and able" to embrace it, giving Burt a chance to be "successful, even more successful than Billy Graham" with his promise of an easy and instant female orgasm, produced, of course, by the male.[46]

For this was Burt's second core philosophy: women should be submissive. Though he placed great importance on a woman's ability to orgasm as part of the sexual key to a couple's relationship, he never wavered from his underlying belief that men gave women orgasms and that while those orgasms could occur in any position, the best one, the most normal one, was missionary. Burt's opinions concerning women's submissive sexual role were tied to his ideas concerning women's submissive social roles, limited to that of wife and a mother, a narrow view many women were vocally challenging in the 1970s.

Burt, however, very much believed passivity was necessary in a good wife. Though Joan Burt was, according to James Burt in *Surgery of Love*, an "accomplished actress and musician and a sought-after professional in real estate" with great "artistic abilities," in his view, a wife needed to give "exclusive attention in her private life to her husband in every and all ways and focuses attention on his wants, needs, [and] goals." Moreover, a wife faced "her children and the world at large as a member of a loving couple; not as an individual." A good wife, Burt believed, "will never at any time in any way in public or private be *critical or demanding* of her husband." If the husband wanted his wife to gain or lose weight, she should oblige. A good wife would also dress the way her husband wanted or wear makeup if he wanted.[47] Burt's ideas about sex were tied to his ideas about women: both in their social and sexual roles, women were to be supine.

Sex as the central part of existence for a couple and a passive yet sexually desirous wife were enhanced by love surgery and were packaged by Burt as sexual ecstasy. But it was not just sexual ecstasy Burt sold with the love surgery package; it was also the ability for a woman to keep her husband. Burt more than once hinted that women who submitted to their husbands' forceful sex and standards of dress stayed married. According to Burt, "For the woman to be beautiful to the man, she must have his interests and needs and desires as her goal and focus attention thereon rather than making any demands or criticisms of her man." Women who did this, as well as who underwent love surgery, achieved "ecstasy in their living and loving permanently until death do us part."[48] As Burt conceived it, love surgery promoted sexual happiness and thus saved marriages. Burt marketed his surgery during a time when it contained added allure: the hope that the surgery and its promised sexual enhancement would reduce a couple's chances of becoming part of the 50 percent who divorced.[49]

Love Surgery Goes National

Published when Americans were much more publicly focused on sex, *Surgery of Love* brought Burt both local and national attention. In September 1975, a month after the publication of *Surgery of Love*, the *Dayton Daily News* wrote a glowing description of the local doctor and his wife and passed an uncritical look at love surgery. In the article, "Local Doctor Develops Corrective Surgery," Burt stated that side effects from love surgery were minimal, and nearly 100 percent of the women who had undergone the surgery were "ecstatic" with the results. Joan Burt chimed in, saying her husband has "given women the opportunity to enjoy sex," adding that she had never had an orgasm before love surgery.[50]

The book provided Burt and the surgery with increased exposure and in 1976 he began offering it as an elective for $1,500 plus hospitalization costs. The two-hour long surgery required five days in the hospital, at least a week of sitting on an inner tube, and six to eight weeks without sex. According to Burt, two hundred women requested the surgery by 1976.[51] But while *Surgery of Love* drew the doctor lots of attention, he wanted more, and a 1970s US Supreme Court decision enabling physicians to advertise more than their hours and specialty helped him.[52] Burt hired a New York City public relations firm to publicize love surgery, and he was featured favorably in *Playboy* and *Playgirl* and in an appearance on the *Phil Donahue Show*.[53] He spent years as a weekly guest on a local radio talk show as the "love surgeon."[54] The plethora of media appearances by Burt resulted in a large number of inquiries into love surgery. Burt, as journalist Demick wrote in 1978, was a capable surgeon with excellent bedside manners. But to the women who sought him out and who went to him for love surgery, he was more than that: he was an "emotional and sexual cult figure."[55] And, with his national publicity, the women who sought out James Burt were now not just from around Dayton but across the country.[56]

Like with Judy and Bruce, who introduced this chapter, Burt routinely told women and men who came to him requesting the surgery what he was going to do, reportedly showing them before and after love surgery diagrams and photographs. He gave, according to Demick, many of the women, as well as their male partners, their first and perhaps only sex counseling, taking time to show them how female orgasm was achieved and how love surgery would better facilitate that orgasm.[57] But what Burt did not tell women, either those who elected to have love surgery or those upon whom he performed the surgery without informing them, was that it was meant to limit sexual positions to just one: missionary. He also downplayed possible complications from the surgery, saying they were "no more than the standard perineorraphy [repair of the perineum] carried out as described in the surgical textbooks."[58]

Burt maintained that the ideal candidate for love surgery was a heterosexual woman who climaxed easily through clitoral manipulation and who wanted but seldom had an orgasm during penetrative sex.[59] Recall from the last chapter that this, according to national polls conducted in the 1970s, would have been most women. In Shere Hite's 1972 survey, only 30 percent of the women who answered said they regularly had an orgasm from coitus without additional direct clitoral stimulation, 44 percent regularly reached orgasm when manually stimulated and 42 percent when orally stimulated, though some women were hampered from even trying the latter by what one woman called feeling "dirty down there."[60] For many women, reaching orgasm during intercourse was not easy. Yet this common inability to orgasm during missionary position intercourse without, as James Burt described it, "gymnastics," or the man or woman touching the clitoris during intercourse, was called "coital anorgasmia" and considered a sexual dysfunction.[61] Burt then not only agreed with Masters and Johnson when they proved the unique importance of the clitoris to female orgasm, he also agreed with them that women who could not achieve "hands-free" missionary position orgasm were suffering from a sexual dysfunction.[62]

In Burt's view, love surgery relieved women of this dysfunction. In the 1970s, Burt presented his ideas regarding sex and love surgery to at least one professional conference, the International Academy of Sex Research. Following the presentation, Ira Reiss, a professor of sociology who later served as president of the academy, approached Burt and suggested to him a less expensive and invasive method for women to achieve orgasm during sex in the missionary position: a two-inch soft cushion that a man attached to the base of his erect penis with elastic straps. During intercourse, this cushion pressed upon the clitoris, something Reiss suggested to Burt was a "far easier solution than surgery for those women who insisted on hands-off coital orgasm." According to Reiss, Burt seemed surprised by his suggestion and, after a pause, told Reiss that it "might work, but you and I both know that most men would never bother to wear such a contraption."[63]

Though Burt wrote *Surgery of Love* largely for the nonmedical reader and marketed both his book and his surgery to this audience, he was, as his presentation at the convention where Reiss confronted him suggests, also trying to convince his medical peers of love surgery's validity. But lack of demonstrable proof that love surgery increased female orgasm blocked his efforts to publish within medical journals. In his effort to begin a more scientifically valid study of the effects of love surgery, Burt developed a postsurgery questionnaire and began sending the twenty-seven-page form to his patients. In 1977, he attended half a dozen sex-therapy organization meetings, claiming that the first one hundred women who responded to his questionnaire were overwhelmingly pleased with the sexual benefits of love surgery.[64] He also tried to be formally placed on the program of the Eastern Association for Sex Therapists to present his findings but was denied.[65] Burt wrote frequently to Frederick Zuspan, a professor of obstetrics and gynecology at Ohio State University and editor of the *American Journal of Obstetrics and Gynecology*, who rejected his articles.[66] With the exception of the International Academy of Sex Research, apparently every medicine or sex therapy journal or conference turned down the research papers he submitted.[67]

Professional Reaction to Burt

Physicians who knew Burt considered him quite technically competent. According to Walter Reiling, president of the local Montgomery County Medical Society in the late 1970s, Burt was no charlatan; indeed, Reiling said Burt truly "believed he was accomplishing some good with his surgery." But Reiling also recalled that around the time Burt published *Surgery of Love* he "seemed to become obsessed with it."[68] Some nurses and doctors were concerned about his obsession with love surgery, in particular his frequent and indiscriminate practice of it.

Traditionally defined as a supportive profession, nurses were largely bound to the authority of the physician in the 1970s. In 1976, in a famous critique of the role of the nurse within the medical system at a time when the majority of doctors and hospital administrators were male, Jo Ann Ashley pointed out that physicians seldom perceived "nurses as anything other than the women with whom they work and nurses relate to physicians not only as nurse to a physician, but as a female to a male," reflecting the dominant and subordinate roles of men and women in the larger culture.[69] Though in the 1970s some nurses began to challenge their subservient role, on a daily level many nurses rarely advocated for their patients because of their limited influence with doctors or hospital administrators.[70] Moreover, the power disparities between doctors and nurses that enabled doctors to not directly speak with nurses also meant that if a nurse offered criticism or reported on something a doctor was doing she knew to be wrong, she risked losing her job.[71]

But despite these professional limitations and risks, at least a few nurses working at St. Elizabeth Medical Center in the 1970s tried to convince physicians and hospital administrators that what Burt was doing to his patients made them very uncomfortable. They witnessed Burt's patients suffer with postsurgery complications such as difficulty urinating after love surgery: for some patients, the urethra had been moved further into the vagina, resulting in infections.[72] Beatrice Busse worked as a nurse-anesthetist at St. Elizabeth Medical Center in the 1970s. She claimed Burt performed love surgery on every one of his obstetrics patients during that decade and nurses complained that, unless Burt killed someone, it seemed unlikely the hospital would do anything to stop him.[73] Carol Brewer, a nurse at St. Elizabeth's from 1963 to 1974, recalled overhearing another nurse say "if someone were left lying, dying in the gutter, they'd rather be allowed to die peacefully in the gutter than to be butchered to death by Burt or to be saved and rescued by him to live in agony." Brewer worked in the children's section of the hospital, and nurses attending Burt's patients frequently asked her for child-size catheters. The nurses who sought the small devices did so while complaining about how tightly Burt had stitched up his patients.[74]

During interviews and testimonies they gave later on, nurses recalled how they complained to each other and to the director of nursing at St. Elizabeth's in the late 1970s. Many of the nurses, especially the ones in the operating room or who attended to Burt's patients, were appalled.[75] A few nurses went beyond complaining to their peers. Nancy Goodman, who occasionally worked as an obstetrics nurse during her tenure at St. Elizabeth's from 1972 to 1976, protested to E. C. Kuhbander, the chief administrator at the hospital, about Burt. She believed Burt overmedicated his patients and that the surgery he did to repair episiotomies was different enough to warrant a special consent form. But she recalled being told that the hospital could do nothing to stop the doctor. Kuhbander, Goodman later said, informed her that the administration had "spent hours—hundreds of hours" discussing Burt, even bringing the issue of his unorthodox surgery before their attorneys, who informed them that "because of the restraint of trade issue," because Burt did not have privileges at any other local hospital, "he could sue the hospital." According to Goodman, Kuhbander supported and understood her concern, but "he wasn't sure anything could be done."[76]

In 1975, a state law went into effect that required doctors to report to the Ohio State Medical Board colleagues who were practicing medicine below the standard. Many physicians labeled it the "snitch provision."[77] And, according to Kuhbander, the chief administrator for St. Elizabeth's in the late 1970s to whom Goodman complained, a fellow physician needed to "snitch" on Burt for the hospital to do something. Goodman recalled

Kuhbander telling her, "I cannot get one physician in this town to stand up and say to me that what Jim Burt is doing is outside of current medical practice." If just one did so, he told Goodman, then "we could do something."[78]

But while they did not speak out publicly, some of Burt's fellow gynecologists in Dayton were concerned after examining some of Burt's patients. These women's genitals looked entirely different, they reported. The opening of the vagina was smaller and had been moved closer to the clitoris. During intercourse, the labia minora of these women were pulled inside the vagina. The women's genitals "were completely disfigured," one doctor recounted, with "their vaginas looking like funnels." Moreover, some of the reconstructed women had been sewn up so tightly they had to be cut to have intercourse. Another problem, these physicians pointed out, and one that Burt merely hinted at, was that reconstructed women were too small for vaginal childbirth. For a baby to be delivered vaginally, love surgery had to be undone through an extensive episiotomy. The primary concern, however, for many of Burt's peers was Burt's lack of selectivity for love surgery; Burt himself admitted turning down only three women.[79]

Some doctors, like some nurses who knew of Burt's work, tried to do something out of the public view. Barbara Demick, who interviewed Burt in 1978 for the *Real Paper*, also interviewed another local doctor regarding Burt. But though the physician complained to Demick, the doctor refused to be quoted by name. This physician told Demick about how several doctors were appalled when they saw that Burt had scheduled a nineteen-year-old woman, who had only been married for a year and weighed less than one hundred pounds, for love surgery. "It's inconceivable," the doctor told Demick, "that this operation is recommended for women who plan to have babies." Burt, according to the doctor, "has such a manipulative way with women" it was "almost like a seduction." The woman scheduled for surgery, the doctor recalled, was "young, timid, and scared, and she thought—and he made her believe—she was sexually inadequate because she couldn't climax at the *exact* same time as her husband." Like this particular young woman, "women who think they're inadequate are very susceptible," the doctor told Demick. These women were "generally low-to-middle income people," who trusted Burt, who in turn charged them one hundred dollars an hour for consultation. "It's like selling a cancer patient Laetrile," the doctor complained.[80] Laetrile is an alternative, supposedly miraculous, cancer treatment drug banned in the United States, that in 1977 the FDA commissioner stated was not just ineffective as cancer treatment but also highly likely to result in cyanide poisoning. That the physician chose to compare Burt's work with Laetrile is, perhaps, a telling statement on how this doctor felt about the surgery—or at the very least was evocative of the time.[81]

The doctor who spoke on condition of anonymity to Demick was probably one of a group of five gynecologists in Dayton who attempted to work within the medical review system to restrict Burt's ability to practice love surgery. She may have been Donne Holden, a gynecologist who had moved to the area in 1976, who years later was remembered as leading the charge against Burt; in 1989, Holden spoke on record with a national medical journal regarding the Burt affair. As Holden later recalled she became concerned after a young woman who "was Catholic and wanted four or five babies" came to her for another opinion about love surgery. If she had undergone love surgery, Holden questioned her ability to then have a vaginal delivery. The woman told Holden that Burt had told her he could fix her inability to climax at the exact time as her husband through love surgery; Holden convinced her to seek additional opinions from other Dayton gynecologists. After telling her that love surgery "shouldn't have been recommended," Holden was able to convince the young woman to cancel the surgery and write a letter to the medical society and St. Elizabeth's regarding Burt. Holden then gathered letters from the other gynecologists who saw her and sent the young woman's letter along with her own letter to the medical society and the hospital.[82]

Walter Reiling Jr., a physician and then-president of the county medical society, recalled that he had always disapproved of the surgery, as it was unnecessary for health reasons, "but so is breast augmentation." He had assumed "women had requested it."[83] So when Holden and the four gynecologists complained that Burt was perhaps aggressively pushing the surgery, the society decided to examine Burt's practice. As part of their look into Burt, the society asked the dean of the Wright State University School of Medicine in Dayton to review Burt's book, *Surgery of Love*. The dean called the book "poorly written" and "medically unfounded" and further stated that a "rebuttal to the author would only add dignity to its existence."[84]

Burt knew about the society's investigation into his surgery and in an April 1978 letter threatened to sue the society for slander if they formed a policy critical of it.[85] In July 1978, the society labeled love surgery as "undocumented by ordinary standards of scientific reporting" and "not a generally gynecologically accepted procedure," the results of which had not been duplicated by other physicians and which had been described in only "nonscientific literature." The county medical society sent their statement to local hospitals, including St. Elizabeth.[86] The society further published its statement in one of the local newspapers, the *Journal Herald*, on October 22, 1980, a little more than two years later. And Richard Tapia, the society's executive director, later claimed he had engaged in discussions regarding Burt at least three times with an Ohio State Medical Board investigator in the early 1980s, with no response.[87] Though the county medical society claimed it told them about Burt and its conclusions, the state board later stated it had no record of their complaint.[88]

Part of the reason Dayton doctors were hesitant to confront Burt may have been economic. Doctors were afraid of legal retaliation from Burt directly or through his patients. And their fears were well founded, for Burt was a litigious fellow. In addition to his 1978 threat to sue the Montgomery County Medical Society, at Burt's urging, perhaps two women during the late 1970s sued other gynecologists for undoing their love surgeries.[89] One of these women, local gynecologists told each other, wanted the surgery removed, but her husband did not and, with Burt's encouragement, he sued the doctor. "It's almost pathological," one doctor complained to journalist Barbara Demick in 1978. "He's always been a Johnny-out-of-step, so he attacks other professionals—he just says we're the ones who are wrong. He's just a menace here. And he's a slick and shrewd person with a very powerful full-time attorney."[90]

Fear of lawsuits kept many quiet. Nevertheless, years later, Donne Holden defended the actions she and her peers took against Burt. "What were we supposed to do, tell the board that Dr. Burt had suggested something to patients we disagreed with?" During an interview in 1989, Holden remembered that in the late 1970s the licensing board was largely toothless, so she and the other doctors worked behind the scenes to limit Burt's ability to operate, keeping him from obtaining full privileges at area hospitals. "That was very aggressive for the time," Holden stated.[91]

In 1978, Burt became so involved with promoting and performing love surgery that he essentially halted his obstetrics practice.[92] The negative reaction to love surgery by his medical peers disappointed him and made him even more preoccupied about proving the validity of his surgery. Indeed, Barbara Demick, the journalist who interviewed him in 1978, called him a touch paranoid in his perception of how others saw him.[93] His paranoia was no doubt fueled by the negative publicity he started receiving. Just when Burt's self-generated promotion had started making him and his surgery better known, some not so flattering stories had begun to appear. In April 1978, the national medical magazine *Medical World News* interviewed Burt, described his surgery and his various attempts to convince sex therapists of its legitimacy, and provided as much space to those speaking out against the surgery as to Burt's attempts to justify it. Interviewed by the magazine at the Eastern Association for Sex Therapy meeting in New York City, which had for the second year in a row denied him a place on the program, Burt acknowledged, hesitatingly, that most sex therapists were not impressed by the surgery. But, he said, this was because "pelvic surgeons rarely think about sexual function, and sex therapists don't think of surgery for women at all."[94]

None of Burt's patients were interviewed for the article, but several non-Dayton sex therapists and physicians were, and they were unanimous in their thoughts on Burt. Diane Fordney, a sex therapist and associate professor of obstetrics at the State University of New York at Stony Brook, called Burt a "nice person" but said "he is a zealot, and that makes him dangerous." Moreover, from a philosophical view, Fordney called the suggestion that a woman rearrange her genitals to meet a "male-induced and-desired goal" a "sexist, woman-reducing process." Selig Neubardt, an assistant clinical professor of obstetrics and gynecology at Albert Einstein College of Medicine in New York, essentially agreed, saying, "Dr. Burt wants to build everyone a vagina to please himself." The operation, Neubardt concluded, was "lousy," but if it or any other surgery was presented honestly and openly and "a woman chooses it anyway, then it is okay." Though the *Medical World News* contacted the Montgomery County Medical Society in Dayton for a local view of the city's love doctor, the president of the society declined to comment.[95]

Illustrating the Benefits of Love Surgery

Presumably still stinging from the *Medical World News* article, later that year Burt agreed to the interview with Barbara Demick from the *Real Paper*, though he was at first hesitant because of "the distortionist drivel that's come out from people who haven't talked to the patients and who have refused my research paper." Demick asked Burt whether he felt discouraged by the poor reception love surgery had received from sex therapists and other physicians. Burt told Demick he was not discouraged, he was "disgusted." He continued, saying he "expected scientifically minded people to be scientifically and intellectually honest." He accused sex therapists of demanding more "proof of my surgery than for any of their own work because they are afraid I'll take their $100-an-hour counseling fees away."[96] Indeed, Burt believed that the underlying reason other physicians and sex therapists rejected his surgery was because of their fear that the surgery would take away clients. Few couples, he stated, "could afford the expense" of "direct personal consultation with professional therapists."[97] Since sex was the basis of all marital problems, according to Burt, couples should spend their money on surgically altering the woman, a much more cost-effective approach.

To Demick, it was clear Burt considered himself more than just a good surgeon. There was, she wrote, "a Grand Concept behind all this—and it is no less presumptuous than the surgery itself." For, as Burt saw it, he was simplifying the problem of treating sexual malfunction by surgically correcting what he believed were physiological problems. Not that the mind was unimportant, he told Demick, "but it's like trying to win a race with a lousy car no matter how good a driver you are." As he explained, good sex treatment was physical and psychological and love surgery provided both. As Burt explained to Demick, after the surgery the women underwent a "dramatic attitude change." They were, he said, more positive and "nicer to their husbands." One can, he attested, see the benefits of the surgery "when the women come back into the office after their surgery—in their faces, in their dress, in their posture and bearing, in their lack of bitchiness. . . . They have a much greater ability to look at the roses instead of the thorns."[98]

In addition to Judy, whose story began this chapter, Demick interviewed seven other women who elected to have love surgery and were happy with the results. Another patient, Pat, reiterated Judy's enthusiasm for the surgery, and for the doctor who invented it, saying, "I've never had a doctor as kind." Before going to Burt, sex had been painful, but the other doctors she went to kept telling her it was all in her head. Then she went to Burt. Her appointment with him was at two in the afternoon; two hours later she was in surgery. Before love surgery, she told Demick, "all I was good for was pleasing my husband, I felt like I wasn't a woman. But since, my life has just gotten better. If another woman can do it [climax] once in five minutes, I can do it twice."[99]

Like Judy and Pat, twenty-year-old Kathy was self-conscious during her interview. Demick spoke with Kathy alongside Jim, her forty-one-year-old live-in boyfriend and father of her one-year-old child. "Sex felt good," she told Demick, but she reached orgasm only once in a while, and often she faked it. Her lack of orgasm fed into her insecurity. Jim's mother suggested they see her physician, and, after meeting Burt and discussing the surgery, Jim paid for Kathy to have it. "It cost me 1,500 dollars," Jim told Demick. "I could have bought me a car for that, but why shouldn't I spend it on her cause I enjoy her a lot more." Jim further told Demick that after the surgery Kathy was "much firmer and our bodies are much closer together during sex." Now he no longer had to worry about foreplay "or even try for her to enjoy herself." A man, he said, "feels like he ain't much of a man, like she might be seeing other men. Now, why would she when she's getting satisfied at home?" Love surgery was, he said, "one of the greatest things I've ever seen for saving a relationship."[100]

Demick interviewed four more of Burt's happy patients. Dolores told Demick she no longer popped Valium all day. Dolores's boyfriend added that her "vagina feels like a velvet glove." Minnie, the only African American woman interviewed, said that sex had been painful and that love surgery probably saved her marriage. Beverly, a nurse in her midthirties, underwent love surgery because she wanted to climax "without a whole lot of fooling around." But the patient who most impressed Demick was nearly twice Beverly's age. Ernestine was sixty-two, a retired second-grade school teacher from a suburb of Dayton. With jet-black hair and wearing a "chic pale green silk, she is a striking figure," Demick wrote, whose "self-assured comments" lacked the "traumatic overtones" of the other women. Before having love surgery, Ernestine had been married for forty years and had experienced her last orgasm in 1942, the year she gave birth to her first child. After reading about love surgery in the local newspaper, she decided to have it. Now, she told Demick, she and her husband "are as happy as two bugs in a rug. We enjoy our sex life more than when we were newlyweds." Ernestine echoed Burt, saying that after the surgery, a woman "feels like a better person, she's nicer to people. . . . And my husband's much nicer to me." Since the surgery, her husband had given her three mink coats and a new Monte Carlo, even though she admitted she did not have a driver's license.[101]

All eight of the women were glowing in their praise for Burt and love surgery. Not one consulted with another doctor about love surgery before undergoing it; indeed, they largely felt other doctors had abused them and that Burt was the first one to take them seriously. Nor had any of the women or their partners sought sex counseling, and none of the women even hinted to Demick that the person in the relationship with the sexual "problem" might have been the man. Demick further noted that nearly all of the women had married young, with little knowledge or experience about sex before marriage, and, with the exception of Ernestine, they all had experienced either marital or sexual traumas in their lives. But they were all absolutely convinced that surgery had saved their relationships and believed love surgery necessary, regardless of price—especially compelling to Demick, since she noted none of the women were rich. "Whether or not Burt's love surgery has physiological merit, there is more than enough to indicate a potent placebo effect," she concluded.[102] The women Demick interviewed espoused exactly the benefits from the surgery Burt had in *Surgery of Love*: greater marital happiness, even marital salvation. But the women were also championing the other benefit of love surgery Burt had expressed in his book: female submissiveness.

In the years after the publication of *Surgery of Love*, however, Burt began marketing love surgery as female sexual empowerment, and for this his wife was very important. Burt promoted Joan Burt as a successful love surgery recipient, saying that Joan, who claimed to never have had an orgasm prior to love surgery, following the surgery had "climaxed in elevators from the Southampton Princess in Bermuda to the Kuilima in Hawaii more than many women do in their entire lives."[103]

Joan Burt's appearance further promoted the benefits of love surgery: she was young, in her early thirties, with platinum blonde hair. Demick described her as "a bubbling, colorful figure, richly garbed with diamonds and flouncing ruffles." To further market the positive effects of love surgery to women outside of her husband's practice, Joan Burt joined the local chapter of the National Organization for Women, declaring love surgery a feminist option. "If women can indeed be made the sexual equals of men, why shouldn't they have that choice?" she asked Demick. Using this reasoning, Joan Burt and a lawyer went to the Ohio Civil Rights Commission to attempt to force insurance companies to pay for love surgery. Companies such as Blue Cross–Blue Shield paid for the hospital portion of the bill for love surgery but were less consistent in their payment of Burt. "They pay in full for impotent men to get silicone implants," argued Joan Burt, "so why not do the same for women?" As she told Barbara Demick, "we have to stop treating the penis as a special sex symbol."[104]

Clitoral Mutilation, American Style

Though Joan Burt argued for love surgery as a woman's sexual right, many feminists disagreed. In June 1978, the Boston Women's Health Book Collective, the authors of the important feminist health book *Our Bodies, Ourselves*, sent copies of the *Medical World News* article on Burt to 250 women's health organizations across the United States as part of their monthly mailing. Along with the article, the collective enclosed a letter, saying they were "appalled by the vaginal and clitoral mutilation recommended by Dr. James C. Burt." To suggest, the letter continued, "that women need vaginal surgery because they do not have orgasm with each penile-vaginal intercourse is to inflict upon women male fantasies and assumptions about female sexuality." The collective urged "all medical professionals and their organizations to take a stand condemning this practice and to bring pressure on Dr. Burt to stop performing this surgery." Additionally, the Women's Community Health Center in Cambridge, Massachusetts, also sent letters to women's health centers in an effort to end love surgery.[105] The center in Cambridge, a feminist self-help health collective founded in 1974, had recently begun extending their work from well-woman gynecological care and education to working more actively with other Boston health groups as well as national groups, focusing on issues within the women's movement.[106] This was apparently one of the issues they considered within their growing spectrum of concerns, and their action was especially noteworthy since in 1978 the collective was battling a lack of funding, state licensing regulations, and antiabortion publicity.[107]

Other activists also criticized Burt and his surgery. Carol Downer, one of the founders of the women's self-help gynecology movement, noted in 1980 "some therapists refer women for female circumcision (clitoridotomy) to have their clitoral hoods removed so that they can be more sensitive to the thrusts of the penis." Though this statement implies more than one physician was practicing female circumcision, which was the case, Downer explicitly called attention to "one gynecologist, James Burt of Dayton, Ohio," for his development of "a two-hour operation for surgically redesigning the vagina, referred to as the 'reborn Burt vagina.'"[108]

Similar warnings about Burt appeared in feminist health texts as well, such as the 1980 *Women in the Health System*.[109] Additionally, feminist publications criticized Burt and his surgery. In the July 31, 1978, issue of *off our backs*, under the title "Vaginal Mutilation American Style," author Tacie Dejanikus referred to the Dayton, Ohio, gynecologist "Dr. Burton [*sic*]," calling his surgery "one of the latest and grossest practices in a long line of tampering with women's bodies." Burt claimed, Dejanikus wrote, that the surgery "made the clitoris more accessible to direct penile stimulation so that a woman can have more frequent and intense orgasms in intercourse." It was not even known, however, noted Dejanikus, "if the surgery is effective even if it weren't unnecessary mutilation."[110] Two months later, in the October 1978 issue, the *National NOW Times* also briefly drew attention to Burt and his surgery, again quoting the information in the *off our backs* article on his belief that his surgery enabled women to have more and better orgasms.[111]

While in 1978 feminist health activists in Boston were disavowing the merits of love surgery and articles questioning Burt appeared in feminist publications from Denver to Rochester, the Dayton-area NOW Chapter and the Dayton Women's Center expressed concern yet were not active in opposing Burt or his love surgery. During the 1970s, Dayton had a fairly robust feminist network.[112] Though some women were quite active in these groups, small membership numbers, declining activism by the late 1970s, and personal and ideological conflicts beset them; by 1980, the Women's Center and the local chapter of NOW had both folded.[113] Thus, these groups were perhaps unable to do much more in 1978 than to monitor Burt.

National women's health activists were a core mobilization group against Burt, as exemplified by Downer and the two Boston-area groups, and some in the growing feminist antipornography movement joined them. While feminists in the late 1960s and early 1970s challenged the limited roles of women socially, by the mid-1970s, some began to challenge the limited roles of women in the media as well, with particular focus on images conflating female sexuality and violence. As scholar Carolyn Bronstein noted in her examination of the feminist antipornography movement in the United States, these activists "connected their insights about real-world media effects to a new body of radical feminist theory that revealed heterosexuality as an institution and ideology that created and maintained male supremacy."[114] Historian Christine Stansell argued that though women's liberation largely slowed as a movement alongside the end of the New Left in the 1970s, feminism spread. Women's liberation morphed into body politics, and, like the movement for abortion rights, reached across generations. Following the publication in 1975 of Susan Brownmiller's *Against Our Will*, which argued that rape was enmeshed with normal male behavior, many women began calling for an overhaul of rape laws and a reexamination of ideas about rape in society. The antipornography movement emerged from this furor. As legal scholar and antipornography activist Catherine MacKinnon stressed, "Pornography is the theory, rape is the practice." With antifeminism on the rise, it became more culturally and politically palatable to establish a rape crisis center or hotline, both of which maintained women as vulnerable to male violence, than to confront structures of inequality, as the earlier women's liberation movement had done.[115]

Historian Jane Gerhard noted many women became frustrated with the sexual revolution that seemed to limit them to passivity or *Playboy* bunnies.[116] In addition, both a realization of male violence against women and the rapid growth of the commercial sex industry in the 1970s brought a focus, alongside the critique of heterosexuality, on pornography, according to Bronstein.[117] As antipornography activist Beverly LaBelle noted in the late 1970s, though some women began mobilizing against pornography earlier, it was the 1976 film *Snuff* that set a larger feminist antipornography movement into action.[118] Two years after the release of the film, which earned notoriety for the supposedly actual violent murder of a woman as part of the culmination of a man's orgasm, more than five thousand women from across the country traveled to San Francisco for a conference, "Feminist Perspectives on Pornography," organized by Women against Violence in Pornography and Media.[119] After 1978, Women against Pornography groups spread across the country.[120] As antipornography activist Laura Lederer wrote in the introduction to the 1980 book *Take Back the Night: Women on Pornography*, "Pornography is the ideology of a culture which promotes and condones rape, woman-battering, and other crimes of violence against women."[121]

According to Bronstein, though the original antipornography movement was concerned with a spectrum of media depictions of sexual violence against women, by the late 1970s much of the movement became focused upon such images just within pornography.[122] The idea of sexual violence, however, was extended publicly by at least two activists to love surgery as a violent creation of a sexual woman. In 1979, at the Women against Pornography conference in New York City, activist Janice Raymond spoke out against Burt in her speech, "The Medical Creation of the Pornographic Woman."[123] That same year, in a speech she gave in Denver, Robin Morgan also criticized Burt, though she placed him in California. As Morgan told those assembled at the National Conference on Violence against Women in early October 1979:

> Anyone here hear of love surgery? Well, moving right along in the category of 'If-the-shoe-doesn't-fit-then-change-the-foot' category: Rather than change male attitudes toward women . . . a California gynecologist—male—has come up with a wonderful solution. Noting that 70 to 80 percent of American women are pre-orgasmic, as we would call them, or as they would call them, frigid; because American men seem to refuse to understand the basic clitoral anatomy, this particular doctor has decided that rather than going to the trouble of teaching men how to be halfway, decent, courteous lovers—which might begin with even locating the clitoris—that what you do is simply move the

clitoris [*sic*]. I'm quite serious. Since most men are, according to his research into sexual practices, interested in penile insertion into the vagina, then what you do is simply move the clitoris down nearer to the vagina. Then there might actually be some clitoral stimulation. Now this goes so much into the atrocity area, beyond even plastic surgery, enforced beauty standards, silicone breast transplants.[124]

For Morgan and Raymond, love surgery was a surgical sexually violent act on the female body, a means by which a male doctor transformed the female body into an instrument for male sexual pleasure.

Falling Out of Love

Between the late 1970s and the late 1980s, a number of people—former patients, nurses who worked alongside James Burt in the operating room, gynecologists in Dayton, the Montgomery County Medical Society, and the hospital where he most often operated, St. Elizabeth Medical Center—all to a certain extent either tried to end Burt's practice of love surgery or to at least restrict his ability to practice it. The hospital, for example, began insisting in 1979 that Burt use a special consent form to be signed by women before they underwent "female coital area reconstruction." The form called the surgery "not documented," "not a generally accepted procedure," one that was "as yet not duplicated by other investigators" and considered "an unproven, non-standard practice of gynecology."[125] Despite being considered by other physicians as outside the standard of medical care, Burt's practice of love surgery seemed impervious to lawsuits. Though malpractice suits in general rose dramatically in the 1970s, they remained uncommon, so perhaps it is not surprising that between 1976 and 1986 only nine women sued Burt for malpractice.[126] None of the suits went to trial.[127] Indeed, though many of Burt's patients experienced problems following surgery, including urinary incontinence, urinary tract, vaginal, and bladder infections, chronic yeast infections, and pain during, or even inability to have, intercourse because of a near-closure of the vaginal entrance, a successful lawsuit did not go forward against him until the late 1980s.

The woman who brought that suit was Janet Phillips. Phillips first went to Burt in early 1981 for relief of her painful cramps, excessive bleeding, and back pain when she menstruated.[128] All of this concerned her enough to seek medical attention, and Phillips chose Burt because he had hours after she was off work and his office was close to her home.[129] In August 1981, Burt's case notes stated he discussed performing both a hysterectomy and love surgery with Phillips, and that she seemed interested in the latter.[130] Phillips would later dispute this claim, recalling that she did not discuss, let alone consent to, anything other than a total hysterectomy, though she did sign and date all of the consent forms, including the special one required by St. Elizabeth Medical Center for love surgery.[131] Phillips was in the hospital for eleven days following her surgery and in so much pain she could not get out of bed.[132] Even after she left the hospital, she remained in pain and ceased to be able to control her bladder; she was not even aware she needed to urinate and sometimes urinated down her leg. She battled infections for a year. When she asked Burt, he told her she needed more time to heal. A year after her surgery, she recalled still feeling rawness in her vagina and external genitals, including her clitoris and called sex painful; even wearing clothes caused her pain.[133]

Though Burt and Phillips disagreed on much of her case, they both agreed she stopped seeing him in 1984. But Burt had scared Phillips by telling her another physician might hurt her if he tried to examine her, so she did not seek another physician's advice right away.[134] In December 1985, Phillips finally sought another physician's attention because of her chronic urinary stress incontinence.[135] It was after this examination that Janet Phillips first learned the extent of her surgery: she had been circumcised, with a good deal of scar tissue in the clitoral area, her labia had been removed, and her urine was collecting in a little pouch that resulted from the operation. The physician also told Phillips her vagina had been redirected.[136] To better help her understand what had been done to her, he drew pictures of typical female genitals and then contrasted them with her genitals.[137]

Soon after, Phillips sought legal advice, hiring a local attorney, Mary Lee Sambol. On April 4, 1986, she filed a malpractice suit against James Burt.[138] Though Phillips was the first malpractice case against Burt that Sambol took, other former patients now approached her and she took several more on as clients.[139] But Sambol also began going public against Burt in other ways; according to Sambol, she complained to the AMA, the Montgomery County Medical Society, the *Dayton Daily News*, and to St. Elizabeth.[140]

Phillips's case finally went to trial in 1991.[141] It was not Phillips's lawsuit, however, which ultimately forced the end of Burt's practice of love surgery. Rather, it was one of Sambol's letters that resulted in a CBS television report that aired on Saturday, October 29, 1988. Burt issued a statement the day before the show stating that the claim he had "performed experimental surgery for 22 years without patients' consent and authorization" was "totally false and untrue." St. Elizabeth Medical Center, which was also negatively portrayed, issued in their statement that "the procedure, though controversial, is a combination of medically accepted procedures."[142]

Both Burt and several of the women suing him appeared on the CBS show, *West 57th*, with the women appearing as angry, depressed, but compelling victims, and Burt portrayed as a vile manipulator. Though reporter

Karen Burnes interviewed Burt as well as the women, she quite obviously appeared more sympathetic toward the four women, among them Janet Phillips, and their stories of not being asked or told about love surgery and the complications of the surgery with which they now lived.[143]

Burnes introduced the program as an "extremely disturbing and, in some cases, shocking" story about "a group of women, a doctor and a hospital." This introduction was followed by all four women briefly condemning Burt and stating how they felt they had been, as Phillips said, Burt's "guinea pig[s]." After this introduction, Burnes's voice-over then followed Burt as he went into his clinic, stating "twenty-two years ago, he began to surgically alter the anatomy of women." Burnes continued, telling her viewers that

> Burt has spent these last years trying to perfect his technique while women were asleep under anesthesia. He does this, he says, to make women "better sex partners," and he's called it "love surgery." But some women call him a butcher. Dr. Burt has been sued repeatedly for performing an operation that no other doctor has ever done. He remains in practice for reasons which we will explain, and he remains convinced that women are born with their sexual organs in the wrong place.

With that as her setup, Burnes was then seen sitting with Burt and Burt agreeing that he considered himself a pioneer. The show, with rapid cuts in topic and in who was being interviewed, then turned to Burnes speaking with Bradley Busacco, a gynecologist in Cincinnati, who had seen some of Burt's former patients. Busacco told Burnes, "I hate to use the term 'Frankenstein,' but it's almost like we're creating a new anatomy here, and in order to do that, some are falling by the wayside." Burnes, in a voice-over, told the audience that some of Burt's former patients sought out Busacco when doctors in Dayton refused to treat them and that Busacco had never seen a comparable surgery, nor could he find any medical benefit for it. According to Burnes, "when he spoke off-camera, Dr. Busacco expressed horror and outrage. Before he appeared on-camera, the doctors in his community told him to keep quiet. He agreed to talk to us despite that, and despite his fear of legal repercussions."[144]

When Burnes next challenged Burt about the specifics of his surgery, she gave little room for him to speak. Burnes, asking why he circumcised women, challenged Burt by telling him female circumcision was a "procedure that in Africa is considered punishment." Burt disagreed. Burnes, however, interrupted Burt to say, "Sorry, it's considered a form of punishment to women in Africa." Following this tense exchange, Busacco then told viewers that while perhaps removing the clitoral foreskin would make a woman more sensitive, this may not be desirable. Phillips reiterated this point, by saying "the hood that he cuts off from over the clitoris is there for a reason, for protection.

And it's easier for me to understand how important that is because now mine is exposed. And to wear jeans, if you get bumped there, if you're—during sex, foreplay—if you're touched rough, it is very painful." Cheryl Sexton added that when she got the bill for circumcision, she thought, "Heaven's, this is—I've gotten a man's bill." Sexton further told Burnes that she felt as though Burt had "just taken everything from me."[145]

What happened to these four women, as the introduction noted, could "happen to anyone," a theme brought forward again at the conclusion of the show. Burnes asked Busacco whether the women who went to Burt were naïve. He responded that they were to some degree "but no more than most patients who come in the office." An unscrupulous physician "could take advantage of the majority of patients who walk into your office." The *West 57th* segment ended with a voice-over from Burnes, who told her audience, "Dr. James Burt continues to practice, and the system continues to let him. He believes he has made a contribution to mankind, and that one day history will vindicate him. No matter what, he says, he'll fight to keep his work alive."[146]

Despite this declaration by Burt, the television show accomplished what Dayton gynecologists, nurses, and patients had been unable to do: prompt the only entity with the power to take away Burt's license into action. On Thursday, December 8, 1988, the Ohio State Medical Board sent Burt a letter notifying him that the board "intends to determine whether or not to limit, revoke, suspend, refuse to register or reinstate your certificate to practice medicine" based on his performing surgery that "was actually far more extensive than merely closing the episiotomy" on women and that he performed this surgery without their informed consent. The board issued forty-one violations against Burt, charging him with offenses such as gross immorality, overprescribing pain killers, and performing unnecessary surgery without informed consent. While five of the violations regarded his practice of love surgery in general, thirty-six of the violations referred to individual, though unnamed, patients. Many of the cases dated from the 1970s, though there were a number from the 1980s. The board called Burt's surgeries "unproven" and "not scientifically validated with respect to safety and efficacy, and were thus experimental or investigational."[147]

Burt did not wait to see what the board's actions would be regarding his ability to practice. On January 12, 1989, he closed his medical practice.[148] Later that month, he voluntarily gave up his license, effective immediately and enforceable throughout the United States.[149] Burt's attorney, Earl Moore, told the local newspaper that by avoiding the hearing, his client would not have to produce evidence and testimony which would then become public information and thus available to former patients suing him.[150] But, even as he surrendered his license, Burt admitted no wrongdoing and defended love surgery.[151] Far from admitting guilt, two days after he surrendered his license, Burt announced he would stay in Dayton and promote love surgery, saying he would teach other doctors who wanted to learn and would now spend his time writing for medical journals about the surgery. Through his attorney, Burt contended he had received teaching offers, though Moore declined to name the schools.[152] Though I am unsure whether Burt taught any other physician how to perform love surgery, some of his former patients succeeded in their lawsuits against him. While they never received financial remuneration from him, many ultimately did from St. Elizabeth Medical Center.[153]

Conclusion

Genital Geographies

When most Americans hear the term "female circumcision," they typically do not place its practice in the context of the United States, nor do they label it a medical procedure. Despite the long history of various clitoral surgeries, the notoriety of James Burt, and the contemporary use of female circumcision in the United States, probably most Americans, upon hearing the term, envision the practice generically as African. This is most likely because, in this country, by far the most popular attention on the procedures labeled under the term female circumcision have been in an African context. Though published accounts in the medical literature of female circumcision as practiced on the African continent had occurred decades prior, and while activists like Fran Hosken in the 1970s worked to bring the issue of female circumcision—what she described as misogynistic mutilation—forward, it was not until the early 1990s when the issue aroused a good deal of public attention in the United States.[1]

During the 1990s, A. M. Rosenthal covered the topic extensively in the *New York Times*, writing numerous opinion pieces about "female genital torture" as practiced in certain African countries and within certain immigrant communities in the United States.[2] Additional articles appeared during this decade in the American lay and medical press decrying the procedures as practiced both abroad and domestically by immigrants, labeling them as human rights violations.[3] A particular loud voice was that of the novelist Alice Walker, who researched female circumcision for her 1992 novel, *Possessing the Secret of Joy*.[4] In 1993 she, together with filmmaker Pratibha Parmar, produced a book and a movie documenting their view of female circumcision in Africa, *Warrior Marks: Female Genital Mutilation and the Sexual Blinding of Women*. In this book, Walker wrote about her surprise to discover that "women are often blamed for their own sexual mutilation." Their genitals were seen as "unclean" and "monstrous" unless they were circumcised. "The activity of the unmutilated female vulva frightens men and . . . the clitoris challenges male authority." It must, Walker wrote, be "destroyed."[5]

Walker and others argued to stop using the term "female circumcision," as they believed it was unclear and not encompassing the extent of the various procedures and to instead use "female genital mutilation." Spurred on by such reports and activism, Representative Patricia Schroeder introduced legislation in the US Congress outlawing female genital mutilation in America. Her legislation passed in October 1996. In addition to making the practice illegal, with the possibility of up to five years in prison for someone convicted of performing circumcision on a girl under eighteen, Congress also directed federal authorities to tell new immigrant parents from countries where circumcision was commonly practiced that they, too, could face prison if they arranged circumcision for their daughters.[6]

Though Walker's and similar critiques did not go unchallenged—one reviewer of Walker and Parmar's film, for example, called it "problematic" and lacking in an understanding of the cultural context of the practices— here I want to again stress that the concern with female circumcision or female genital mutilation raised by Rosenthal, Walker, and others largely focused on the practices as African, or, put another way, as distinctly not American practices, even when they occurred in America.[7] While at times those who argued against the practices in their African context referred to the procedures in an American or European context as well, the references were largely cursory—a few paragraphs at most pointing out that, historically, these procedures were not isolated to Africa. To illustrate, in their classic *Ms.* article from 1980, Robin Morgan and Gloria Steinem listed occurrences of female circumcision and clitoridectomy in the United States as well as in England. After describing some of the practices next to a photo of a seven-year old African girl who, the caption noted, had just been circumcised, they stated that for readers who were just learning about this custom "it is vital that we immediately recognize the connection between these patriarchal practices and our own." Morgan and Steinem then described how "Western 19th-century medical texts also proclaim surgical mutilation as accepted treatment for 'nymphomania,' 'hysteria,' 'masturbation,' and other nonconforming behavior."[8] With these short ruminations about the historical practice of using female circumcision and clitoridectomy to treat certain conditions within an American and European context, Morgan and Steinem and others tried to make a transcultural link between the practices, but they largely failed to do so because they focused on the practices as limited to a moment in history—typically that of the (seemingly sexually repressed) late nineteenth-century Victorian era. The historical moment was framed as barbaric in its treatment of women, but a barbarism the West had overcome, the implication being that those in Africa who continued these practices had not.

While there is no evidence the four surgeries that have over the years been grouped under the names female circumcision and clitoridectomy occurred on the same scale in the United States as they did and still do in parts of Africa and the Middle East, I am also uncertain how commonly they were performed in America. Because of the relative ease in performing these procedures, they were often accomplished in a physician's office in a short amount of time: they were quick procedures that provided women and girls in the United States a surgical method for sexual acceptability. Some critics of female circumcision as it occurs in parts of Africa and the Middle East stress that the practices are wrong because the intention is to control female sexual behavior: specifically, they charge, to make girls and women more eligible for marriage by making them less interested in sex and thus less likely to have sex before marriage or to betray their spouses once married. This control of female sexuality was the link others, like Morgan and Steinem, attempted to make between the practices in the United States and Africa but failed to do so because the American and European context they used was confined to a short and specific moment in the past. By looking at the long and continued use of female circumcision and clitoridectomy in the United States since the mid-nineteenth century, one can more easily see that these procedures were used in their American context to control the sexual behavior of women and girls. American physicians practiced—and some families and women sought—female circumcision and clitoridectomy to direct sexual behavior to that which was culturally regarded as a correct level or direction of sexual response or desire. So although I am uncertain how many women and girls lost all or part of their clitoris in the United States, what I am certain of is that clitoridectomy and female circumcision were used to direct their sexual behavior.

The practice of female circumcision (as well as cutting on other parts of the female genitalia) to "improve" female anatomy for increased orgasm potential did not end when James Burt gave up his medical license in 1989; as I noted at the beginning of this book, many believe the number of women seeking female genital cosmetic surgeries, which include clitoral unhooding, are on the rise. Not everyone following this trend is pleased. In addition to questioning the medical, physiological, and cultural advisability of surgeries labeled as female genital cosmetic surgeries, others have questioned why this set of genital procedures are legally and more culturally acceptable in the United States (and European countries) while another set, labeled as female genital mutilation or female genital cutting, are not.[9] While the federal law passed in 1996 prohibits female circumcision only for those under eighteen, more than a dozen states have their own laws forbidding these so-called cultural procedures, with several states explicitly forbidding any female, regardless of age, from undergoing them. The federal law, however, does not disallow all genital cutting; rather it allows genital cutting for reasons of health.[10] But, as traced in this book, surgical interventions on the clitoris have long been made in the name of health.

Though the federal law banning the practice of female circumcision in the United States passed nearly two decades ago, whether physicians can—or should—perform procedures regarded as cultural and often labeled in this country as female genital mutilation remains a highly charged issue in the United States. In 2010, when the American Academy of Pediatrics updated its 1998 statement regarding female genital mutilation, its authors added a provision at the end suggesting a "ritual clitoral nick," a procedure described as "not physically harmful," could be offered by physicians practicing in immigrant communities as a "compromise" that could build trust, "save some girls from undergoing disfiguring and life-threatening procedures in their native countries, and play a role in the eventual eradication of FGC [female genital cutting]."[11] Harborview Medical Center in Seattle had offered a similar superficial nick in 1996. Home to an increasing population of people from Somalia, the hospital came up with what they considered a procedure their physicians could perform—a small cut in the clitoral prepuce—and that they hoped would be acceptable to parents requesting their daughter be cut.[12] Fourteen years later, when the American Academy of Pediatricians suggested a similar option for pediatricians, the reaction was again quick, strong, and negative; one of the many e-letters that appeared in 2010 on the website for *Pediatrics* summarized the sentiment of many: "Are you out of your mind?"[13] The academy quickly backed away from the clitoral nick, stating that the organization "reaffirms its strong opposition to FGC and counsels its members not to perform such procedures." In its revocation of the clitoral nick, the academy stated that it did not "endorse the practice of offering a 'clitoral nick,'" something the retraction noted was "forbidden under federal law."[14]

But are there differences—essential differences, ones that go beyond the age of the person being cut—between so-called female genital mutilation or cutting and so-called female genital cosmetic surgeries, including clitoral unhooding? Whenever I have talked about my work on the history of the various medical procedures that fall under the heading of female circumcision and clitoridectomy, I am always asked some sort of variation of this question. Americans believe the practices somehow cannot be equivalent. I spent a quarter at Northwestern University in a seminar with a dozen engaged undergraduate students grappling with this idea of difference. How does race and geography play into the perceived (or perhaps hoped-for) difference? How do ideas of legitimacy—medical versus cultural—factor into this difference? How do ideas about gender roles, conceptions about "appropriate" and "deviant" female sexual behavior, and normative cultural (and medical) ideas of genitals? And, finally, how does one factor in the issues of age and consent, both of which are central in popular accounts in the United States about procedures labeled as female genital mutilation?

Months after this class ended, a student said to me, "You know, I still haven't decided how I feel about FGC." I taught the class in part to enable me to finally decide how I felt about the difference between so-called female genital cutting and so-called female genital cosmetic surgeries. I have been asked this question of difference a lot over the years, and I had largely backed off answering it, saying I was interested in the history of the procedures in the United States as medical therapies. I owe it to a fourth-year medical student at Northwestern for saying something that made me realize why I had backed off this question of difference for so long and why I found it so troubling: because, from my vantage point, it was the wrong question.[15]

It is the desire to find a difference that I find so troubling, and I find it troubling because it presumes the practices as performed in the United States were historical anomalies, that they were not embedded historical practices in the United States: without the historical context, the search for difference is superficial and thus meaningless. The question, then, should not be what are the differences, but, rather, as I have explored in this book, how are they part of America's own cultural and medical history? Though this book is, to date, the fullest accounting of these practices in the United States, I am of course not the only one aware that they occurred, and continue to occur, and I end with a brief mention by a handful of Seattle physicians. In a letter to the *New England Journal of Medicine* in 1995 in response to an article about considering female circumcision a public health concern, three doctors from the University of Washington in Seattle noted the complexity of the issue. "As health providers for refugees, we work with many Ethiopian and Eritrean women who underwent this form of circumcision as infants, just as their brothers were circumcised" and who, upon coming here, "are surprised at the refusal of outsiders to recognize this practice." Those who seek to end the practice of female circumcision among immigrants in the United States, they concluded, "must acknowledge that a variety of practices exist" in the United States, "including a practice that not only is equivalent to male circumcision but has also been used by U.S. physicians to treat frigidity in adults."[16] Examining the history of medical ideas about and interventions on the clitoris allows us to see that the therapy being rendered was not evidence-based medicine but rather culturally based medicine, a therapy that supported cultural ideas about acceptable female sexual behavior and bodily norms. An acknowledgment of the diverse purported therapeutic reasons for the practice of clitoral cutting since the nineteenth century in the United States is, as the Seattle physicians suggested nearly twenty years ago, imperative to understanding the similarities, the differences, and the future of female circumcision, female genital mutilation, and clitoral unhooding.

Appendix

The Clitoris in Anatomy and Gynecology Texts

I examined more than 150 anatomy texts (published between 1859 and 1981) and more than 100 gynecology texts (published between 1870 and 1981) for their representations of the clitoris. All of the texts I examined are listed below. I found the anatomy texts at three major medical school libraries, the Galter Health Sciences Library at Northwestern University, the John Crerar Library at the University of Chicago, and the Ebling Library for the Health Sciences at the University of Wisconsin–Madison, and I found the gynecology texts in the medical libraries at Northwestern and the University of Chicago. I purposely looked at the books on the shelves of major medical school libraries under the assumption they were thus fairly standard. In addition to the books I found at these three libraries, I looked at two specifically about female genital anatomy at the Countway Library of Medicine, Harvard Medical School: Netter, *Major Anatomy of the Female Genital Tract*; and Smout and Jacoby, *Gynaecological and Obstetrical Anatomy*. I obtained photocopies of Furneaux, *Philips' Anatomical Model of the Female Human Body*; and Giles, *Anatomy and Physiology of the Female Generative Organs and of Pregnancy* (1910) from the University of California, San Francisco, Archives and Special Collections. I examined only anatomy and gynecology texts written in English and published either in the United States or Great Britain.

Not all the gynecology texts had entries for the clitoris; for example, Bender's 1909 *Medical Gynecology* did not list the clitoris in the index. Another book mentioned the clitoris but only regarding the pathology of carcinoma, considered "unusual" in this organ.[1] What I quickly discovered was that specific texts—texts on surgery, texts on specific diseases like tuberculosis or cancer, and texts principally dealing with topics such as menstruation or childbirth—often did not mention the clitoris.[2] For this reason, I examined only general gynecology texts (though as the twentieth century progressed, gynecology texts increasingly combined with obstetric texts as these two specialties merged).[3]

As I note in my introduction, not all physicians would have agreed with these texts, and there was then (as today) a difference between textbook-recommended practice and actual clinical practice, so I am using these texts as a proxy for medical understanding of the clitoris during this time. Additionally, many of these texts (especially the gynecology texts) were quite sexist in their comments about not just female sexuality but also issues dealing with, for example, reproductive functions. Finally, as I note in my introduction, and I here again stress, that these texts often suggested that the clitoris was the sexual equivalent of the penis does not mean these texts conferred equivalency as regards sexual autonomy.

Anatomy Texts

Anatomical Chromographs of the Human Male and Human Female. Detroit: Parke, Davis, 1958.

Anderson, Paul D. *Clinical Anatomy and Physiology for Allied Health Sciences*. Philadelphia: W. B. Saunders, 1976.

Anson, Barry J. *An Atlas of Human Anatomy*. 2nd ed. Philadelphia: W. B. Saunders, 1963.

Anthony, Catherine Parker. *Structure and Function of the Body*. 5th ed. St. Louis, MO: C. V. Mosby, 1976.

———. *Textbook of Anatomy and Physiology*. 4th ed. St. Louis, MO: C. V. Mosby, 1955.

Anthony, Catherine Parker, and Gary A. Thibodeau. *Structure and Function of the Body*. 6th ed. St. Louis, MO: C. V. Mosby, 1980.

Bailliere's Atlas of Female Anatomy. Revised by Katharine F. Armstrong. 4th ed. London: Bailliere, Tindall and Cox, 1952.

Brantigan, Otto C. *Clinical Anatomy*. New York: McGraw Hill, 1963.

Boolootian, Richard A. *Elements of Human Anatomy and Physiology*. St. Paul, MN: West, 1976.

Callender, Curie Latimer. *Callender's Surgical Anatomy*. Edited by Barry J. Anson and Walter G. Maddock. 3rd ed. Philadelphia: W. B. Saunders, 1952.

———. *Callender's Surgical Anatomy*. Edited by Barry J. Anson and Walter G. Maddock. 4th ed., Philadelphia: W. B. Saunders, 1958.

Christensen, John B., and Ira Rockwood Telford. *Synopsis of Gross Anatomy*. New York: Harper and Row, 1966.

Christian, William Gay. *A Textbook of Anatomy for Nurses*. St. Louis, MO: C. V. Mosby, 1917.*

Crafts, Roger C. *A Textbook of Human Anatomy*. New York: John Wiley and Sons, 1966.

———. *A Textbook of Human Anatomy*. 2nd ed. New York: John Wiley and Sons, 1979.

Crouch, James E. *Functional Human Anatomy*. 2nd ed. Philadelphia: Lea and Febiger, 1975.

Cunningham, D. J. *Cunningham's Manual of Practical Anatomy*. Edited by James Couper Brash. 12th ed. London: Oxford University Press, 1958.

———. *Cunningham's Manual of Practical Anatomy*. Edited by G. J. Romanes. Vol. 2. 14th ed. New York: Oxford University Press, 1977.

———. *Cunningham's Text-Book of Anatomy*. Edited by J. C. Brash and E. B. Jamieson. 7th ed. New York: Oxford University Press, 1937.*

———. *Cunningham's Text-Book of Anatomy.* Edited by James Couper Brash. 9th ed. London: Oxford University Press, 1951.

———. *Cunningham's Text-Book of Anatomy.* Edited by G. J. Romanes. 11th ed. London: Oxford University Press, 1972.

Dawson, Helen L. *Basic Human Anatomy.* New York: Appleton-Century-Crofts, 1966.

Dickinson, Robert Latou. *Human Sex Anatomy: A Topographical Hand Atlas.* 2nd ed. Baltimore: Williams and Wilkins, 1949.

Ellis, Harold. *Clinical Anatomy: A Revision and Applied Anatomy for Clinical Students.* 5th rev. ed. London: Blackwell Scientific, 1971.

Figge, Frank H., ed. *Atlas of Human Anatomy.* New York: Hafner Press, 1974.

Francis, Carl C. *Introduction to Human Anatomy.* St. Louis, MO: C. V. Mosby, 1949.

———. *Introduction to Human Anatomy.* 3rd ed. St. Louis, MO: C. V. Mosby, 1959.

———. *Introduction to Human Anatomy.* 5th ed. St. Louis, MO: C. V. Mosby, 1968.

Furneaux, William S. *Dr. Minder's Anatomical Manikin of the Human Body.* Revised by Ethel Mayer. New York: American Thermo-Ware, 191?

———. *Philips' Anatomical Model of the Female Human Body.* London: George Philip and Son, 1904.

Gardner, Ernest, and Donald J. Gray, and Ronan O'Rahilly. *Anatomy: A Regional Study of Human Structure.* Philadelphia: W. B. Saunders, 1960.

———. *Anatomy: A Regional Study of Human Structure.* 2nd ed. Philadelphia: W. B. Saunders, 1963.

———. *Anatomy: A Regional Study of Human Structure.* 3rd ed. Philadelphia: W. B. Saunders, 1969.

———. *Anatomy: A Regional Study of Human Structure.* 4th ed. Philadelphia: W. B. Saunders, 1975.

Gardner, Weston D., and William A. Osburn. *Structure of the Human Body.* Philadelphia: W. B. Saunders, 1967.

Giles, Arthur E. *Anatomy and Physiology of the Female Generative Organs and of Pregnancy.* London: Bailliere, Tindall and Cox, 1909.*

———. *Anatomy and Physiology of the Female Generative Organs and of Pregnancy.* 3rd ed. New York: Paul B. Hoeber, 1910.

Grant, J. C. Boileau. *An Atlas of Anatomy by Regions.* Vol. 1. Baltimore: Williams and Wilkins, 1943.*

———. *An Atlas of Anatomy by Regions.* 3rd ed. Baltimore: Williams and Wilkins, 1951.

———. *An Atlas of Anatomy by Regions.* 4th ed. Baltimore: Williams and Wilkins, 1956.

———. *An Atlas of Anatomy by Regions.* 5th ed. Baltimore: Williams and Wilkins, 1962.

———. *An Atlas of Anatomy by Regions.* 6th ed. Baltimore: Williams and Wilkins, 1972.

———. *Grant's Atlas of Anatomy.* Edited by James E. Anderson. 7th ed. Baltimore: Williams and Wilkins, 1978.

———. *Grant's Method of Anatomy.* Edited by John V. Basmajian. 8th ed. Baltimore: Williams and Wilkins, 1971.

———. *Grant's Method of Anatomy.* Edited by John V. Basmajian. 9th ed. Baltimore: Williams and Wilkins, 1975.

———. *Grant's Method of Anatomy.* Edited by John V. Basmajian. 10th ed. Baltimore: Williams and Wilkins, 1980.

———. *Method of Anatomy: Descriptive and Deductive.* Baltimore: Williams and Wilkins, 1937.*

———. *Method of Anatomy: Descriptive and Deductive.* 2nd ed. Baltimore: Williams and Wilkins, 1940.*

———. *Method of Anatomy: Descriptive and Deductive.* 3rd ed. Baltimore: Williams and Wilkins, 1944.*

———. *Method of Anatomy: Descriptive and Deductive.* 4th ed. Baltimore: Williams and Wilkins, 1948.

———. *Method of Anatomy: Descriptive and Deductive.* 6th ed. Baltimore: Williams and Wilkins, 1958.

Gray, Henry. *Anatomy: Descriptive and Surgical.* Philadelphia: Blanchard and Lea, 1859.

———. *Anatomy: Descriptive and Surgical.* 2nd American edition from the revised and enlarged London ed. Philadelphia: Blanchard and Lea, 1862.

———. *Anatomy: Descriptive and Surgical.* New American edition from the 5th English ed. Philadelphia: Henry C. Lea, 1870.

———. *Anatomy: Descriptive and Surgical.* New American edition from the 8th English ed. Philadelphia: Henry C. Lea, 1878.*

———. *Anatomy: Descriptive and Surgical.* Edited by T. Pickering Pick. New American edition from the 10th English ed. Philadelphia: Lea and Sons, 1883.*

———. *Anatomy, Descriptive and Surgical.* Edited by T. Pickering Pick and William W. Keen. New American edition from the 11th English ed. Philadelphia: Lea Brothers, 1887.

———. *Anatomy: Descriptive and Surgical.* Edited by T. Pickering Pick. New American edition from the 13th English ed. Philadelphia: Lea Brothers, 1893.*

———. *Anatomy: Descriptive and Surgical.* Edited by T. Pickering Pick. New American edition from the 13th English ed. Philadelphia: Lea Brothers, 1897.

———. *Anatomy: Descriptive and Surgical.* Edited by T. Pickering Pick and Robert Howden. Revised American edition from the 15th English ed. Philadelphia: Lea and Febiger, 1901.*

———. *Anatomy: Descriptive and Surgical.* Edited by Pick and Howden. 16th ed. New American ed. Revised and reedited by John Chalmers DaCosta. Philadelphia: Lea Brothers, 1905.

———. *Anatomy: Descriptive and Surgical.* Edited by John Chalmers DeCosta and Edward Anthony Spitzka. 17th ed. Philadelphia: Lea and Febiger, 1908.*

———. *Anatomy: Descriptive and Applied.* Edited by Edward Anthony Spitzka. 18th ed. Philadelphia: Lea and Febiger, 1910.

———. *Anatomy: Descriptive and Applied.* Edited by Edward Anthony Spitzka. New American edition from the 18th English ed. Philadelphia: Lea and Febiger, 1913.

———. *Anatomy of the Human Body.* Edited by Warren H. Lewis. 20th ed. Philadelphia: Lea and Febiger, 1918.*

———. *Anatomy of the Human Body.* Edited by Warren H. Lewis. 21st ed. Philadelphia: Lea and Febiger, 1924.*

———. *Anatomy of the Human Body.* Edited by Warren H. Lewis. 22nd ed. Philadelphia: Lea and Febiger, 1930.*

———. *Anatomy of the Human Body.* Edited by Warren H. Lewis. 23rd ed. Philadelphia: Lea and Febiger, 1936.*

———. *Anatomy of the Human Body.* Edited by Warren H. Lewis. 24th ed. Philadelphia: Lea and Febiger, 1942.*

————. *Anatomy of the Human Body.* Edited by Charles Mayo Goss. 25th ed. Philadelphia: Lea and Febiger, 1948.

————. *Anatomy of the Human Body.* Edited by Charles Mayo Goss. 26th ed. Philadelphia: Lea and Febiger, 1954.

————. *Anatomy of the Human Body.* Edited by Charles Mayo Goss. 27th ed. Philadelphia: Lea and Febiger, 1959.

————. *Anatomy of the Human Body.* Edited by Charles Mayo Goss. 28th ed. Philadelphia: Lea and Febiger, 1966.

————. *Gray's Anatomy.* Edited by Charles Mayo Goss. 29th ed. Philadelphia: Lea and Febiger, 1973.

Grobler, N. J. *Textbook of Clinical Anatomy.* Vol. 1. New York: Elsevier Scientific, 1977.

Hamilton, W. J. *Textbook of Human Anatomy.* London: MacMillan, 1956.

————. *Textbook of Human Anatomy.* 2nd ed. St. Louis, MO: C. V. Mosby, 1976.

Hart, D. Barry. *Atlas of Female Pelvic Anatomy.* New York: D. Appleton, 1884.*

Harvey, B. C. H. *Simple Lessons in Human Anatomy.* Chicago: American Medical Association, 1931.*

Hickman, Cleveland Pendleton. *Functional Human Anatomy.* New York: Prentice Hall, 1940.*

Hollinshead, W. Henry. *Textbook of Anatomy.* 2nd ed. New York: Harper and Row, 1967.

————. *Textbook of Anatomy.* 3rd ed. New York: Harper and Row, 1974.

Howell, A. Brazier. *Gross Anatomy: A Brief Systematic Presentation of the Macroscopic Structure of the Human Body.* New York: D. Appleton-Century, 1939.*

Jacob, Stanley W., and Clarice Ashworth Francone. *Structure and Function in Man.* Philadelphia: W. B. Saunders, 1965.

————. *Structure and Function in Man.* 2nd ed. Philadelphia: W. B. Saunders, 1970.

————. *Structure and Function in Man.* 3rd ed. Philadelphia: W. B. Saunders, 1974.

Jacob, Francone, and Walter J. Lossow. *Structure and Function in Man.* 4th ed. Philadelphia: W. B. Saunders, 1978.

Jung, Frederic Theodore, Anna Ruth Benjamin, and Elizabeth Carpenters Earle. *Anatomy and Physiology.* Philadelphia: F. A. Davis, 1939.*

Jung, Frederic Theodore, and Elizabeth Carpenters Earle. *Anatomy and Physiology.* 3rd ed. Philadelphia: F. A. Davis, 1950.

Kimber, Diana Clifford. *Kimber-Gray-Stackpole's Anatomy and Physiology.* Edited by Marjorie A. Miller and Lutie C. Leavell. 16th ed. New York: Macmillan, 1972.

Kimber, Diana Clifford, and Carolyn Elizabeth Gray. *Anatomy and Physiology.* Revised by Caroline E. Stackpole and Lutie C. Leavell. 13th ed. New York: Macmillan, 1955.

————. *Textbook of Anatomy and Physiology.* 6th ed. New York: Macmillan, 1925.*

Kimber, Diana Clifford, Carolyn Elizabeth Gray, and Caroline Emorette Stackpole. *Anatomy and Physiology.* Revised by Lutie C. Leavell and Marjorie A. Miller. 15th ed. New York: Macmillan, 1966.

————. *Textbook of Anatomy and Physiology.* 11th ed. New York: Macmillan, 1942.*

————. *Textbook of Anatomy and Physiology.* 12th ed. New York: Macmillan, 1948.

King, Barry G., and Mary Jane Showers. *Human Anatomy and Physiology.* 6th ed. Philadelphia: W. B. Saunders, 1969.

Knox, James P. *Physicians' Anatomical Aid.* Chicago: W. P. H., 192?

188 ❧ APPENDIX

Last, R. J. *Anatomy: Regional and Applied.* 3rd ed. Boston: Little, Brown, 1963.
———. *Anatomy: Regional and Applied.* 6th ed. Boston: Little, Brown, 1978.
Lumley, J. S. P., J. L. Craven, and J. T. Aitken. *Essential Anatomy and Some Clinical Applications.* Edinburgh: Churchill Livingstone, 1975.
Mainland, Donald. *Anatomy As a Basis for Medical and Dental Practice.* New York: Paul B. Hoeber, 1945.*
Marshall, Clyde, and Edgar L. Lazier. *An Introduction to Human Anatomy.* 3rd ed. Philadelphia: W. B. Saunders, 1946.
———. *An Introduction to Human Anatomy.* 4th ed. Philadelphia: W. B. Saunders, 1955.
McClintic, J. Robert. *Basic Anatomy and Physiology of the Human Body.* 2nd ed. New York: John Wiley and Sons, 1980.
Mitchell, G. A. G., and E. L. Patterson, *Basic Anatomy.* Baltimore: Williams and Wilkins, 1954.
Morris, Henry. *Morris's Human Anatomy: A Complete Systematic Treatise.* 2nd ed. Philadelphia: P. Blakiston's Sons, 1898.*
———. *Morris's Human Anatomy: A Complete Systematic Treatise by English and American Authors.* Edited by C. M. Jackson. 5th rev. ed. Philadelphia: P. Blakiston's Sons, 1914.*
———. *Morris's Human Anatomy: A Complete Systematic Treatise by English and American Authors.* Edited by C. M. Jackson. 9th rev. ed. Philadelphia: P. Blakiston's Sons, 1933.*
———. *Morris's Human Anatomy: A Complete Systematic Treatise.* Edited by J. Parsons Schaeffer. 10th ed. Philadelphia: Blakiston, 1942.*
———. *Morris' Human Anatomy: A Complete Systematic Treatise.* Edited by Barry J. Anson. 12th ed. New York: Blakiston/McGraw-Hill, 1966.
Morris, Henry, and J. Playfair McMurrich. *Morris's Human Anatomy: A Complete Systematic Treatise by English and American Authors.* 4th ed. Philadelphia: P. Blakiston's Son, 1907.*
Netter, Frank H., ed. *The CIBA Collection of Medical Illustrations: Reproductive System.* New York: Ernest Oppenheimer CIBA Pharmaceutical, 1965.
———. *Major Anatomy of the Female Genital Tract.* Summit, NJ: CIBA Pharmaceutical Products, 1948.
Pace, Donald M., and Benjamin W. McCashland, and Paul A. Landolt. *Physiology and Anatomy.* New York: Thomas Y. Crowell, 1965.
Pansky, Ben, and Earl Lawrence. *Review of Gross Anatomy: A Dynamic Approach.* New York: MacMillan, 1964.
Pansky, Ben. *Review of Gross Anatomy: Text and Illustrations.* 4th ed. New York: Macmillan, 1979.
Piersol, George A. *Human Anatomy: Including Structure and Development and Practical Considerations.* 4th ed. Philadelphia: J. B. Lippincott, 1913.*
———. *Human Anatomy: Including Structure and Development and Practical Considerations.* Edited by Thomas Dwight. 8th ed. Philadelphia: J. B. Lippincott, 1923.*
———. *Piersol's Human Anatomy: Including Structure and Development and Practical Considerations.* Edited by G. Carl Huber. 9th ed. Philadelphia: J. B. Lippincott, 1930.*

Pitzman, Marsh. *The Fundamentals of Human Anatomy: Including Its Borderland Districts, from the Viewpoint of a Practitioner*. St. Louis, MO: C. V. Mosby, 1920.*

Ross, Janet S., and Kathleen J. W. Wilson. *Foundations of Anatomy and Physiology*. Baltimore: Williams and Wilkins, 1963.

Savage, Henry. *The Surgical, Surgical Pathology, and Surgical Anatomy of the Female Pelvic Organs*. 3rd ed. New York: William Wood, 1880.*

Scott, James Henderson, and Andrew Derat Dixon. *Anatomy for Students of Dentistry*. 2nd ed. Edinburgh: E. & S. Livingstone, 1966.

Simkins, Cleveland S. *Functional Human Anatomy: An Introduction Into the Fabric of the Human Body*. Dubuque, IA: W. M. C. Brown, 1949.

Sinclair, David. *An Introduction to Functional Anatomy*. Springfield, IL: Charles C. Thomas, 1957.

———. *An Introduction to Functional Anatomy*, 2nd ed. Oxford: Blackwell Scientific, 1961.

———. *An Introduction to Functional Anatomy*, 3rd ed. Oxford: Blackwell Scientific, 1966.

Smout, C. F. V. *Basic Anatomy and Physiology*. London: Edward Arnold, 1962.

Smout, C. F. V., and F. Jacoby. *Gynaecological and Obstetrical Anatomy and Functional Histology*. 3rd ed. London: Edward Arnold, 1953.

Snell, Richard S. *Atlas of Clinical Anatomy*. Boston: Little, Brown, 1978.

———. *Clinical Anatomy for Medical Students*. Little, Brown, 1973.

Sobotta, Johannes. *Atlas of Human Anatomy*. Vol. 2. Philadelphia: W. B. Saunders, 1906.*

———. *Atlas of Human Anatomy*. Vol. 2. New York: G. E. Stechert, 1909.*

———. *Atlas of Human Anatomy*. Vol. 2. New York: G. E. Stechert, 1928.*

Spalteholz, Werner. *Hand-Atlas of Human Anatomy*. Translated by Lewellys F. Barker. Vol. 3. 4th ed. Philadelphia: J. B. Lippincott, 1923.*

———. *Hand-Atlas of Human Anatomy*. Translated by Lewellys F. Barker. Vol. 2. 5th ed. Philadelphia: J. B. Lippincott, 1925.*

Spence, Alexander P., and Elliott B. Mason. *Human Anatomy and Physiology*. Menlo Park, CA: Benjamin/Cummings, 1979.

Stibbe, Edward P. *Aids to Anatomy*. Baltimore: Williams and Wilkins, 1940.*

———, ed. *Practical Anatomy by Six Teachers*. London: Edward Arnold, 1932.*

Taylor, Norman Burke, and Margaret G. McPhedran. *Basic Physiology and Anatomy*. New York: G. P. Putnam's Sons, 1965.

Terry, Robert James. *An Introduction to the Study of Human Anatomy*. New York: Macmillan, 1929.*

Thompson, Edward T., and Adaline C. Hayden. *Anatomy for the Medical Record Librarian*. Chicago: Physician's Record, 1956.

Tobin, Charles E., ed. *Shearer's Manual of Human Dissection*. 4th ed. New York: Blakiston/McGraw-Hill, 1961.

Tobin, Charles E., and Peter Ng. *Visual Principles of Elementary Human Anatomy*. Philadelphia: F. A. Davis, 1965.

Toldt, Carl. *An Atlas of Human Anatomy for Students and Physicians*. Vol. 2. 2nd ed. New York: Macmillan, 1944.*

Von Bardeleben, Karl, and Heinr. Haeckel. *Atlas of Applied (Topographical) Human Anatomy*. New York: Rebman, 1906.*

Williams, Jesse Feiring. *A Textbook of Anatomy and Physiology for Schools of Nursing, Normal Schools, and Colleges.* Philadelphia: W. B. Saunders, 1923.*
———. *A Textbook of Anatomy and Physiology.* 6th ed. Philadelphia: W. B. Saunders, 1939.*
Wilson, Doris Burda, and Wilfred J. Wilson. *Human Anatomy.* New York: Oxford University Press, 1978.
Wischnitzer, Saul. *Outline of Human Anatomy.* Springfield, IL: Charles C. Thomas, 1972.
Woodburne, Russell T. *Essentials of Human Anatomy.* 2nd ed. New York: Oxford University Press, 1961.
———. *Essentials of Human Anatomy.* 3rd ed. New York: Oxford University Press, 1965.
———. *Essentials of Human Anatomy.* 6th ed. New York: Oxford University Press, 1978.
Zuckerman, Solly. *A New System of Anatomy.* New York: Oxford University Press, 1961.

Gynecology Texts

Adair, Fred L. *Obstetrics and Gynecology.* Vol. 2. Philadelphia: Lea and Febiger, 1940.
Atkinson, William B. *The Therapeutics of Gynecology and Obstetrics.* Philadelphia: D. G. Brinton, 1880.
Baird, Dugald, ed. *Combined Textbook of Obstetrics and Gynecology for Students and Practitioners.* 7th ed. Edinburgh: E. & S. Livingston, 1962.
———. *Combined Textbook of Obstetrics and Gynecology for Students and Practitioners.* 8th ed. Edinburgh: E. & S. Livingstone, 1969.
Bandler, Samuel Wyllis. *Medical Gynecology.* 2nd ed. Philadelphia: W. B. Saunders, 1909.
Barber, David, H. Fields, and Sherwin A. Kaufman. *Quick Reference to OB-GYN Procedures.* 2nd ed. Philadelphia: J. B. Lippincott, 1979.
Barber, Hugh R. K., and Edward A. Graber. *Quick Reference to OB-GYN Procedures.* Philadelphia: J. B. Lippincott, 1969.
Barbour, A. H. F., and B. P. Watson. *Gynecological and Diagnosis and Pathology.* 3rd ed. Edinburgh: W. Green and Son, 1922.
Barnes, Robert. *A Clinical History of Medical and Surgical Disease of Women.* 2nd ed. Philadelphia: Henry C. Lea, 1878.
Beacham, Daniel Winston, and Woodard Davis Beacham. *Synopsis of Gynecology.* 9th ed. St. Louis, MO: C. V. Mosby, 1977.
Behrman, Samuel J., and John R. G. Gosling. *Fundamentals of Gynecology.* New York: Oxford University Press, 1966.
Bell, W. Blair. *The Principles of Gynecology: A Manual for Students and Practitioners.* 3rd ed. London: Bailliere, Tindall and Cox, 1919.
Bender, Samuel Wyllis. *Medical Gynecology.* Philadelphia: W. B. Saunders, 1909.
Benson, Ralph C. *Current Obstetric and Gynecological Diagnosis and Treatment.* Los Altos, CA: Lange Medical, 1976.
———. *Current Obstetric and Gynecological Diagnosis and Treatment.* 2nd ed. Los Altos, CA: Lange Medical, 1978.
———. *Handbook of Obstetrics and Gynecology.* Los Altos, CA: Lange Medical, 1964.

———. *Handbook of Obstetrics and Gynecology.* 2nd ed. Los Altos, CA: Lange Medical, 1966.

———. *Handbook of Obstetrics and Gynecology.* 6th ed. Los Altos, CA: Lange Medical, 1977.

———. *Handbook of Obstetrics and Gynecology.* 7th ed. Los Altos, CA: Lange Medical, 1980.

Berkeley, Comyns, and Victor Bonney. *A Guide to Gynecology in General Practice.* 2nd ed. London: Frowde, 1919.

———. *A Textbook of Gynecological Surgery.* 3rd ed. London: Cassell, 1935.

Blech, Gustavus M. *The Practitioner's Guide to the Diagnosis and Treatment of Diseases of Women.* Chicago: M. Robertson, 1903.

Brewer, John I. *Gynecology: The Teachings of John I. Brewer.* New York: Tomas Nelson and Sons, 1950.

———. *Textbook of Gynecology.* Baltimore: Williams and Wilkins, 1953.

Brewer, John I., and Edwin J. DeCosta. *Textbook of Gynecology.* 4th ed. Baltimore: Williams and Wilkins, 1967.

Byford, Henry T. *Manual of Gynecology.* Philadelphia: P. Blakiston, Son, 1895.

———. *Manual of Gynecology.* 3rd rev. ed. Philadelphia: P. Blakiston, Son, 1902.

Cameron, J. Lyle. *Gynecological Operations.* London: Oxford University Press, 1941.

Caplan, Ronald M., and William J. Sweeney. *Advances in Obstetrics and Gynecology.* Baltimore: Williams and Wilkins, 1978.

Castallo, Mario A. *The Mechanics of Obstetrics.* Philadelphia: F. A. Davis, 1949.

Crossen, Harry Sturgeon, and Robert James Crossen. *Diseases of Women.* St. Louis, MO: C. V. Mosby, 1944.

———. *Operative Gynecology.* 5th ed. St. Louis, MO: C. V. Mosby, 1938.

Crossen, Robert James. *Diseases of Women.* St. Louis, C. V. Mosby, 1953.

Curtis, Arthur Hale. *Gynecological Diagnosis.* Philadelphia: W. B. Saunders, 1929.

———. *A Textbook of Gynecology.* Philadelphia: W. B. Saunders, 1931.

———. *A Textbook of Gynecology.* 2nd ed. Philadelphia: W. B. Saunders, 1936.

———. *A Textbook of Gynecology.* 3rd ed. Philadelphia: W. B. Saunders, 1938.

———. *A Textbook of Gynecology.* 4th ed. Philadelphia: W. B. Saunders, 1942.

———. *A Textbook of Gynecology.* 5th ed. Philadelphia: W. B. Saunders, 1946.

Curtis, Arthur Hale, and John William Huffman. *A Textbook of Gynecology.* 6th ed. Philadelphia: W. B. Saunders, 1950.

Danforth, David N., ed. *Textbook of Obstetrics and Gynecology.* New York: Harper and Row, 1966.

———. *Textbook of Obstetrics and Gynecology.* 2nd ed. New York: Harper and Row, 1971.

———. *Obstetrics and Gynecology.* 3rd ed. New York: Harper and Row, 1977.

DeLee, Joseph B., and J. P. Greenhill. *Principles and Practice of Obstetrics.* Philadelphia: W. B. Saunders, 1947.

Dewhurst, C. J. *Integrated Obstetrics and Gynaecology for Postgraduates.* 2nd ed. London: Blackwell Scientific, 1976.

Dilts, P. V., Jr., J. W. Greene Jr., and J. W. Roddick Jr. *Core Studies in Obstetrics and Gynecology.* Baltimore: Williams and Wilkins, 1971.

Dougherty, Cary M. *Surgical Pathology of Gynecologic Disease.* New York: Harper and Row, 1968.

Dudley, E. C. *Diseases of Women: A Treatise on the Principles and Practice of Gynecology for Students and Practitioners.* Philadelphia: Lea Brothers, 1898.

——. *The Principles and Practice of Gynecology.* 3rd ed. Philadelphia: Lea Brothers, 1902.

——. *The Principles and Practice of Gynecology.* 5th ed. Philadelphia: Lea Brothers, 1908.

Fox, H., and F. A. Langley, eds. *Postgraduate Obstetrics and Gynecology.* Oxford: Pergamon Press, 1973.

Fritsch, Heinrich. *The Diseases of Women: A Manual for Physicians and Students.* New York: William Wood, 1883.

Everett, Houston. *Gynecological and Obstetrical Urology.* 2nd ed. Baltimore: Williams and Wilkins, 1947.

Gallabin, Alfred Lewis. *A Handbook of the Diseases of Women.* Philadelphia: P. Blakiston, Son, 1882.

Glass, Robert H. *Office Gynecology.* 2nd ed. Baltimore: Williams and Wilkins, 1981.

Gompel, C., and S. G. Silverberg. *Pathology in Gynecology and Obstetrics.* Philadelphia: J. B. Lippincott, 1969.

Graber, Edward A. *Gynecologic Endocrinology.* Philadelphia: J. B. Lippincott, 1961.

Green, Charles M. *Case Histories in Diseases of Women.* Boston: W. M. Leonard, 1915.

Greene, Thomas H., Jr. *Gynecology: Essentials of Clinical Practice.* Boston: Little, Brown, 1971.

Greenhill, J. P. *Obstetrics.* 13th ed. Philadelphia: W. B. Saunders, 1965.

——. *Office Gynecology.* 9th ed. Chicago: Year Book Medical, 1971.

——. *Surgical Gynecology: Including Important Obstetric Operations.* Chicago: Year Book Medical, 1963.

Hall, J. Edward. *Applied Gynecologic Pathology.* New York: Appleton-Century-Crofts, 1963.

Hamblen, E. C. *Endocrinology of Woman.* Springfield, IL: Charles C. Thomas, 1945.

Hart, D. Berry, and A. H. Barbor. *Manual of Gynecology.* New York: William Wood, 1883.

Heardman, Helen. *Physiotherapy in Obstetrics and Gynecology.* Edinburgh: E. & S. Livingston, 1951.

Henry, W. O. *A Physician's Practical Gynecology.* Lincoln, NE: Review Press, 1902.

Jeffcoate, T. N. A. *Principles of Gynaecology.* 3rd ed. New York: Appleton-Century-Crofts, 1967.

Kelly, Howard A. *Gynecology.* New York: D. Appleton, 1928.

——. *Medical Gynecology.* New York: D. Appleton, 1908.

Kelly, Howard A., and Charles P. Nobel. *Gynecology and Abdominal Surgery.* Vol. 1. Philadelphia: W. B. Saunders, 1907.

Kerr, J. M. Munro. *Combined Textbook of Obstetrics and Gynecology.* Baltimore: William and Wilkins, 1946.

Kimbrough, Robert A., ed. *Gynecology.* Philadelphia: J. B. Lippincott, 1965.

Kisch, E. Heinrich. *The Sexual Life of Woman.* New York: Rebman, 1910.

Kistner, Robert W. *Gynecology: Principles and Practice.* 2nd ed. Chicago: Year Book Medical, 1973.

——. *Gynecology: Principals and Practice.* 3rd ed. Chicago: Year Book Medical Publications, 1979.

Kraus, Frederick T. *Gynecologic Pathology.* St. Louis, MO: C. V. Mosby, 1967.

La Vake, Rae Thornton. *A Handbook of Clinical Gynecology and Obstetrics.* St. Louis, MO: C. V. Mosby, 1928.

Lewis, T. L. T. *Progress in Clinical Obstetrics and Gynecology.* 2nd ed. London: J. A. Churchill, 1964.

Macleod, Douglas, and John Hawkins. *Bonney's Gynecological Surgery.* 7th ed. New York: Harper and Row, 1964.

Marcuse, Peter. *Diagnostic Pathology in Gynecology and Obstetrics.* New York: Harper and Row, 1966.

May, Charles Henry. *May's Diseases of Women.* Edited Leonard S. Rau. 2nd ed. Philadelphia: Lea Brothers, 1890.

Miller, C. Jeff. *An Introduction to Gynecology.* 2nd ed. St. Louis, MO: C. V. Mosby, 1934.

Morrill, C. *The Physiology of Woman and Her Disease from Infancy to Old Age.* 8th ed. Boston: James Campbell, 1870.

Novak, Edmund R., Georgeanna Seegar Jones, and Howard W. Jones Jr. *Novak's Textbook of Gynecology.* 9th ed. Baltimore: Williams and Wilkins, 1975.

Novak, Edmund R., and J. Donald Woodruff. *Novak's Gynecologic and Obstetric Pathology with Clinical and Endocrine Relations.* 5th ed. Philadelphia: W. B. Saunders, 1962.

————. *Novak's Gynecologic and Obstetric Pathology.* 7th ed. Philadelphia: W. B. Saunders, 1974.

————. *Novak's Gynecologic and Obstetric Pathology.* 8th ed. Philadelphia: W. B. Saunders, 1979.

Novak, Josef. *Gynecological Therapy.* New York: McGraw-Hill, 1960.

————. *Novak's Textbook of Gynecology.* Edited by Howard W. Jones Jr. and Georgeanna Seegar Jones. 10th ed. Baltimore: Williams and Wilkins, 1981.

Novak, Josef, and Edmund R. Novak. *Gynecologic and Obstetric Pathology with Clinical and Endocrine Relations.* 4th ed. Philadelphia: W. B. Saunders, 1958.

Philipp, Elliot E. *Obstetrics and Gynaecology: Combined for Students.* London: H. K. Lewis, 1962.

Philipp, Elliot E., Josephine Barnes, and Michael Newton, eds. *Scientific Foundations of Obstetrics and Gynaecology.* Philadelphia: F. A. Davis, 1970.

————. *Scientific Foundations of Obstetrics and Gynaecology,* 2nd ed. London: William Heinemann Medical Books, 1977.

Pryor, William R. *Gynaecology: A Textbook for Students and a Guide for Practitioners.* New York: D. Appleton, 1903.

Ramon de Alvarez, Russell, ed. *Textbook of Gynecology.* Philadelphia: Lea & Febiger, 1977.

Reed, Charles A. *Diseases of Women: Medical and Surgical Gynecology.* New York: D. Appleton, 1913.

Reich, Walter J., and Mitchell J. Nechtow. *Pitfalls in Gynecologic Diagnosis and Surgery.* New York: McGraw-Hill, 1962.

Robinson, Byron. *Landmarks in Gynecology.* Vol. 1. Detroit: George S. Davis, 1894.

Rogers, Joseph. *Endocrine and Metabolic Aspects of Gynecology.* Philadelphia: W. B. Saunders, 1963.

Romney, Seymour L., Mary Jane Gray, A. Brian Little, James A. Merrill, E. J. Quilligan, and Richard Stander. *Gynecology and Obstetrics: The Health Care of Women.* New York: McGraw Hill, 1975.

———. *Gynecology and Obstetrics: The Health Care of Women.* 2nd ed. New York: McGraw-Hill, 1981.

Roques, Frederick W., John Beattie, and Joseph Wrigley, eds. *Diseases of Women by Ten Teachers.* 10th ed. London: Edward Arnold, 1959.

Shaw, Wilfred. *Shaw's Textbook of Operative Gynecology.* Revised by John Howkins. 2nd ed. Edinburgh: E. & S. Livingstone, 1960.

Shirodkar, V. N. *Contributions to Obstetrics and Gynecology.* Edinburgh: E. & S. Livingstone, 1960.

Skene, Alexander J. C. *Treatise on the Diseases of Women for the Use of Students and Practitioners.* New York: D. Appleton, 1890.

Stallworthy, John, and Gordon Bourne. *Recent Advances in Obstetrics and Gynecology.* London: J. A. Churchill, 1966.

Stewart, Felicia Hance, Gary K. Stewart, Felicia Jane Guest, and Robert A. Hatcher. *My Body, My Health: The Concerned Woman's Guide to Gynecology.* Clinician's Edition. New York: John Wiley and Sons, 1979.

Stoddard, F. Jackson. *Case Studies in Obstetrics and Gynecology.* Philadelphia: W. B. Saunders, 1964.

Sturgis, Somers H., and Doris Menzer-Benaron. *The Gynecologic Patient: A Psycho-Endocrine Study.* New York: Grune and Stratton, 1962.

Tait, Lawson. *Diseases of Women.* New York: William Wood, 1879.

Taylor, E. Stewart. *Essentials of Gynecology.* 4th ed. Philadelphia: Lea and Febiger, 1969.

Titus, Paul. *The Management of Obstetric Difficulties.* Revised by J. Robert Wilson. 5th ed. St. Louis, MO: C. V. Mosby, 1955.

Townsend, Lance. *Obstetrics for Students.* London: Melbourne University Press, 1964.

Webster, J. Clarence. *A Text-book of Diseases of Women.* Philadelphia: W. B. Saunders, 1907.

Wilson, J. Robert, Clayton T. Beecham, and Elsie Reid Carrington. *Obstetrics and Gynecology.* 5th ed. St Louis: C. V. Mosby, 1975.

Young, James. *A Text-Book of Gynecology for Students and Practitioners.* 6th rev. ed. London: Adam and Charles Black, 1944.

Notes

Introduction

Epigraph. Laqueur, *Making Sex*, 234.

1. Beasley, "Gynecologists Alarmed by Plastic Surgery Trend."

2. "Otto J. Placik, M.D., F.A.C.S.," *Labiaplastysurgeon.com*, accessed April 24, 2012, http://www.labiaplastysurgeon.com/dr-placik.html.

3. International Society of Cosmetogynecology, accessed April 25, 2012, http://www.iscgyn.com/en/index.php.

4. For examples of popular press coverage, see Singer, "'Recontouring' and Its Critics"; "Nips, Tucks, and . . . Designer Vaginas?" *National Research Center for Women & Families*, August 2007, http://center4research.org/medical-care-for-adults/breast-implants-and-other-cosmetic-procedures/nips-tucks-anddesigner-vaginas/; Rapaport, "Designer Vagina Surgery is a $5,500 Risk"; Childs, "Intimate Operations." For an overview of academic discussion on these surgeries, see Braun, "Female Genital Cosmetic Surgery."

5. Tiefer, "Activism on the Medicalization of Sex and Female Genital Cosmetic Surgery"; American College of Obstetricians and Gynecologists, "Vaginal 'Rejuvenation' and Cosmetic Vaginal Procedures."

6. American College of Obstetricians and Gynecologists, "Vaginal 'Rejuvenation' and Cosmetic Vaginal Procedures," 737. See also the Royal College of Obstetricians and Gynaecologists, "Ethical Considerations in Relation to Female Genital Cosmetic Surgery."

7. Goodman et al., "Large Multicenter Outcome Study."

8. Perry, *Straight Talk about Cosmetic Surgery.*

9. Duffy, "Masturbation and Clitoridectomy."

10. See, for example, Barker-Benfield, "A Historical Perspective on Women's Health Care"; and Barker-Benfield, *The Horrors of the Half-Known Life.* Others often cite the latter when briefly mentioning either clitoridectomy or female circumcision as male hostility toward female bodies. See, for example, Bermosk and Porter, *Women's Health and Human Wholeness.* Though her examination is more about Great Britain than the United States, Ann Dally noted the occurrence of clitoridectomy in the United States, a procedure that, according to Dally, "became a source of deep shame to an emerging profession." Dally, *Women under the Knife*, 160. Wendy Mitchinson found, in her examination of gynecological procedures on mentally ill women in late nineteenth-century Canada, at least one physician who performed surgery on the clitoris. Mitchinson, "Gynecological Operations on Insane Women."

11. See, for example, Morgan and Steinem, "International Crime."

12. In particular, Thomas Laqueur, though others have also written about medical interpretations of the clitoris, including Susan Lawrence and Kae Bendixen, Lisa Jean Moore and Adele C. Clarke, Margaret Gibson, Jennifer Terry, Nancy Tuana, and Darlaine Gardetto. Laqueur, "Amor Veneris"; Lawrence and Bendixen, "His and Hers"; Moore and Clarke, "Clitoral Conventions and Transgressions"; Gibson, "Clitoral Corruption"; Terry, *An American Obsession*; Terry, "Lesbians under the Medical Gaze"; Tuana, "Coming to Understand"; Gardetto, "Engendered Sensations." In addition, for a brief look at the external female genitals in history, see Drenth, *Origin of the World*.

13. Morris, *Naked Woman*, 215. Morris, a zoologist, refers to a physician in Texas in 1937 as advocating for the removal of the clitoris to cure frigidity, but he does not give a reference.

14. Please see the appendix for a discussion regarding the research I conducted using anatomy and gynecology texts, as well as a listing of the texts I examined.

15. Thank you to Joseph Pincus for stressing this point to me. See Gillis, "History of the Patient History"; and Warner, "Uses of Patient Records by Historians" for more on the use of textbooks as normative statements and how they reflect, or do not reflect, clinical practice.

16. Rosse, "Anatomical Atlases." Though both types of anatomy texts, as well as gynecology texts, deal with the seemingly stable human body, none were impervious to cultural forces in how authors represented bodies, and they typically viewed the male body as the standard. See Laqueur, *Making Sex*, and Schiebinger, *Nature's Body*, for more on the two-body frame. Alan Petersen is another scholar who used the two-body frame established by Laqueur when he examined *Gray's Anatomy* beginning with the first edition in 1858. He found the female body to be represented as the lesser body within these texts. Petersen, "Sexing the Body."

17. As Thomas Kuhn pointed out, textbooks are one of the core sources of authority in science. Kuhn, *Structure of Scientific Revolutions*.

18. Laqueur, "Amor Veneris," 97–98.

19. Moore and Clarke, "Clitoral Conventions and Transgressions"; Lawrence and Bendixen, "His and Hers."

20. Dickinson, *Human Sex Anatomy*, 42. The definition of homologous is "corresponding in structure, position, origin, etc." *Dorland's Illustrated Medical Dictionary*, 880.

21. Smout, *Basic Anatomy and Physiology*, 81.

22. Something Moore and Clarke, as well as Lawrence and Bendixen, observed. Moore and Clarke, "Clitoral Conventions and Transgressions"; Lawrence and Bendixen, "His and Hers."

23. Pitzman, *Fundamentals of Human Anatomy*, 146.

24. Spalteholz, *Hand-Atlas of Human Anatomy*, 624; Grant, *Method of Anatomy* (1944), 306; Grant, *Method of Anatomy* (1948), 316; Grant, *Method of Anatomy* (1958), 326.

25. Gardner, Gray, and O'Rahilly, *Anatomy* (1975). For additional examples, see Grant, *Atlas of Anatomy* (1951), figure 203; Grant, *Atlas of Anatomy* (1956), figure 203; Grant, *Atlas of Anatomy* (1962), figure 203.

26. Byford, *Manual of Gynecology* (1902), 19; Miller, *Introduction to Gynecology* (1934), 20–21; Philipp, *Obstetrics and Gynaecology*, 44.

27. Something Lawrence and Bendixen, as well as Moore and Clarke, argued. Lawrence and Bendixen, "His and Hers"; Moore and Clarke, "Clitoral Conventions and Transgressions."

28. Of course, seeing the clitoris as homologous with the penis stems also from evolutionary debates about whether the female orgasm—and the clitoris—was adaptive ("traits that have evolved to serve a particular fitness-enhancing role, and that is why they are prevalent") or exaptation (this term applies to two sorts of traits: "traits that are adapted for one evolutionary function, but were then coopted to service another function" as well as "traits that were correlates of growth or accidental byproducts that were later coopted to serve a role in current reproductive success.") Lloyd, *Case of the Female Orgasm*, 4, 170. For an excellent overview, as well as critique, of this debate, see Lloyd, *Case of the Female Orgasm*. Also see Gould, "Freudian Slip."

29. The only function of the clitoris is sexual, unlike the penis, an organ responsible for three functions: reproductive, excretive, and sexual. Not sharing all of the same functions is another possible reason for the more extensive information given to the penis.

30. Gray, *Anatomy* (1859), 683; Gray, *Anatomy* (1862), 747; Gray, *Anatomy* (1870), 812; Gray, *Anatomy* (1878), 868; Gray, *Anatomy* (1883), 899; Gray, *Anatomy* (1887), 977; Gray, *Anatomy* (1893), 1049; Gray, *Anatomy* (1897), 1165; Gray, *Anatomy* (1901), 1027; Gray, *Anatomy* (1905), 1480; Gray, *Anatomy* (1908), 1494; Gray, *Anatomy* (1913), 1419; Gray, *Anatomy* (1918), 1266; Gray, *Anatomy* (1924), 1276; Gray, *Anatomy* (1930), 1259; Gray, *Anatomy* (1936), 1254; Gray, *Anatomy* (1942), 1285; Gray, *Anatomy* (1948), 1318; Gray, *Anatomy* (1954), 1407; Gray, *Anatomy* (1959), 1381.

31. Mitchell and Patterson, *Basic Anatomy* (1954), 377; Gardner, Gray, and O'Rahilly, *Anatomy* (1960), 631; Gardner, Gray, and O'Rahilly, *Anatomy* (1963), 644; Gardner, Gray, and O'Rahilly, *Anatomy* (1969), 521; Gardner, Gray, and O'Rahilly, *Anatomy* (1975), 505.

32. Dawson, *Basic Human Anatomy*, 260; Christensen and Telford, *Synopsis of Gross Anatomy*, 99.

33. Dickinson, *Human Sex Anatomy*, 42.

34. Bell, *Principles of Gynecology*, 77.

35. Miller, *Introduction to Gynecology*, 20–21.

36. Roques, Beattie, and Wrigley, *Diseases of Women by Ten Teachers*, 5; Benson, *Handbook of Obstetrics and Gynecology* (1977), 4.

37. Behrman and Gosling, *Fundamentals of Gynecology*, 10.

38. Jung, Benjamin, and Earle, *Anatomy and Physiology* (1939), 548.

39. Cunningham, *Cunningham's Text-Book of Anatomy* (1937), 747; Frances, *Introduction to Human Anatomy* (1959), 478; Lumley, Craven, and Aitken, *Essential Anatomy*, 155.

40. Novak and Woodruff, *Novak's Gynecologic and Obstetric Pathology with Clinical and Endocrine Relations* (1962), 9; Greenhill, *Obstetrics* (1965), 67. Fritsch, *Diseases of Women*, 2; Byford, *Manual of Gynecology* (1902), 19; Bell, *Principals of Gynecology*, 77; Miller, *An Introduction to Gynecology*, 20–21.

41. Morris, *Human Anatomy* (1898), 1040.

42. Gardner, Gray, and O'Rahilly, *Anatomy* (1960), 631; Gardner, Gray, and O'Rahilly, *Anatomy* (1963), 644; Gardner, Gray, and O'Rahilly, *Anatomy* (1969), 521; Gardner, Gray, and O'Rahilly, *Anatomy* (1975), 505; Wilson and Wilson, *Human Anatomy*, 384.

43. Morrill, *The Physiology of Woman*, 25; Fritsch, *The Diseases of Women*, 2.

44. Crossen and Crossen, *Diseases of Women*, 98.

45. Spence and Mason, *Human Anatomy and Physiology*, 773; Gardner and Osburn, *Structure of the Human Body*, 381.

46. Jung, Benjamin, and Earle, *Anatomy and Physiology*, 548.

47. Morrill, *Physiology of Woman*, 25.

48. May, *Diseases of Women*, 40–41.

49. Miller, *Introduction to Gynecology* 33; Crossen and Crossen, *Diseases of Women*, 98; Crossen, *Diseases of Women* (1953), 110. Crossen also stated that because the clitoris was so sensitive, clitoridectomy was proposed to relieve "sexual hyperesthesia, but the results were not such as to recommend the operation, and it is now rarely practiced"; Crossen, *Diseases of Women*, 110.

50. Kistner, *Gynecology: Principles and Practice* (1973), 25; Kistner, *Gynecology: Principles and Practice* (1979), 25.

51. Jeffcoate, *Principles of Gynaecology*, 24.

52. Stewart et al., *My Body, My Health*, 8.

53. Beacham and Beacham, *Synopsis of Gynecology* 3.

54. Philipp, Barnes, and Newton, eds. *Scientific Foundations of Obstetrics and Gynaecology* (1977), 70.

55. Philipp, Barnes, and Newton, eds. *Scientific Foundations of Obstetrics and Gynaecology* (1977), 138.

56. Elisabeth Lloyd noted many methodological problems with these studies, including sample sizes, the use of women of similar backgrounds extrapolated to the larger female population, and the reliability of self-reporting. Lloyd, *Case of the Female Orgasm*, 39–41.

57. Ibid., 38.

58. See ibid., esp. 233.

59. I agree with Rachel Maines's assertion that there was only one form of sex regarded as healthy for white middle class women: vaginal, penetrative, and married. But in contrast to her contention that "the role of the clitoris in arousal to orgasm was systematically misunderstood" by physicians "since its function contradicted the androcentric principal that only an erect penis could provide sexual satisfaction to a healthy, normal adult female," the history of surgery on the clitoris shows that physicians understood the role of the clitoris even as they sought to maintain a narrow view of what healthy sex meant. Maines, *Technology of Orgasm*, 9–10.

60. Of course, we must take into consideration the reliability of the physician's description of patients. For more on female patients' voices read through published medical articles and monographs and for how women negotiated with their doctors their mutual understanding of illness, see Theriot, "Negotiating Illness."

61. As Bernard Rudofsky pointed out decades ago, the female body perhaps has never looked "good" until modified. Rudofsky, *Unfashionable Human Body*.

Chapter One

1. Polak, "Case of Nymphomania," 301–2.

2. Laqueur, "Amor Veneris," 91. I am extending Laqueur's argument beyond 1905, where he ends. Though Freud declared the vaginal orgasm as the "healthy" orgasm for mature women to be experiencing in 1905, his view does not appear to have taken a foothold in medical and sexual advice literature until after World War II, an era when psychoanalysis in general became part of the cultural and medical fabric in the United States.

3. Reed, "Doctors, Birth Control, and Social Values," 113.

4. Wallerstein, *Circumcision*, 36. According to Wallerstein, the US Patent Office issued about twenty patents for devices to prevent masturbation, the earliest recorded in 1861 and the latest in 1932. See also Spitz, "Authority and Masturbation," 389. Laqueur, in his history of masturbation, lists the following appliances invented to stop masturbation: "erection alarms, penis cases, sleeping mitts, bed cradles to keep the sheets off the genitals, hobbles to keep girls from spreading their legs." Laqueur, *Solitary Sex*, 46.

5. Warner, "From Specificity to Universalism"; Starr, *Social Transformation of American Medicine*.

6. Roy, "Surgical Gynecology," 185–86.

7. Wilde, "Truth, Trust, and Confidence in Surgery."

8. Morantz-Sanchez, *Conduct Unbecoming a Woman*.

9. Russett, *Sexual Science*.

10. Groneman, *Nymphomania*, xxii.

11. Waiss, "Reflex Neuroses from Adherent Prepuce in the Female," 280.

12. Beebe, "Clitoris," 9.

13. Ibid., 8–12.

14. Robinson, "Clitoris," 22.

15. Pancoast, *Ladies' New Medical Guide*, 56; Melendy, *Perfect Womanhood*, 60.

16. D'Emilio and Freedman, *Intimate Matters*, 266–67.

17. Fellman and Fellman, "Rule of Moderation."

18. Alcott, *Physiology of Marriage*, 120.

19. Guernsey, *Plain Talk on Avoided Subjects*, 92–95.

20. Taylor, *Practical Treatise*, 414; Beebe, "Clitoris," 11.

21. Beebe, "Clitoris," 11.

22. Cooper, "Removing the Clitoris in Cases of Masturbation," 19; Hale, "Two Cases of Imprisoned Clitoris," 446.

23. Abbott, "Importance of Circumcision of the Female," 439.

24. Howe, *Excessive Venery*, 71–72.

25. Smith, "Masturbation in the Female," 78.

26. La Vake, *A Handbook of Clinical Gynecology*, 26.

27. Beebe, "Clitoris," 11.

28. Engelhardt, "Disease of Masturbation," 13; Newman, "Masturbation, Madness," 1–2, 5.

29. Gollaher, "From Ritual to Science," 20.

30. Engelhardt, "Disease of Masturbation," 13–14, 16. For a more thorough discussion of why it became such a force during this time, see Laqueur, *Solitary Sex*. Also see Haller and Haller, *Physician and Sexuality in Victorian America*.

31. Newman, "Masturbation, Madness," 8.

32. Laqueur, *Solitary Sex*, 21, 210, 202.

33. Smith-Rosenberg and Rosenberg, "Female Animal," 121.

34. In the 1953 *Sexual Behavior in the Human Female*, Alfred Kinsey and his coauthors wrote in a footnote that "the dominance of labial and clitoral techniques is widely recognized in both the European and American literature. See, for instance: Anon., Histoire du Vice n.d.: 74. Rosenbaum 1845:137. Moraglia 1897: 5–7. Kisch 1907: 107. Moll 1909: 82; 1912:90. Back 1910: 112–13. Adler 1911:116. Rohleder 1921: 14. Moll 1926(1): 292. Roland 1927:30. Bauer 1929:234. Kelly 1930: 166, 169–70. Dickinson and Beam 1931: 351 (66 per cent of more than 400 cases used vulvar friction). Meagher and Jelliffe 1936: 70. Dearborn in Fishbein and Burgess 1947: 365." Kinsey et al., *Sexual Behavior in the Human Female*, 158.

35. Walkowitz, "Dangerous Sexualities," 370.

36. Sahli, "Sexuality and Woman's Sexual Nature"; Degler, "What Ought to Be and What Was."

37. Beebe, "Clitoris," 9.

38. Bloch, "Sexual Perversion in the Female," 4.

39. Laqueur, *Making Sex*, 227.

40. Gollaher, *Circumcision*, 79–80.

41. Shorter, *From Paralysis to Fatigue*, 20–23.

42. Abbott, "Importance of Circumcision of the Female," 438.

43. Theriot, "Women's Voices in Nineteenth-Century Medical Discourse."

44. Taylor, *Practical Treatise*, 422.

45. Kelly, *Medical Gynecology*, 292.

46. Taylor, *Practical Treatise*, 414, 422.

47. Robinson, "Clitoris," 18–23.

48. Robinson, *Woman*, 289.

49. Miller, *Introduction to Gynecology*, 22.

50. Pryor, *Gynaecology*, 103.

51. Sligh, "Adherent Prepuce in the Female," 217.

52. Bacon, "Adhesions of the Female Prepuce," 278–79.

53. Robinson, *Landmarks in Gynecology*, 5.

54. Kelly and Noble, *Gynecology and Abdominal Surgery*, 810.

55. Reed, *Diseases of Women*, 3.

56. Dudley, *Diseases of Women*, 424.

57. Sligh, "Adherent Prepuce in the Female," 215–16.

58. Sligh, "Adherent Prepuce in the Female," 218.

59. Kelly, *Medical Gynecology*, 298.

60. Hale, "Two Cases of Imprisoned Clitoris," 446.

61. Beebe, "Clitoris," 12.

62. Costain, "Circumcision." For more on the history of female patients insisting on specific treatments during this time, see Leavitt, *Brought to Bed*; Morantz-Sanchez, *Conduct Unbecoming a Woman*; Morantz-Sanchez, "Negotiating Power at the Bedside"; Houck, *Hot and Bothered*; and Marsh and Ronner, *The Fertility Doctor*. See also Powderly, "Patient Consent and Negotiation."

63. Waiss, "Reflex Neuroses from Adherent Prepuce," 281.

64. Kistler, "Rapid Bloodless Circumcision," 1782.

65. Beebe, "Clitoris," 9.

66. Cooper, "Removing the Clitoris in Cases of Masturbation," 17–20.

67. Taylor, *Practical Treatise*, 417.

68. Groneman, *Nymphomania*, xxii.

69. Southwick, *Practical Manual of Gynecology*, 180.

70. Howe, *Excessive Venery*, 108–9; Taylor, *Practical Treatise*, 415.

71. Taylor, *Practical Treatise*, 422.

72. Cooke, *Satan in Society*, 112.

73. Taylor, *Practical Treatise*, 422.

74. "Case of Excessive Masturbation," 141–42. "Lupulin," definition, Drugs.com, accessed July 13, 2013, http://www.drugs.com/dict/lupulin.html.

75. "Case of Excessive Masturbation," 142.

76. Eyer, "Clitoridectomy for the Cure," 259.

77. Eyer, at least in this article, seemed mostly concerned with use of this treatment in girls.

78. Howe, *Excessive Venery*, 110; Bloch, "Sexual Perversion in the Female," 4; Engelmann, "Clitoridectomy," 1.

79. Shorter, *From Paralysis to Fatigue*, 81.

80. "Case of Idiocy in a Female." This article was listed under the Foreign Department, and I believe it came from either France or Germany.

81. Tanner, "On Excision of the Clitoris."

82. Though he did not invent the operation, his work is the most discussed when it comes to the history of clitoridectomy in the West. Many have looked at Brown's work, including Guy, "Clitoris Martyr"; Scull and Favreau, "Chance to Cut Is a Chance to Cure"; Scull and Favreau, "Clitoridectomy Craze"; Black, "Female Genital Mutilation"; and Sheehan, "Victorian Clitoridectomy."

83. Fleming, "Clitoridectomy."

84. Brown, *On the Curability of Certain Forms*, vii. Brown was not, however, consistent in recording the ages or the marital status of all the women upon whom he operated.

85. Brown, *On the Curability of Certain Forms*, 17–18.

86. Fleming, "Clitoridectomy," 1019, 1022. The other major medical publication in Britain, *The Lancet*, however, remained silent during this time, something at least one contemporary observer believes is due to the editor of the *BMJ*, W. O. Markham, having animosity toward Brown based on a charge Markham laid while both were physicians at St. Mary's Hospital in 1858. Markham accused Brown of charging one of the female patients, something prohibited at a voluntary hospital. Though this accusation was dropped, it was just the first regarding improper interactions with patients by Brown. Fraser, "Female Genital Mutilation."

87. As Scull and Favreau noted in their history of Brown and his use of clitoridectomy, his activities raised serious concern about the gentlemanly status physicians were still trying to secure. Medical elites, wrote Scull and Favreau, were "extraordinarily sensitive about behavior that threatened the profession's social standing." Indeed, that Brown aggressively marketed himself to nonphysicians was very troublesome to his peers. Before his book appeared in 1866, Brown sought and received a favorable review in a popular newspaper. Brown, according to Scull and Favreau, appeared to his peers to be seeking public favor ahead and instead of professional approval. Many wrote letters to the *BMJ* with the same sentiments as Robert

Greenhalgh, who stated that Brown's efforts to woo the public were "offensive" and "fraught with considerable danger to the morals of the public and high tone of the profession." This charge was made stronger by the appearance of an article in the *Church Times* endorsing clitoridectomy and urging pastors to recommend it to their parish and by the fact that Brown sent an annual report to numerous nonmedical people. Indeed, one letter to the *BMJ* commented that Brown sent his annual report to "half the nobility in the kingdom" and ended by saying how "astounded" he was at the thought of some "innocent curate going about recommending his easy little operation for 'distressing cases of illness.'" A Provincial F.R.C.P., "Mr. Baker Brown's Operation," 478; Scull and Favreau, "Clitoridectomy Craze," 252–54; Greenhalgh, letter to the editor, 730. Brown's quest for popular approval independent of the approval of his peers raised the specter of quackery among his fellows. Scull and Favreau, "Clitoridectomy Craze," 254.

88. Winslow, letter to the editor, 706.

89. Fleming, "Clitoridectomy," 1026, 1029.

90. Gwillim, "President's Address."

91. "Clitoridectomy," *Southern Journal of the Medical Sciences*, 794.

92. "Dr. Baker Brown of London," 442.

93. Howe, *Excessive Venery*, 110–11.

94. Engelmann, "Clitoridectomy," 2.

95. Ibid., 2.

96. Storer, "On Self Abuse in Woman," 456.

97. Ibid., 422.

98. Wylie, "Amputation of the Clitoris," 722.

99. Frederick, "Nymphomania as a Cause of Excessive Venery," 743–44.

100. Atkinson, *Therapeutics of Gynecology and Obstetrics*, 156.

101. Mills, "Case of Nymphomania," 538–39.

102. Taylor, *Practical Treatise*, 422.

103. Shorter, *From Paralysis to Fatigue*, 208.

104. Engelmann, "Clitoridectomy," 2–7, 11–12.

105. Munde, "Mental Disturbances," 53–55.

106. Mills, "Case of Nymphomania," 534–35.

107. See Groneman, *Nymphomania*, 24–25, for a longer discussion about this patient and Mills.

108. For an interesting look at how kleptomania was also made into a disease to explain aberrant behavior, see Abelson, "Invention of Kleptomania."

Chapter Two

1. Eyer, "Clitoridectomy for the Cure," 259–60.

2. Graetzer, *Practical Pediatrics*, 321.

3. Sauer, *Nursery Guide for Mothers*, 133.

4. For more on "masturbatory insanity" as a diagnosis and its basis in maintaining the asexual child or the sexually controlled adolescent male, see Neuman, "Masturbation, Madness."

5. Egan and Hawkes, "Imperiled and Perilous," 329.

6. Sauer, *Nursery Guide for Mothers*, 133. That girls masturbated more than boys was not a universally accepted opinion.

7. Kerr, *Care and Training of Children*, 221.

8. Meagher, *Study of Masturbation*, 68.

9. Freeman, *Elements of Pediatrics for Medical Students*, 96–97.

10. Holt, *Care and Feeding of Children*, 195–96.

11. Goodhart and Still, *Diseases of Children*, 715.

12. Cooke, *Satan in Society*, 111.

13. Goodhart and Still, *Diseases of Children*, 715.

14. Ibid., 715.

15. Hale, "Two Cases of Imprisoned Clitoris," 448.

16. Willard, *Surgery of Childhood*, 199, 203.

17. Neuman, "Masturbation, Madness."

18. Freeman, *Elements of Pediatrics for Medical Students*.

19. Adair, *Obstetrics and Gynecology*, 485.

20. Kerley, *Treatment of the Diseases of Children*, 434.

21. Smith, *Baby's First Two Years*, 63.

22. Tomes, *Gospel of Germs*.

23. Abbott, "Importance of Circumcision of the Female," 438.

24. Hall, *Adolescence*, 436.

25. Brill, "Masturbation," 98.

26. Pryor, *Gynaecology*, 103.

27. Fischer, *Baby and Growing Child*, 150–51.

28. Morris, "Is Evolution Trying to Do Away with the Clitoris?," 2nd ed., 127.

29. Grandin, "Role of the Clitoris," 145.

30. Cotton, *Medical Diseases of Infancy and Childhood*, 389–90.

31. Graham, *Diseases of Children*, 571.

32. Wilcox, "Phimosis and Adherent Hood of the Clitoris," 339–40.

33. Koplik, *Diseases of Infancy and Childhood*, 807–8.

34. Davison, *Complete Pediatrician*, number 247 (no page numbers in book).

35. Lucas, *Modern Practice of Pediatrics*, 695; Litchfield and Dembo, *Therapeutics of Infancy and Childhood*, 3:2545–46.

36. Freeman, *Elements of Pediatrics for Medical Students*, 96–97.

37. Dudley, *Diseases of Women*; Dudley, *Principles and Practice of Gynecology* (1902); Dudley, *Principles and Practice of Gynecology* (1908).

38. Wilcox, "Phimosis and Adherent Hood of the Clitoris," 340.

39. Green, *Case Histories in Diseases of Women*, 7.

40. Hawkes, "Rational Treatment of Prepuce," 354.

41. Kerley, *Treatment of the Diseases of Children*, 434–35.

42. For boys, this could include urethral rings with spikes inside them that would spear an erect penis, thus presumably encouraging the penis to become less excited and enlarged. See images inserted after p. 43 in Stengers and Van Neck, *Masturbation*. Some physicians, however, disavowed such restraints, increasingly so by the early twentieth century.

43. Litchfield and Dembo, *Therapeutics of Infancy and Childhood*, 2:1729–30. L. Emmett Holt believed that while physically restraining an infant from masturbating may end the practice, "with older children they usually make matters worse." He,

like many of his peers, however, believed that older children needed to be watched, taught self-control, and rewarded for not masturbating. Holt, *Care and Feeding of Children*, 195–96. George M. Tuttle, a St. Louis physician, agreed with this sentiment. Tuttle, *Diseases of Children*.

44. Sauer, *Nursery Guide for Mothers*, 133.

45. Griffith and Mitchell, *Diseases of Infants and Children* (1927), 2:572; Griffith and Mitchell, *Diseases of Infants and Children* (1934), 895–96.

46. Sauer, *From Infancy through Childhood*.

47. Gollaher, *Circumcision*, 100, 104. See his "From Ritual to Science" for more on circumcision's use to prevent masturbation as well on other diseases, ranging from cancer to STDs. Though the focus of this chapter is masturbation through clitoral stimulation, concern also existed at this time for the solitary act when performed by men and boys. Advice to males instructed them to avoid masturbation or their manly energies would be depleted. See Gibbs, "Self Control and Male Sexuality." Doctors noted "peevishness, listlessness, pallor, and headaches in men and boys who practiced the 'secret vice' of masturbation." Wood, "Fashionable Diseases," 223.

48. Gollaher, "From Ritual to Science," 22–23; Sorrells, "History of Circumcision in the United States." The United States was the only country where the overwhelming majority of infant males were circumcised for health reasons, and until the 1950s there was little opposition to routine male circumcision in the United States. Wallerstein, "Circumcision." Ironically, a 1997 study showed that circumcised men masturbated more often than men who were not circumcised. Laumann et al., "Circumcision in the United States." In 1999, the American Academy of Pediatrics (AAP) issued new recommendations stating that the benefits of circumcision were "not significant enough for the AAP to recommend circumcision as a routine procedure." Task Force on Circumcision, American Academy of Pediatrics, "Circumcision Policy Statement" (1999). The AAP revised their guidelines in 2012, however, pointing to some medical benefits for infant male circumcision but still leaving the final decision to the parents. Task Force on Circumcision, American Academy of Pediatrics, "Circumcision Policy Statement" (2012). In addition to the references given above, for more on the history of male circumcision, also see Grossman and Posner, "Circumcision Controversy." For two older historical perspectives, see Conrad, "Side Lights on the History of Circumcision"; and Jacobs, "Circumcision."

49. Burnett, "Clitoris," 202.

50. Walls, "Circumcision," 511.

51. Costain, "Circumcision," 160.

52. Morris, "Circumcision in Girls," 136.

53. Hassler, "Preputial Adhesions in Little Girls," 185.

54. Eskridge, "Why Not Circumcise the Girl," 18–19.

55. Dawson, "Circumcision in the Female," 521.

56. Pratt, "Circumcision of Girls," 385, 392.

57. Rutkow, "Edwin Harley Pratt and Orificial Surgery," 558–63.

58. Hsu, "Orificial Surgery," 7.

59. Rutkow, "Edwin Harley Pratt and Orificial Surgery," 560–63.

60. Meagher, "Quackery de Luxe," 224.

61. Ashton, *Text-Book of the Practice of Gynecology*, 159.

62. Morse, *Case Histories in Pediatrics*, 511.

63. Dudley, *Principles and Practice of Gynecology* (1908), 526.

64. Cooper, "Removing the Clitoris in Cases of Masturbation," 17–20.

65. Sutcliffe, "Excision of the Clitoris," 64.

66. Sutcliffe, "Excision of the Clitoris," 64.

67. Colby, "Mechanical Restraint," 206.

68. Koplik, *Diseases of Infancy and Childhood*, 807–8.

69. Dudley, *Principles and Practice of Gynecology* (1908), 526.

70. Bolling, *Surgery of Childhood*, 355.

71. Meagher, *Study of Masturbation*, 112.

72. Schauffler, *Pediatric Gynecology*, 53.

73. Mason, "Hypertrophy of the Clitoris," 144–46.

74. Holt, *Diseases of Infancy and Childhood*, 746; Holt and Howland, *Diseases of Infancy and Childhood* (1916), 718; Holt and Howland, *Diseases of Infancy and Childhood* (1933), 780; Holt and Howland, *Holt's Diseases of Infancy and Childhood* (1940), 944.

75. Shorter, *From Paralysis to Fatigue*, 45, 201–3.

76. Dennett, *Sex Side of Life*, 14.

77. Newman, "Masturbation, Madness," 13.

78. Laqueur, *Solitary Sex*, 66–69.

79. Holt and Howland, *Holt's Diseases of Infancy and Childhood* (1940), 943.

80. Mitchell, *Mitchell-Nelson Textbook of Pediatrics* (1945), 1018.

81. Schauffler, *Pediatric Gynecology*, 63.

82. Spock, *Common Sense Book*, 303.

83. Schauffler, *Pediatric Gynecology*, 47, 50–51, 53.

84. Mitchell, *Mitchell-Nelson Textbook of Pediatrics* (1945), 1018.

85. Mitchell, *Mitchell-Nelson Textbook of Pediatrics* (1945), 1018.

86. Spock, *Common Sense Book*, 304.

87. Lief, "Sex Education of Medical Students and Doctors," 23.

88. Schauffler, *Pediatric Gynecology*, 52.

89. Schauffler, "Persistent Vaginal Discharge," 645.

90. Levinson, *Pediatric Nursing*, 278.

91. Holt and Howland, *Holt's Diseases of Infancy and Childhood* (1940), 943.

92. Litchfield and Dembo, *Therapeutics of Infancy and Childhood*, 2:1729–30.

93. Mitchell, *Mitchell-Nelson Textbook of Pediatrics* (1945), 1018.

94. Holt and Howland, *Holt's Diseases of Infancy and Childhood* (1940), 944.

95. Parsons and Barling, *Diseases of Infancy and Childhood*, 1365–66.

96. Again, as Thomas Kuhn pointed out, textbooks are one of the core sources of authority in science. Kuhn, *Structure of Scientific Revolutions*.

97. Feibleman, "Natural Causes."

98. Coventry, "Making the Cut."

99. Robinett, *Rape of Innocence*.

100. McDonald, "Circumcision of the Female," 98. This physician also thought it stopped bed-wetting.

101. Council on Scientific Affairs, American Medical Association, "Female Genital Mutilation," 1714. Their reference for this practice is Hanny Lightfoot Klein, who in turn cites Fran Hosken's *WIN News* from 1980–82. Klein, *Prisoners of Ritual*, 180.

Chapter Three

1. Lichtenstein, "'Fairy' and the Lady Lover," 372.
2. Kisch, *Sexual Life of Woman*, 330.
3. Gibson, "Clitoral Corruption," 114.
4. Haller, "Physician versus the Negro." See also Weiner and Hough, *Sex, Sickness, and Slavery*.
5. Horn, "This Norm Which Is Not One."
6. Cole, "Fingerprint Identification and the Criminal Justice System."
7. Terry and Urla, "Introduction."
8. Not all doctors agreed with this. For example, American gynecologist Robert Latou Dickinson in 1902 stated, "All observers agree that there is no change in the outer genitalia in prostitutes" because of their profession. Dickinson, "Hypertrophies of the Labia Minora," 247.
9. Much good historical work has been done on this topic. Kessler, *Lessons from the Intersexed*; Kessler, "Medical Construction of Gender"; Dreger, "Hermaphrodites in Love"; Dreger, *Hermaphrodites and the Medical Invention of Sex*; Fausto-Sterling, *Sexing the Body*; Reis, "Impossible Hermaphrodites"; Reis, *Bodies in Doubt*; and Eder, "Volatility of Sex." See also Kenen, "Scientific Studies of Human Sexual Difference in Interwar America"; Preves, "Sexing the Intersexed"; Preves, *Intersex and Identity*; Epstein, "Either/Or—Neither/Both"; Crouch, "Betwixt and Between"; and Hausman, *Changing Sex*.
10. Horn, "This Norm Which Is Not One," 109.
11. Goodell, "Masturbation in the Female," 226.
12. Dunglison, *Medical Lexicon* (1854), 214.
13. Dunglison, *Medical Lexicon* (1900), 244.
14. Greene, *Lippincott's Medical Dictionary*, 228.
15. "Masturbation," *Boston Medical and Surgical Journal*, 102.
16. Buck, "Hypertrophy of the Clitoris," 22.
17. Gould and Pyle, *Anomalies and Curiosities of Medicine*, 309.
18. Beebe, "Clitoris," 8, 11.
19. Mitchell, *Mitchell-Nelson Textbook of Pediatrics* (1959), 79.
20. Bigelow, "Aggravated Instance of Masturbation," 440.
21. Ashwell, *Practical Treatise on the Diseases Peculiar to Women*, 501.
22. Hor and Sprague, "Case of Nymphomania," 62.
23. Taylor, *Practical Treatise*, 416.
24. Howe, *Excessive Venery*, 71.
25. Kellogg, *Plain Facts for Old and Young*, 199, 286.
26. Platt, "Hypertrophy of the Clitoris," 104.
27. Gallabin, *A Handbook of the Diseases of Women*, 333–34.
28. Winckel, *Diseases of Women: A Handbook for Physicians' Students*, 32.
29. Dickinson, "Hypertrophies of the Labia Minora," 238.
30. See Auchincloss, "Expiration of Enlarged Clitoris"; Bainbridge, "Case of Enlarged Clitoris"; Dawson, "Hypertrophy of the Clitoris"; Bumstead, "Hypertrophied Clitoris"; Potter, "Case of Enormous Hypertrophy of Clitoris"; Helmuth, *A Dozen Cases of Clinical Surgery*; Kelly, "Elephantiasis of the Clitoris"; Buck, "Hypertrophy of the Clitoris."

31. Dawson, "Hypertrophy of the Clitoris," 97.

32. Buck, "Hypertrophy of the Clitoris," 22.

33. Keating, *Clinical Gynecology, Medical and Surgical*, 242.

34. Dudley, *Principles and Practice of Gynecology* (1908), 526.

35. Clark, *Treatise on the Medical and Surgical Diseases of Women*, 46.

36. Ballantyne, "Malformations of the Genital Organs in Woman," 97.

37. "Removal of Hypertrophied Clitoris by Excision," *Medical Press*.

38. Madden, *Clinical Gynecology*, 62.

39. Curtis, *A Textbook of Gynecology* (1938), 20.

40. Miller, *An Introduction to Gynecology*, 20.

41. Fritsch, *Diseases of Women*, 2; Crossen and Crossen, *Diseases of Women*, 98; Young, *A Text-Book of Gynecology for Students and Practitioners*, 3.

42. Tait, *Diseases of Women* (1879), 28.

43. Berkeley and Bonney, *Guide to Gynecology in General Practice* (1919), 268.

44. Smith, "Masturbation in the Female," 77.

45. Dickinson and Pierson, "Average Sex Life of American Women," 1113.

46. Dickinson, *Human Sex Anatomy*.

47. Dickinson and Pierson, "Average Sex Life of American Women," 1113; emphasis in original.

48. Dickinson, *Human Sex Anatomy*, 45, 53. Kinsey asked female students at Indiana University in private about the length of their clitorises. Gathorne-Hardy, *Sex the Measure of All Things*, 132. Kinsey also tried to measure them himself on the women he interviewed. He noted clitorises as long as three inches, and some women in peep shows had four-inch clitorises. Bullough, *Science in the Bedroom*, 185.

49. Dickinson and Pierson, "Average Sex Life of American Women," 1115–16.

50. Howell, *Gross Anatomy*, 372.

51. Gray, *Anatomy* (1893), 1049; Giles, *Anatomy and Physiology of the Female Generative Organs* (1909), 11.

52. Grant, *Atlas of Anatomy* (1943), 119.

53. Helmuth, *A Dozen Cases of Clinical Surgery*, 5.

54. Birn, Pillay, and Holtz, *Textbook of International Health*.

55. Dewees, *Treatise on the Diseases of Females*, 25.

56. Clark, *Treatise on the Medical and Surgical Diseases of Women*, 46.

57. Winckel, *Diseases of Women*, 32.

58. Dudley, *Principles and Practice of Gynecology* (1908), 526.

59. Kelly and Noble, *Gynecology and Abdominal Surgery*, 810.

60. Knott, "Normal Ovariotomy," 34–35.

61. Bovee, *Practice of Gynecology*, 64–65. Bovee, it should be noted, believed that if Caucasian women masturbated, they too would suffer a "moderate degree of hypertrophy" of the labia (64).

62. See Schiebinger, *Nature's Body*.

63. Buck, "Hypertrophy of the Clitoris," 22–23.

64. Dudley, *Principles and Practice of Gynecology* (1908), 526.

65. Bovee, *Practice of Gynecology*, 64–65.

66. Morris, "Is Evolution Trying to Do Away with the Clitoris?," 1st ed., 126–28; emphasis in original.

67. Keating, *Clinical Gynecology, Medical and Surgical,* 242.

68. Matas, "Surgical Peculiarities of the Negro," 492.

69. Haller, *Outcasts from Evolution;* Schiebinger, *Nature's Body.*

70. Byrd and Clayton, *African American Health Dilemma.*

71. Spongberg, "Are Small Penises Necessary for Civilization?"

72. Haller, *Outcasts from Evolution,* 51.

73. "Genital Peculiarities of the Negro," *Atlanta Journal-Record of Medicine,* 842.

74. Giddings, "Last Taboo."

75. Guy-Sheftall, "Body Politic," 359.

76. Hoffman, "Race Traits and Tendencies of the American Negro," 202; emphasis in original.

77. Roberts, "Paradox of Silence and Display," 42, 44–45. See also Omolade, "Hearts of Darkness." Omolade notes that, in the early twentieth century, some African American women broke from their community's paternal restraints and "were castigated for seeming to reflect the truth of the white man's views of black women as whorish and loose," something epitomized by the blues (374).

78. Greenlee-Donnell, "White Man Has Got Hattie."

79. As Deborah Willis noted in the introduction to a book she recently edited about Baartman, many of the facts of Baartman's life have become both distorted and mythologized; indeed, scholars cannot even agree on the spelling of her name. Willis, "Introduction."

80. Hobson, *Venus in the Dark,* 1.

81. Ibid., 17, 46. Gould, "Hottentot Venus"; Sharpley-Whiting, *Black Venus;* Fields, *Intimate Affair;* and Fields, "From Black Venus to Blonde Venus."

82. Gould, "Hottentot Venus," 294, 299.

83. Gilman, *Difference and Pathology.* Gilman also noted that though black men were seen as sexually primitive as well, their genitals did not become the focus of dissections (89).

84. Magubane, "Which Bodies Matter?," 47–61.

85. The forty-eight texts, with the exception of Smith, *Anatomical Atlas,* are indicated by an asterisk in the appendix listing the anatomy texts I examined for other parts of this book.

86. Literature scholar Siobhan Somerville, in her article on the intersections of racism and the homosexual body, noted that comparative anatomists in the late nineteenth century "repeatedly located racial difference through the sexual characteristics of the female body." The *American Journal of Obstetrics,* she wrote, "was a frequent forum for these debates." However, after looking through several volumes (at random) published between 1877 and 1906 of this journal, I only found one such discussion: the one in the 1877 volume cited by Somerville. Somerville, "Scientific Racism and the Emergence of the Homosexual Body," 251. I looked through nine other volumes: vol. 15 (July–October 1882), vol. 18 (1885), vol. 21 (1888), vol. 24 (January–June 1891), vol. 28 (July–December 1893), vol. 32 (July–December 1895), vol. 39 (January–June 1899), vol. 49 (January–June 1904), and vol. 54 (July–December 1906). Vol. 32 had one article that spoke about "unusually large and well developed" labia but without a reference to race. It was, rather, a report of unusual things seen that year at Methodist Hospital in Philadelphia by the gynecologist-author. Shoemaker, "Malformations of Female Genitalia," 216. My search, being

random, however, does not mean that such discussion did not happen—though I do wonder how frequently they occurred in this journal.

I searched for the following terms in IndexCat, with the number of "hits" in parenthesis: Negro and clitoris (0); warm climates and clitoris (0); warm climates and genitals (0); tropical climates and clitoris (0); tropical and genitals (2, neither relevant, both about nontropical cases of elephantiasis in the 1930s); southern and clitoris (0); southern and genitals (0); African and clitoris (0); African and genitals (1 related): Drennan, "Pudenda of South African Bushwoman"; black and clitoris (0); Negress and clitoris (0); negress and clitoris (0); Negress and genitals (2 related): Parrish, "Tumors of Left Labium"; and Moseley, "Elephantiasis Arabum." Search done on April 10, 2012. Of course, my lack of finding other possibly relevant articles may indicate that such articles were indexed in a manner outside of the search terms I used.

87. "Genital Peculiarities of the Negro," *Atlanta Journal-Record of Medicine*, 842.

88. Schumann, "Observations on the Comparative Anatomy of the Female Genitalia."

89. Turnispeed, "Some Facts in Regard to the Anatomical Difference," 32.

90. Editorial note, *American Journal of Obstetrics*, 33.

91. Hyatt, "Note on the Normal Anatomy of the Vulvo-Vaginal Orifice," 254, 256.

92. Editorial note, *American Journal of Obstetrics* (April 1877), 256–58.

93. Fort, "Some Corroborative Facts in Regard to the Anatomical Difference," 259.

94. Savitt, *Race and Medicine.*

95. Parrish, "Tumors of Left Labium," 229. The infant died shortly after birth; Parrish did not attend to her during her labor. Of further interest is that one doctor asked another to go see this young woman—did he do so out of medical curiosity or perhaps concern? Regardless, several medical men were involved in her care.

96. Moseley and Morison, "Elephantiasis Arabum," 462–63.

97. Kelly, "Elephantiasis of the Clitoris," 227–30.

98. Moseley and Morison, "Elephantiasis Arabum," 462.

99. Hoffman, "Vital Statistics of the Negro," 534.

100. See, for example, Zimmerman, "A Comparative Study of Syphilis"; and Reverby, *Examining Tuskegee.*

101. Helmuth, *A Dozen Cases of Clinical Surgery*, 6.

102. Crenner, "Race and Medical Practice," 823, 835.

103. Crenner, "Race and Medical Practice."

104. Savitt, *Race and Medicine.*

105. Byrd and Clayton, *African American Health Dilemma.* See also Beardsley, "Race as a Factor in Health."

106. Dickinson, "Hypertrophies of the Labia Minora," 231, 234–35.

107. Gilman, *Difference and Pathology*, 89.

108. Collins, *Black Sexual Politics*, 193, 198.

109. Somerville, "Scientific Racism and the Emergence of the Homosexual Body."

110. Terry, *American Obsession*, 36.

111. Bland, "Trial by Sexology?"; Beccalossi, *Female Sex Inversion.*

112. Gibson, "Clitoral Corruption," 116. Bullough and Voght, "Homosexuality and Its Confusion."

113. See for example Foucault, *History of Sexuality*; and Katz, *Invention of Heterosexuality*.

114. Terry, *American Obsession*, 40–42. See also Hansen, "American Physicians' 'Discovery' of Homosexuals, 1880–1900."

115. Terry, "Anxious Slippages.'"

116. Terry, *American Obsession*, 70, 74–75, 77–78. Chauncey, "From Sexual Inversion to Homosexuality."

117. Parke, *Human Sexuality*, 319.

118. Smith-Rosenberg, *Disorderly Conduct*.

119. Terry, "Anxious Slippages," 129.

120. Laqueur, *Making Sex*.

121. Gardetto, "Engendered Sensations," 101. Some doctors viewed the large clitoris as a sign of lesbianism. Ambroise Paré in 1573 equated a large clitoris with "tribadism" and recommended removing the organ. The British doctor Nicholas Culpepper a century later similarly saw them as connected and recommended the organ's amputation. Traub, "Psychomorphology of the Clitoris," 314.

122. Terry, *American Obsession*, 86.

123. Terry, "Anxious Slippages" 129.

124. Wise, "Case of Sexual Perversion," 89–90. See Gamwell and Tomes, *Madness in America*, for a longer discussion about ideas concerning madness and sexual behavior.

125. Gibson, "Clitoral Corruption," 122.

126. Parvin, "Nymphomania and Masturbation," 51.

127. The text further noted the organ could be removed without risk. *Dr. Groves' Reproductive Physiology*, 21.

128. Somerville, "Scientific Racism and the Emergence of the Homosexual Body."

129. Beccalossi, *Female Sex Inversion*, 107. See also her article, "Female Same-Sex Desires."

130. Gibson, "Clitoral Corruption," 124.

131. Bigelow, "Aggravated Instance of Masturbation in the Female," 436–37.

132. Terry, "Anxious Slippages," 135.

133. Freud, "Three Essays on the Theory of Sexuality," 195.

134. Young-Bruehl, *Freud on Women*, 19, 24, 28.

135. Freud, *New Introductory Lectures on Psycho-Analysis*, 172.

136. Creed, "Lesbian Bodies," 116.

137. Traub, "The Psychomorphology of the Clitoris," 301–2.

138. Terry, *American Obsession*, 69.

139. Potter, *Strange Loves*, 149.

140. Caprio, *Female Homosexuality*, 20.

141. Kelly, *Sexual Feeling in Women*, 149.

142. As Erin Carlston pointed out in her essay on lesbians and doctors in the interwar period, though there was an increase in medical writings about lesbianism, medicine did not necessarily define how those women saw themselves. Carlston, "Finer Differentiation."

143. Terry, "Anxious Slippages," 138. Terry is not the only scholar to have examined this study. Heather Lee Miller also briefly discusses it in "Sexologists Examine Lesbians and Prostitutes."

144. Terry, "Anxious Slippages," 139; Terry, *American Obsession*, 198.

145. Terry, "Anxious Slippages," 139.

146. Terry, "Anxious Slippages"; Terry, *American Obsession*.

147. Terry, *American Obsession*, 178–79, 186, 190–91, 196, 198, 203; Henry, *Sex Variants*; Haller, *Outcasts from Evolution*.

148. Dickinson, "Gynecology of Homosexuality," in Henry, *Sex Variants*, 1047, 1086, 1088, 1083, 1108, 1094–95, 1083, 1108, 1085, 1092–93, 1096, 1088–89, 1093–94.

149. Terry, "Anxious Slippages."

150. Dickinson, "Gynecology of Homosexuality," 1095–97.

151. Ibid., 1102, 1110, 1125.

152. Terry, *American Obsession*, 204–5.

153. Ibid., 243.

154. Barkan, *Retreat of Scientific Racism.*

155. Terry, *American Obsession*, 207–8.

156. Dickinson, "Gynecology of Homosexuality," 1079, 1047, 1080–81; emphasis in original.

157. Terry, "Anxious Slippages," 151.

Chapter Four

1. Bernardy, "Report of Cases of Aneroticism in Women," 51.

2. Ibid.

3. I did find one instance where a physician removed the entire clitoris. This 1901 case was apparently done to stop the woman from masturbating as much as it was to assist in marital relations. During the late nineteenth century, Clement Cleveland examined a patient who complained to her doctor of unpleasant marital relations. Eighteen and married to a man ten years her senior, the woman confessed to her doctor that she masturbated. Cleveland labeled the woman "excessively nervous and excitable" and upon physical examination discovered a large clitoris. Believing the organ to be hindering her marital relations, Cleveland performed a clitoridectomy. The woman's relations with her husband, the doctor reported, "vastly improved." Though Cleveland wrote that the woman's sexual relations with her husband improved, other aspects of their relationship had not, as the doctor also reported that the woman attempted to shoot her husband and then ran away to China. I note this example, however, as a good case to show how marital relations were considered to be serious enough to warrant a surgical intervention when relations were unsatisfactory for the woman. Cleveland, "Amputation of the Clitoris," 722–23.

4. Schauffler, *Pediatric Gynecology*, 50.

5. Walkowitz, "Dangerous Sexualities," 370.

6. Rothman, *Hands and Hearts*, 103, 245–46.

7. Celello, *Making Marriage Work.*

8. Jordan, *Little Problems of Married Life*, 20.

9. Coontz, *Marriage, a History.*

10. Degler, "What Ought To Be and What Was." Like many eras, there was diversity of thought on sexuality and sexual behavior in the late nineteenth century. Free lovers, for instance, were never a large percentage of the population, but their existence

means that one cannot write off the era as completely shunning sexuality outside marriage. See Battan, "World Made Flesh." Moreover, some women within the free love movement challenged the idea that sexual drive was purely a male attribute. See DuBois and Gordon, "Seeking Ecstasy on the Battlefield"; Stearns and Stearns, "Victorian Sexuality"; and Sahli, "Sexuality and Woman's Sexual Nature"; for a more thorough discussion of the complexities of sexuality in the late nineteenth century. Also see D'Emilio and Freedman, *Intimate Matters*, for more about the history of sexuality in the United States. For an early twentieth-century perspective, see Lindsey and Evans, *Companionate Marriage*. Lindsey believed sex with birth control was vital to a healthy marriage and advocated for nonprocreative sex as a means to save marriage, restoring sex to "wholesome sense and sanity" (154). Many thought he advocated unmarried sex or trial marriage, something he denied (see his preface).

11. Smith, "Dating of the American Sexual Revolution," 330; D'Emilio and Freedman, *Intimate Matters*, 266–67.

12. Guernsey, *Plain Talk on Avoided Subjects*, 95–96.

13. Fellman and Fellman, "Rule of Moderation," 251.

14. Kent, *Sexual Neuroses*, 21.

15. Perry thought that if women's "rights were properly attended to at home there would be less talk of women's rights at the ballot-box and less violation of the civil code." Apparently, American women owe a good deal to bad sex at the turn of the last century. Perry, "Sexual Hunger," 6.

16. Kolischer, "Sexual Frigidity in Women," 416.

17. Griswold, "Some Observations on the Physiology," 449.

18. Sahli, "Sexuality and Woman's Sexual Nature," 83; Degler, "What Ought to Be and What Was," 471.

19. Haller and Haller, *Physician and Sexuality in Victorian America*, 97; Gordon, "From an Unfortunate Necessity," 64–66.

20. Groves, *Marriage Crisis*, 1.

21. Celello, *Making Marriage Work*.

22. Collins, *Doctor Looks at Marriage and Medicine*, 15. The term "keelson," according to *Merriam-Webster*, is "a longitudinal structure running above and fastened to the keel of a ship in order to stiffen and strengthen its framework." *Merriam-Webster OnLine*, s.v. "keelson," accessed April 8, 2014, http://www.merriam-webster.com/dictionary/keelson.

23. Wortis, "Counseling in the Premarital Interview," 86.

24. Stone, "Marriage Education and Marriage Counseling," 38–39, 50.

25. Jung, "Course in Modern Marriage," 43, 50.

26. Simmons, *Making Marriage Modern*, 185.

27. Stone, "Marriage Education and Marriage Counseling," 38–39, 50.

28. Mudd and Rose, "Development of Marriage Counsel," 40–41.

29. Stone, "Marriage Education and Marriage Counseling," 38–39, 50.

30. Schroeder, "Background Factors in Divorce," 72.

31. Celello, *Making Marriage Work*, 37–38. As Celello detailed in her book, these clinics were mostly interested in educating those who were young, white, and middle class, and some of the marriage education movement's strongest proponents had eugenic beliefs.

32. Davis, *Factors in the Sex Life*, 63, 66.

33. Hamilton, *Research in Marriage*, 147.
34. Neuhaus, "Importance of Being Orgasmic."
35. Walters, *Primers for Prudery*, 11.
36. Willman, *Married Life*, 51.
37. Malchow, *Sexual Life*, 70.
38. Neuhaus, "Importance of Being Orgasmic," 454.
39. Simmons, *Making Marriage Modern*, 183.
40. Neuhaus, "Importance of Being Orgasmic," 460.
41. Simmons, *Making Marriage Modern*, 184.
42. Van de Velde, *Ideal Marriage*, 6.
43. Simmons, *Making Marriage Modern*, 188.
44. Exner, *Sexual Side of Marriage*, 34; emphasis in original.
45. Duvall and Hill, *When You Marry*, 128, 131.
46. Exner, *Sexual Side of Marriage*, 34, 113.
47. Van de Velde, *Ideal Marriage*, 165.
48. Neuhaus, "Importance of Being Orgasmic," 457.
49. Van de Velde, *Ideal Marriage*, 169. In a 1914 paper, W. C. Rivers called cunnilingus "manifestly utilitarian, the purpose served, besides the obvious one of excitation, being that of lubricating the genitals." Rivers, a British physician, noted the work of Havelock Ellis, who stated that "the number of women who find the cunnilingus agreeable" is great. Rivers, "New Theory of Kissing," 255, 262.
50. Costler and Willy, *Encyclopedia of Sexual Knowledge*, 190.
51. Van de Velde, *Ideal Marriage*, 145.
52. Gordon, "From an Unfortunate Necessity."
53. Ibid.
54. Stone and Stone, *Marriage Manual*, 53.
55. Arden, *Handbook for Husbands and Wives*, 27.
56. Butterfield, *Sex Life in Marriage*, 98.
57. Everett, *Hygiene of Marriage*, 126.
58. Rutgers, *How to Attain and Practice the Ideal Sex Life*, 256.
59. Duvall and Hill, *When You Marry*, 138.
60. Harris, *Essays on Marriage*, 120, 123.
61. Everett, *Hygiene of Marriage*, 127; emphasis in original.
62. Long, *Sane Sex Life*, 124–25. Long also encouraged wives, when they are not able to engage in intercourse, to "take *his* penis in *her* hand and 'play with it' till he *spent*" (125; emphasis in original).
63. Neuhaus, "Importance of Being Orgasmic," 457.
64. Exner, *Sexual Side of Marriage*, 116–17.
65. Both men (twenty) and women (eight) also listed fellatio. Hamilton, *Research in Marriage*, 178.
66. Ibid., xi, 174–75, 178.
67. M.D., New York, "Masturbation in Women," 1564.
68. Everett, *Hygiene of Marriage*, 123.
69. Dickinson, *Thousand Marriages*, vii, ix, x, 4, xv, 38–39. Dickinson saw three hundred of these women for more than a decade. The average ages of the women in this study was between thirty-one and thirty-five, and most were white and middle class (21).

70. Ibid., 79–80, 62, 107, 66, 63.

71. Dickinson, "Medical Analysis of *A Thousand Marriages*," 529–35.

72. Simmons, *Making Marriage Modern*; Celello, *Making Marriage Work*.

73. May, *Great Expectations*, 90–108.

74. Ullman, *Sex Seen*, 97, Celello, *Making Marriage Work*. See Peter Laipson for a discussion of the sexual scripts directing male performance and making the man the responsible member in charge of orgasm for both himself and his wife. Laipson, "Kiss without Shame."

75. Dickinson, *Thousand Marriages*, 130.

76. Hamilton, *Research in Marriage*, 157.

77. Robinson, *Woman*, 235.

78. Neuhaus, "Importance of Being Orgasmic"; Bullough, *Science in the Bedroom.* Simmons, *Making Marriage Modern*; Celello, *Making Marriage Work*.

79. Dickinson, *Thousand Marriages*, 129.

80. Starr, *Social Transformation of American Medicine*; Rosenberg, *Care of Strangers*; Numbers, "The Fall and Rise of America's Medical Profession."

81. Iiams, "Female Circumcision," 171–73.

82. Martensen, "Physiology as Destiny," 1213.

83. Bacon, "Adhesions of the Female Prepuce," 278–79; Taylor, *Practical Treatise*, 414.

84. Taylor, *Practical Treatise*, 414.

85. Bacon, "Adhesions of the Female Prepuce," 278–79.

86. Arden, *Handbook for Husbands and Wives*, 14.

87. Morris, "Is Evolution Trying to Do Away with the Clitoris?," 2nd ed., 130.

88. Bernardy, "One of the Causes of Aneroticism in Women," 426–32.

89. Ibid., 426–28.

90. Clark, *Emotional Adjustment in Marriage*, 218.

91. Alfred C. Kinsey, Individual Variation Lecture, lecture 8, Spring 1940 (February 28, 1940), Alfred C. Kinsey Collection. According to Kinsey biographer James H. Jones, this condition was perhaps what prevented Clara Kinsey from reaching orgasm during intercourse with her husband early in their marriage. Jones stated that the Kinseys consulted a local physician, Dr. Thomas Reed, who, after diagnosing Clara Kinsey's condition as an adherent clitoris, "performed the necessary surgery, which consisted of pulling back the veil of connective tissue over the clitoris and performing a blunt dissection under local anesthetic." Jones wrote that Alfred Kinsey told one of his female students the name of the doctor who broke up his wife's clitoral adhesions for a three dollar fee, thus enabling her clitoris to protrude from its hood and receive more direct stimulation during penetrative intercourse. Jones, *Alfred C. Kinsey*, 236, 334, 356. However, in his biography of Alfred Kinsey, published a year later, Jonathan Gathorne-Hardy noted that if, as Jones contended, Clara Kinsey had her adherent clitoris freed, this would not have corrected what Jones claimed was the initial reason for their visit to Reed, which was a difficulty in penetration. But Gathorne-Hardy also noted that this "may well have been an additional problem." Gathorne-Hardy, *Sex the Measure of All Things*, 468. I could not find evidence for what procedure (if indeed any) Clara Kinsey underwent.

92. Duvall and Hill, *When You Marry*, 140–41.

93. Abbott, "Importance of Circumcision of the Female," 438–39. In the book *Strange Loves: A Study in Sexual Abnormalities*, the word "circumcision" in the index stated that it was the "removal of the foreskin, or portion of clitoris." Potter, *Strange Loves*, 241.

94. Waiss, "Reflex Neuroses from Adherent Prepuce in the Female," 279, 282–83.

95. Stewart, "Circumcision of the Preputium Clitoridis," 216–17.

96. Lane, "Remarkable Results following Female Circumcision," 155–56. Lane also noted how circumcision stopped bed-wetting, and he called on physicians to not be shy about looking to the condition of the clitoris "in any obscure condition in the female" (156).

97. Lewis, "Gynecologic Consideration of the Sexual Act," 225.

98. Ibid., 224.

99. Hollander, "51st Landmark Article," 228–29.

100. Lewis, "Gynecologic Consideration of the Sexual Act," 226–27.

101. Curtis, *Textbook of Gynecology* (1938), 20.

102. Curtis, *Textbook of Gynecology* (1942), 1946.

103. Exner, *Sexual Side of Marriage*, 116–17.

Chapter Five

1. Kroger, "Psychosomatic Aspects of Frigidity and Impotence," 386–87, 394.

2. Ibid., 387.

3. Ibid., 389.

4. Hale, *Rise and Crisis of Psychoanalysis*.

5. Lewis, *Prescriptions for Heterosexuality*; Gerhard, *Desiring Revolution*.

6. Gerhard, *Desiring Revolution*; Neuhaus, "Importance of Being Orgasmic."

7. Gould, "Freudian Slip," 18.

8. Historian Rachel Maines wrote that the vaginal orgasm had become by the 1930s the "dominant paradigm of normative female sexuality" and that it persisted "well into the 1970s." Maines, *Technology of Orgasm*, 112. In her article and book on the medical enforcement of heterosexuality during the Cold War, historian Carolyn Herbst Lewis argued that the vaginal orgasm theory was the "dominant narrative on 'normal' female sexuality" and there was "little dissent" from physicians "well into the 1960s." Lewis, "Waking Sleeping Beauty," 86–87; Lewis, *Prescription for Heterosexuality*, 41.

9. Laqueur, "Amor Veneris," 92.

10. Hale, *Beginnings of Psychoanalysis*, 15, 25.

11. Bullough, *Science in the Bedroom*, 90.

12. Gay, *Freud*, 501–2.

13. Harding, "Introduction," 6.

14. Hale, *Beginnings of Psychoanalysis*, 15, 25.

15. Freud, "Three Essays on the Theory of Sexuality," 221.

16. Gay, *Freud*, 515–19. Clara Thompson later challenged this theory as not being an envy of the penis but rather envy of the position of power in society held by those with a penis. Thompson, "Penis Envy in Women"; and Thompson, "Some Effects of the Derogatory Attitude towards Female Sexuality."

17. Freud, "On the Sexual Theories of Children," 217.

18. Gay, *Freud*, 515–19.

19. Freud, "On the Sexual Theories of Children," 217–18; Gay, *Freud*, 515–19.

20. And it also created a latency period between female sexual identities, a moment that created additional instability in their sexual development to maturity. Those analysts who strove to further Freud's ideas worked to solve this concern by making heterosexuality essential to the female body. Gerhard, *Desiring Revolution*, 30–31.

21. Gay, *Freud*, 517–19. Karen Horney and Helene Deutsch both came up with other ideas for the development of female sexuality, though both ultimately believed women were dependent upon men to be fully awakened to healthy and normal heterosexuality. For a larger discussion, see Gerhard, *Desiring Revolution*; Buhle, *Feminism and Its Discontents*; and Gay, *Freud*. See Bennett, "Critical Clitoridectomy," for a discussion on psychoanalyst theorists' inability to embrace the clitoris as an autonomous site of female sexual agency.

22. Scholes, *Semiotics and Interpretation*, 137.

23. According to Gay, psychoanalysts concerned with this theory "did not yet have sufficient clinical or experimental information about the female orgasm to question Freud's thesis" that women needed to graduate from clitoral to vaginal pleasure to reach sexual maturity. But this is doubtful, given how physicians understood the clitoris during this time. Gay, *Freud*, 185, 502, 519. See also Laqueur, "Amor Veneris," for his argument that, prior to 1905, "no one thought there was any other sort of female orgasm than the clitoral sort" (91).

24. Laqueur, "Amor Veneris," 94.

25. Appignanesi and Forrester, *Freud's Women*, 425–27. Freud's writings on women, Gay stated, were "just another demonstration just how over determined his ideas were." Gay, *Freud*, 502.

26. Laqueur, "Amor Veneris," 94.

27. Kinsey et al., *Sexual Behavior in the Human Female*, 584.

28. Hale, *Rise and Crisis of Psychoanalysis*, 181, 304, 177, 225, 397.

29. Burnham, "Psychoanalysis and American Medicine."

30. Gerhard, *Desiring Revolution*.

31. Robie, *Art of Love*, 100.

32. Reich, "The Function of Orgasm," 1148; Fine, *History of Psychoanalysis*, 208.

33. Faulkner and Pruitt, *Dear Dr. Menninger*, 153–57.

34. Gerhard, *Desiring Revolution*, 39–40.

35. Buhle, *Feminism and Its Discontents*, 214.

36. Hitschmann and Bergler, *Frigidity in Women*, 45; Gerhard, "Revisiting 'The Myth of the Vaginal Orgasm,'" 457.

37. Hitschmann and Bergler, *Frigidity in Women*, 4, 20.

38. Gerhard, *Desiring Revolution*, 40–43. Gerhard posited that Freudian views of female sexuality, especially the vaginal orgasm theory, were strongest in the 1940s.

39. Zaretsky, *Secrets of the Soul*, 130, 276.

40. Engel, *American Therapy*, 43. Engel maintained that the general openness of American society to "heresy and innovation" was why the United States was "so receptive to psychoanalytic theory" (14).

41. Buhle, *Feminism and Its Discontents*, 170–71.

42. Laqueur, *Making Sex*, 73.
43. Hale, *Rise and Crisis of Psychoanalysis*, 9, 82, 187, 211–12, 214, 276, 382. However, few became psychoanalysts, even during the 1950s, with a small core group of only several hundred, according to historian John C. Burnham. Burnham, *Paths into American Culture*.
44. Bullough, *Science in the Bedroom*, 148, 85–86.
45. Burnham, *Paths into American Culture*, 99.
46. Hale, *Rise and Crisis of Psychoanalysis*, 9, 82, 187, 211–12, 214, 276, 382.
47. Zaretsky, *Secrets of the Soul*, 276–77. See also Gerhard, *Desiring Revolution*, for a discussion of how Helene Deutsch and Karen Horney also reworked Freud's ideas in ways that more positively reflected female experience and valued female sexuality.
48. Buhle, *Feminism and Its Discontents*, 171.
49. May, *Homeward Bound*.
50. Evans, *Born for Liberty*.
51. As Joanne Meyerowitz argued, "while no serious historian can deny the conservatism of the postwar era or the myriad constraints that women encountered, an unrelenting focus on women's subordination erases much of the history of the postwar years," and it "tends to downplay women's agency and to portray women primarily as victims." Meyerowitz, "Introduction," 1–2, 4. See other recent works examining the dynamic quality of American women and families in the 1950s, such as Weiss, *To Have and to Hold*.
52. Hamilton, "Frigidity in the Female," 1041–42.
53. Lewis, "Waking Sleeping Beauty," 90.
54. Gerhard, "Revisiting 'The Myth of the Vaginal Orgasm,'" 454, 458. See also Gerhard, *Desiring Revolution*. Looking at the history of the social constructions of the clitoris and female orgasm, Darlaine Gardetto suggested that doctors linked the "clitoris and female orgasm to gender by implying that the clitoris was an organ that threatened 'real womanhood.'" She asserted that the clitoral/vaginal orgasm debate during the twentieth century was an extension of a much longer discourse among doctors about what to make of women seemingly having two separate sexual organs. Gardetto, "Engendered Sensations," 3, 8.
55. Kroger and Freed, *Psychosomatic Gynecology*, 299.
56. Greenhill, "Frigidity in Women," 146.
57. Lundberg and Farnham, *Modern Woman*, v, 7, 270, 266.
58. Gordon, *Moral Property of Women*, 255–57, 265, 267–69, 270–71.
59. Robinson, *Power of Sexual Surrender*, 23, 32, 62, 61, 99. But note here that Robinson says clitoral sensitivity "often diminishes," indicating that it may not cease.
60. Bergler, "Problem of Frigidity," 571–73, 581.
61. Robinson, *Power of Sexual Surrender*, 23, 32, 62, 61, 99.
62. Hamilton, "Frigidity in the Female," 1040, 1046, 1041.
63. Lewis, "Waking Sleeping Beauty," 101.
64. Bergler, "Problem of Frigidity," 581.
65. Hamilton, "Frigidity in the Female," 1040, 1046, 1041.
66. Hitschmann and Bergler, *Frigidity in Women*, 3.
67. Rutherford et al., "Psychosomatic Testings in Frigidity and Infertility," 72–74.
68. Lundberg and Farnham, *Modern Woman*, v, 7, 270, 266.
69. Podolsky, "Causes and the Management," 265.

70. Ibid.
71. Lundberg and Farnham, *Modern Woman*, v, 7, 270, 266.
72. Kroger and Freed, "Psychosomatic Aspects of Frigidity and Impotence," 526.
73. Bergler and Kroger, "Dynamic Significance," 715.
74. Bergler, "Some A-typical Forms of Impotence and Frigidity," 43.
75. Greenhill, "Frigidity in Women," 145.
76. Hamilton, "Frigidity in the Female," 1040.
77. Rosen, "Male Response to Frigidity," 135.
78. Bergler and Kroger, "Sexual Behavior," 167–68.
79. Kroger and Freed, *Psychosomatic Gynecology*, 295.
80. Bergler, "Some A-typical Forms of Impotence and Frigidity," 43–44.
81. Bergler, "Newer Genetic Investigations on Impotence and Frigidity," 57.
82. Ibid.
83. Marmor, "Some Considerations concerning Orgasm in the Female," 240. On Marmor being a psychiatrist in Los Angeles, see "Judd Marmor," *American Medical Directory* (1955), 239.
84. Gay, *Freud*, 185, 502, 519. Karen Horney's work in particular was a direct challenge to the penis envy theory and thus a more subtle challenge to the vaginal orgasm theory, as was the work of Melanie Klein. See Gerhard, *Desiring Revolution*, for a longer discussion of their work.
85. In his biography of Alfred Kinsey, historian James Jones noted that scientists were "embroiled in heated debate on the clitoral versus the vaginal orgasm." Jones, *Alfred C. Kinsey*, 694. Carol Groneman, in her history of nymphomania, briefly indicated this debate when she noted that "supporters and detractors" of the vaginal orgasm, particularly Kinsey, debated the vaginal orgasm theory in professional journals during this time. However, she further noted that the public was not so engaged until the work of William Masters and Virginia Johnson "substantially undermined" the vaginal orgasm theory in 1966. I tentatively agree with Groneman that the vaginal orgasm theory was popularly reported upon and even popularly embraced. Groneman, *Nymphomania*, 91. And in her history of the medical enforcement of heterosexuality, Carolyn Herbst Lewis noted there were "voices of dissent within the medical profession that challenged what was quickly becoming the dominant position on the matter." Lewis, *Prescriptions for Heterosexuality*, 53.
86. According to Kroger and Bergler, proponents of the clitoral orgasm theory often combined it with the "vagueness theory, . . . which assumes that orgasm in women involves the whole nervous system without differentiating between clitoric and vaginal orgasm. The 'vagueness theory' of female orgasm fallaciously interprets the fact that the vagina has few nerves, and conveniently overlooks the other fact that orgasm is cortically regulated." Bergler and Kroger, "Dynamic Significance," 712.
87. "Frigidity in Women," *Minnesota Medicine*, 1880.
88. Rutherford et al., "Frigidity in Women," 78.
89. The vaginal orgasm as the route to mature and healthy female sexuality may have come to prevail within psychoanalysis, but it did not go unchallenged during the 1920s and 1930s, in particular but not exclusively by women within the discipline. Many women, like Melanie Klein, were actively engaged in the field in the 1920s; indeed, in 1929, the majority of new trainees were women, and their presence influenced the field. But as psychoanalysis became more institutionalized within

medicine and medical school as part of the growth of psychiatry, fewer and fewer women became analysts because fewer women were admitted to medical school. This dominance of men resulted in the tone of psychoanalysis reflecting the idea that men were dominant and women were passive, a tone that gained particular strength following World War II. Zaretsky, *Secrets of the Soul.*

90. McGuire and Steinhilber, "Sexual Frigidity," 418–19.

91. Moore, "Frigidity in Women," 571–72.

92. Deutsch, *Psychology of Women,* 80–81. See also Bonaparte, *Female Sexuality.*

93. Moore, "Frigidity in Women," 571–72.

94. Fine, *History of Psychoanalysis,* 211.

95. Moore, "Frigidity in Women," 571–72.

96. See Jane Gerhard, *Desiring Revolution,* for a discussion of how Helene Deutsch and Karen Horney also reworked Freud's ideas in ways that more positively reflected female experience and valued their sexuality.

97. Fine, *History of Psychoanalysis,* 212.

98. Glenn and Kaplan, "Types of Orgasm in Women."

99. Moore, "Frigidity in Women," 574.

100. Lewis, "Waking Sleeping Beauty," 91; emphasis in original.

101. In a letter to Kroger and Freed, B. Morales "stressed the need for clarifying terminology" regarding frigidity. According to Morales, frigidity was the "complete and absolute absence of pleasurable response to erotic stimuli of any kind." A woman, then, was seemingly not frigid if she experienced a clitoral orgasm. Kroger and Freed, *Psychosomatic Gynecology,* 297, 312.

102. "Frigidity in Women," *Minnesota Medicine,* 1881.

103. Novak, *Gynecological Therapy,* 59.

104. Alexander Lowen, the executive director of the Institute for Bio-Energetic Analysis in New York City, noted at a symposium held in the late 1950s addressing frigidity in women that "probably no fiction has been more exploited in our culture than the idea that a woman who does not have sexual relations is frigid." Lowen, "Frigidity," 258. This lack of uniformity of meaning is further reflected in dictionary definitions. For example, a 1958 dictionary of psychoanalytic terms defined frigidity as "an abnormal lack of sexual feeling" and most often used in reference to women. English and English, *Comprehensive Dictionary of Psychological and Psychoanalytical Terms,* 217. Further, a dictionary of psychology in 1964 defined frigidity as the "absence of normal sexual desire, especially with reference to a woman," which was "often a symptom of mental disorder." Drever, *Dictionary of Psychology,* 103.

105. Bergler, "Problem of Frigidity," 569.

106. "Frigidity in Women," *Minnesota Medicine,* 1881.

107. McGuire and Steinhilber, "Sexual Frigidity," 416.

108. Layman, Rozan, and Kurland, "Frigidity in the Female," 103–4.

109. Bergler, "Newer Genetic Investigations on Impotence and Frigidity," 58.

110. Ritmiller and Nicodemus, "Frigidity in the Female," 1214; emphasis in original.

111. Layman, Rozan, and Kurland, "Frigidity in the Female," 103–4.

112. Greenhill, "Frigidity in Women," 145.

113. Ritmiller and Nicodemus, "Frigidity in the Female," 1214.

114. Brady, "Brevital-Relaxation Treatment of Frigidity."

115. Stoddard, *Case Studies in Obstetrics and Gynecology*, 169.

116. Rutherford, "Problem of Pelvic Dis-ease," 156.

117. Odlum, "Revision Corner," 737.

118. If none were found, Greenhill, like Rutherford, felt safe to "assume that emotional problems are present which interfere with adequate sexual response." Greenhill, "Frigidity in Women," 146.

119. Novak, *Gynecological Therapy*, 59.

120. Kupperman, "Hormonal Aspects of Frigidity."

121. Curtis and Huffman, *Textbook of Gynecology*, 97.

122. Physical treatment of the female body for (hopefully pleasurable) hetero-sexual intercourse was not limited to the clitoris; Carolyn Herbst Lewis, for example, noted that physicians often ruptured a woman's hymen to enable vaginal penetra-tion. Lewis, *Prescriptions for Heterosexuality*.

123. The "frigidity ointment" consisted of "Camphor 6 per cent, Menthol 3 per cent, Oleoresin capsicum ⅛ per cent, Petroleum ½ ounce." Hudgins, "Doctor as Marital Counselor," 478. Information on Hudgins being an obstetrician gynecologist found in *American Medical Directory* (1961), 2087.

124. Podolsky, "Sexual Frigidity in Women," 459, 464.

125. In her later analysis, Buhle spent a few paragraphs on how those who advo-cated for the prominence of the vaginal orgasm enjoyed an only "unstable lead." Buhle, *Feminism and Its Discontents*, 215.

126. Rutherford et al., "Frigidity in Women," 78.

127. Bergler and Kroger, "Dynamic Significance," 711.

128. Glenn and Kaplan, "Types of Orgasm in Women." See Balint, "On the Termination of Analysis."

129. Glenn and Kaplan, "Types of Orgasm in Women."

130. Brill, *Basic Principles of Psychoanalysis*.

131. Fodor and Gaynor, *Freud*, 142.

132. English and English, *Comprehensive Dictionary of Psychological*, 91.

133. Bergler and Kroger, "Dynamic Significance," 713.

134. Hitschmann and Bergler, "Frigidity in Women," 52.

135. Bergler, "Newer Genetic Investigations on Impotence and Frigidity," 56; emphasis in original.

136. Bergler, *Unhappy Marriage and Divorce*, 94.

137. Hitschmann and Bergler, "Frigidity in Women," 45, 52.

138. *The New Georgia Encyclopedia*, s.v. "G. Lombard Kelly (1890–1972)," accessed July 15, 2011, http://www.georgiaencyclopedia.org/nge/Article.jsp?id=h-2668.

139. Hitschmann and Bergler, "Frigidity in Women," 45–46.

140. Ibid., 49–50.

141. Bergler and Kroger, "Dynamic Significance," 713.

142. Ibid., 712.

143. In response to *Sexual Behavior in the Human Female*, *JAMA* took the unusual step of commissioning two reviews by two people "widely known in their fields." The reviewers, like many others, were critical of his nonrepresentational population. But the first reviewer also questioned Kinsey's "understanding of such psychosexual phe-nomena as 'vaginal orgasm,'" because Kinsey seemed to lack "awareness of the fact

that we are dealing with a complex psychobiological phenomenon" in female sexual response. Review of *Sexual Behavior in the Human Female*, 1045.

144. Bergler and Kroger, "Sexual Behavior," 167–68. In 1954, Bergler and Kroger published *Kinsey's Myth of Female Sexuality*. The reviewer in *JAMA* stated that the book "abounds in criticism and refutation" of Kinsey's work, making much of "the vaginal orgasm" while also claiming that Kinsey's "disregard" for it was due to his "lack of knowledge of the anatomy and physiology of the vaginal walls." While stating that the "average reader" would find *Kinsey's Myth* "difficult to read," the *JAMA* reviewer recommended it to practitioners. "Since the subject of sex behavior in the human female is now so prominently before the profession and the public, physicians, other scientists, and public health workers who have read the Kinsey reports should also read this critical commentary on his work." Review of *Kinsey's Myth of Female Sexuality*, 1390.

145. Hamilton, "Frigidity in the Female," 1040.

146. Robinson, *Power of Sexual Surrender*, 23, 32, 62, 61, 99.

147. Jones, *Alfred C. Kinsey*; Gathorne-Hardy, *Sex the Measure of All Things*; Gould, "Of Wasps and WASPS."

148. Kinsey et al., *Sexual Behavior in the Human Female*, 568.

149. Kinsey interviewed nearly eight thousand women but did not use all of the interviews because 915 were taken from a prison population. They differed so much from the other interviews that he believed they skewed the entire study. Nor did he include the 934 nonwhite women they interviewed because the sample was not large enough to warrant comparisons with the larger white group. Kinsey et al., *Sexual Behavior in the Human Female*, 3, 6, 22.

The core of Kinsey's research was the personal interview. From 1938 through 1956, he, along with his three associates, Wardell Pomeroy, Clyde Martin, and Paul Gebhard, interviewed eighteen thousand men and women on sex for about two hours each. Kinsey worked to ensure the validity of the information obtained in the interview by assuring absolute confidentiality, by being a sympathetic, nonjudgmental interviewer, and by inventing a coding system to record information quickly. The sample used for his research was not truly random and relied on volunteers (it was also heavily composed of midwesterners, prison inmates, and gay men and lesbian women), but Kinsey stuck to his volunteer base instead of trying to coax full reports out of randomly selected people. Robinson, *Modernization of Sex*.

150. Kinsey et al., *Sexual Behavior in the Human Female*, 358, 361–63, 375, 12.

151. Ibid., 282, 358, 361–63, 375, 12.

152. Jones, *Alfred C. Kinsey*, 694.

153. Kinsey et al., *Sexual Behavior in the Human Female*, 574–80.

154. Ibid., 576, 582. Kinsey had become close friends with Robert L. Dickinson and was apparently influenced by his older friend regarding female sexuality. Terry, *American Obsession*, 302–3.

155. Kinsey et al., *Sexual Behavior in the Human Female*, 582, 584. Robinson, *Modernization of Sex*, 47.

156. Gathorne-Hardy, *Sex the Measure of All Things*, 159. According to Gathorne-Hardy, "One of the most noticeable things in both the *Male* and *Female* volumes is Kinsey's unconcealed hostility to, and contempt for, psychoanalysis and in particular Freudian psychoanalysis." Kinsey labeled it "philosophy," and he meant it as pejorative

222   NOTES TO PP. 112–113

term, according to Gathorne-Hardy, who also argued that Kinsey's hostility was more "intense than mere criticism of their science would warrant" and that it "also had a profound emotional and irrational base. . . . He was frightened of them" (252–53).

157. Risen, *History of Psychoanalysis*, 484. Risen also claims Kinsey failed to understand Freud's ideas.

158. Gathorne-Hardy, *Sex the Measure of All Things*; Jones, *Alfred C. Kinsey*.

159. Hale, *Rise and Crisis of Psychoanalysis*, 297. Fellow scientists also criticized Kinsey, specifically regarding his nonrandom volunteer sample. Because his book made assumptions and editorialized freely, people found it easy to attack. The center of the assault was primarily from moralists who thought Kinsey threatened American feminine wholesomeness. Bullough, *Science in the Bedroom*, 175, 180–81. Despite, or perhaps as a result of, the controversy, the female report sold faster than the male report, with the publisher putting out the sixth edition, printing 185,000 copies two weeks after the original came off the press. Gathorne-Hardy, *Sex the Measure of All Things*, 401. Many ministers cried the loudest; Billy Graham, for example, worried that "it is impossible to estimate the damage this book will do to the already deteriorating morals of America." Jones, *Alfred C. Kinsey*, 720.

160. Historians John D'Emilio and Estelle Freedman stated that Kinsey "disputed the Freudian emphasis on the vaginal orgasm," but it was not until Masters and Johnson, and, perhaps more importantly, feminists in the late 1960s, when the questioning of the vaginal orgasm really began in earnest. D'Emilio and Freedman, *Intimate Matters*, 312. Kinsey was also noted as the person responsible for closing "the file on the vagina" as the sexual organ in women. Appignanesi and Forrester, *Freud's Women*, 425. Janice Irvine went even further by arguing that Alfred Kinsey and Albert Ellis "initially posited" the idea of the clitoral orgasm in the 1950s. Irvine, *Disorders of Desire*, 162.

161. Ellis, *Psychology of Sex*, 348–49.

162. Liswood, *Marriage Doctor Speaks Her Mind about Sex*, 15, 73.

163. Wiener, *Albert Ellis*; Reiss, *Insider's View of Sexual Science since Kinsey*. Albert Ellis went on to found Rational-Emotive Therapy, which emphasized, among other principles, taking responsibility for changing personal disturbances rather than looking for them in hidden feelings. In addition to denouncing the vaginal orgasm as a myth, Ellis also promoted sexual liberalism more broadly in the 1950s. Ibid. Ellis, who began researching human sexuality in the 1940s, was one of the founders in 1957 of the Society for the Scientific Study of Sexuality. Reiss, *Insider's View of Sexual Science since Kinsey*.

164. Ellis, "Is Vaginal Orgasm a Myth?," 155–62; emphasis in original. Decades later, Ellis noted that the vaginal orgasm theory had been a dominant one but that he had not believed in it. He called this article "pioneering" and in need of "little revision." In the late 1990s, Ellis wrote, "The Freudians have been routed in the vaginal primacy war. I hope that they gracefully stop this nonsense and go home." *Albert Ellis Reader*, 7–8. His challenge to the vaginal orgasm theory was not the only one he made to the practice of psychoanalysis; in 1949, he published a paper questioning psychoanalytic research as not consistently conforming to "some of the simplest and most accepted requisites of scientific research." Ellis, "Towards the Improvement of Psychoanalytic Research," 124.

165. Kleegman, "Frigidity in Women," 243–46.

166. Rado, "Sexual Anesthesia in the Female," 251.

167. Ellis, "Guilt, Shame, and Frigidity," 259–61.

168. Ellis, *American Sexual Tragedy*, 96–99.

169. Kleegman, "Frigidity in Women," 243–46.

170. Marmor, "Some Considerations Concerning Orgasm in the Female," 245.

171. Liswood, *Marriage Doctor Speaks Her Mind about Sex*, 37, 68–69, 74–75.

172. Kleegman, "Frigidity in Women," 243–46.

173. Hardenbergh, "Psychology of Female Sex Experience." Similarly, Myrtle Mann Gillett, a school psychologist in Pennsylvania, wrote in 1950 that though there had been "much discussion" regarding frigidity in women as defined by Kroger and Freed, what women "actually think about the whole matter is somewhat at variance, sometimes, with the opinions or assumptions of many workers who are trying to ameliorate conditions." Noting that her position as a school psychologist gave her an opportunity to hear from the mothers who brought in their children for psychological examinations, she learned of these women's "restless un-happiness." Gillett proceeded to outline the normality of 151 women whom she had seen and who had been labeled as frigid. Gillett found that, for these women, their lack of orgasmic inclination was based on the state of their marriage or their relationship with their husbands. Rude, inconsiderate, unkind, and impatient husbands did not ignite these women's interests in sex or enable orgasm, Gillett noted. "Before calling a woman 'frigid,' we need to know whether or not there is love and trust, thoughtfulness and unselfishness in all of the marriage relationship," she stressed. If, Gillett wrote, Kroger and Freed were correct that "75% of United States women 'are more or less sexually anesthetized' then something must be radically wrong." Normal people, Gillett continued, "do not try and be unhappy, and no scientific person would consider 75% of our American women abnormal." Gillett, "Normal Frigidity in Women," 29–31. Shere Hite, in her 1976 report, would find similar sentiments among women.

174. Rado, "Sexual Anesthesia in the Female," 251.

175. Ford and Beach, *Patterns of Sexual Behavior*, 21–25.

176. Ellis, *Psychology of Sex*, 348–49.

177. Liswood, *Marriage Doctor Speaks Her Mind about Sex*, 69.

178. Kelly, "Operations on Clitoris for Frigidity," 908.

179. Ibid. Kelly's letter was in response to the editorial answer to a letter sent in by Frank Hyde, which I will discuss shortly. Hyde, "Frigidity and the Clitoris," 546.

180. Kelly, "Operations on Clitoris for Frigidity," 908.

181. Small, "Frigidity and the Clitoris," 680.

182. Liswood, *Marriage Doctor Speaks Her Mind about Sex*, 13, 15, 25, 33, 37.

183. Ibid., 40. Liswood recommended cleaning underneath the foreskin of the clitoris to remove smegma and prevent smell. She advised using a "small piece of cotton, put some surgical lubricating jelly on it, and forcibly remove this whitish-looking discharge from underneath the foreskin of the clitoris" (47). This recommendation was one Jessamyn Neuhaus describes as constructing the female body as "problematic" and in need of maintenance so that men would not be disgusted and stray. Neuhaus, "Importance of Being Orgasmic," 464.

184. Liswood, *Marriage Doctor Speaks Her Mind about Sex*, 71–72.

185. Kleegman, "Frigidity in Women," 243–46.

186. Ibid.
187. Masters and Johnson, "Sexual Response Cycles of the Human Male and Female."
188. "Participants," in *Sex and Behavior*, xii, xi.
189. Masters and Johnson, "Sexual Response Cycles of the Human Male and Female," 528–29.
190. Liswood, *Marriage Doctor Speaks Her Mind about Sex*, 75.
191. Rado, "Sexual Anesthesia in the Female," 251.
192. Ellis, *American Sexual Tragedy*, 104–5; emphasis in original.
193. Rado, "Sexual Anesthesia in the Female," 251.
194. Lewis, *Prescriptions for Heterosexuality*.
195. Kroger, "Psychosomatic Aspects of Frigidity and Impotence," 394.
196. Kroger and Freed, "Psychosomatic Aspects of Frigidity and Impotence," 530.
197. Kroger and Freed, *Psychosomatic Gynecology*, 306; Kroger, *Psychosomatic Obstetrics, Gynecology and Endocrinology* (1962), 306.
198. Stoddard, *Case Studies in Obstetrics and Gynecology*, 169.
199. Curtis and Huffman, *Textbook of Gynecology*, 97.
200. Smith, "Circumcision in Women," 680.
201. Hyde, "Frigidity and the Clitoris" 546.
202. McDonald, "Circumcision of the Female," 98–99. McDonald also noted that circumcision of little girls ended masturbating, bed-wetting, and irritability.
203. Wollman, "Hooded Clitoris."
204. Clark, "Adhesions between the Clitoris and Prepuce."
205. Tyrer, *Sex Satisfaction and Happy Marriage*, 119.
206. Rathmann, "Female Circumcision," 115–17. His definitions again highlight the imprecise definition of frigidity.
207. Ibid., 115–16.
208. Ibid., 117.
209. Ibid., 117–20.
210. Elting and Isenberg, *The Consumer's Guide to Successful Surgery*, 274.
211. Semmens, "Clitoral Surgery," 169, 220.

Chapter Six

1. Kellison, "Circumcision for Women," 76.
2. Ibid., 124; Kellison, "$100 Surgery," 52.
3. Kellison, "Circumcision for Women," 124.
4. Wallerstein, *Circumcision*, 182–83, 185.
5. Haldane, "Clitoral Circumcision," 47; Burt and Burt, *Surgery of Love*.
6. Brody, "Blue Shield Acts to Curb Payment."
7. Ryan, "Surgical Intervention in the Treatment," 238.
8. Graber and Graber, "You and Your Sexuality," 83.
9. Clark, "Adhesions between the Clitoris and Prepuce," 235.
10. Graber and Graber, "You and Your Sexuality," 83; Hartman and Fithian, *Treatment of Sexual Dysfunction*, 70–71; Clark, "Adhesions between the Clitoris and Prepuce," 235.

11. Graber and Graber, "You and Your Sexuality," 83.

12. Haldane, "Clitoral Circumcision," 47.

13. Isenberg and Elting, "Guide to Sexual Surgery," 104.

14. Crist, "Female Circumcision," 77.

15. Haldane, "Clitoral Circumcision," 45.

16. Isenberg and Elting, "Guide to Sexual Surgery," 104.

17. Crist, "Female Circumcision," 77.

18. Wollman, "Hooded Clitoris," 4.

19. Kellison, "Circumcision for Women," 76; Haldane, "Clitoral Circumcision," 45.

20. Haldane, "Clitoral Circumcision," 45.

21. Wollman, "Hooded Clitoris," 3–4.

22. Walden, "MD Feedback," 6.

23. Schultz, "Female Circumcision," 54.

24. Maier, *Masters of Sex*, 66–67, 73, 97.

25. Bullough, *Science in the Bedroom*, 197–200.

26. Maier, *Masters of Sex*, 91.

27. Bullough, *Science in the Bedroom*, 197–200.

28. Maier, *Masters of Sex*, 103–4.

29. Masters and Johnson, *Human Sexual Response*, 3, 8, 11–13, 20–21.

30. Jackson, "Sex Research and the Construction of Sexuality," 44.

31. Robinson, *Modernization of Sex*, 121, 132, 136, 140–41, 158.

32. Ussher, "Biology as Destiny," 19.

33. Robinson, *Modernization of Sex*. For more on the idea that Masters and Johnson may have also had a class bias in their research sample leading to a clitoral bias, see Robinson, *Modernization of Sex*, 133–37. Also see Elisabeth Lloyd's critique of Masters and Johnson's vaginal sex model, as a result of their selection of female subjects. Lloyd, *Case of the Female Orgasm*.

34. Bullough, *Science in the Bedroom*, 200–202.

35. Masters and Johnson, *Human Sexual Response*, 63–65; Jackson, "Sex Research and the Construction of Sexuality," 44.

36. As Robinson stressed, their critique of the "'phallic fantasy' is among their most impressive achievements" and allowed Masters and Johnson to argue that female sexuality is not a "pale replica of that of men." Robinson, *Modernization of Sex*, 151–53, 157.

37. Masters and Johnson, *Human Sexual Response*, 45, 47–50, 56, 66–67.

38. Ibid., 66–67, 138.

39. Maier, *Masters of Sex*, 153.

40. Masters and Johnson, *Human Sexual Response*, 138.

41. Maier, *Masters of Sex*, 144. They did have a chapter in the 1961 *Encyclopedia of Sexual Behavior*. See Masters and Johnson, "Orgasm, Anatomy of the Female."

42. Masters and Johnson, "Sexual Response Cycle of the Human Female: The Clitoris," 248–57.

43. Maier, *Masters of Sex*, 151, 173, 174, 211.

44. See, for example, D'Emilio and Freedman, *Intimate Matters*.

45. Groneman, *Nymphomania*, 91.

46. D'Emilio and Freedman, *Intimate Matters*, 300, 305, 306.

47. Bailey, *Sex in the Heartland*, 5–7.

48. Maier, *Masters of Sex*, 174.

49. Bullough, *Science in the Bedroom*, 203–4.

50. Fine, *History of Psychoanalysis*, 214.

51. Bullough, *Science in the Bedroom*, 203.

52. Fine, *History of Psychoanalysis*, 214.

53. Sherfey, "Evolution and Nature of Female Sexuality."

54. Sherfey, *Nature and Evolution of Female Sexuality*, 14; emphasis in the original.

55. Ibid., 15.

56. Ibid., 16–17.

57. Ibid., 17–18.

58. Sherfey, "Evolution and Nature of Female Sexuality," 84. "In the process of performing the invaluable service of bringing Masters and Johnson's bad news about Freudian 'vaginal orgasm' to the psychiatric community," Elisabeth Lloyd argued, Sherfey "seems to have been overly impressed by the indirect method of attaining orgasm during intercourse, described by Masters and Johnson." Recall that Masters and Johnson selected for their study only women who could reach orgasm this way. Lloyd, *Case of the Female Orgasm*, 93.

59. Sherfey, "Evolution and Nature of Female Sexuality," 34, 36; emphasis in original. Following the publication of their book, Masters and Johnson were asked to present their findings to the biannual meeting of psychoanalysts a few months later. According to Sherfey, Masters told her they went to the meeting prepared for strong resistance to their work, but "it seemed that all of them had read" her article and instead of being resistant, those attending the meeting were "eager to explore the implications of the work." Sherfey later wrote that, in addition to Masters's comment to her, she received further evidence of her article's "acceptance" in letters congratulating her, and not one "denouncing the article or arguing with its chief positions." Sherfey, *Nature and Evolution of Female Sexuality*, 18.

Sherfey's essay resulted in the American Psychoanalytic Association organizing a special panel to discuss her paper, and the work of Masters and Johnson, and to devote an issue to the panel's reply to Sherfey. As the editor of the *Journal of the American Psychoanalytic Association* noted, the panel resulted from "the interest aroused" by Sherfey's article, and, in addition to the responses from the panel, the journal asked for papers from others. Editor's note, "Mary Jane Sherfey." Not all of the articles in the July 1968 issue of the journal were complimentary of Sherfey's work, however. Marcel Heiman, a psychiatrist at Mount Sinai Hospital in New York, for example, stated that Sherfey's conclusion that all embryos begin life as female had "completely misunderstood and misinterpreted the facts established by embryology." Heiman, "Discussion," 415. Similarly, psychoanalyst Judith Kestenberg found that Sherfey's "attempts to reformulate psychoanalytic theory with new advances in biology" failed because she misinterpreted "certain biological data" and disregarded "the cornerstones of psychoanalysis—understanding of the unconscious." Kestenberg, "Discussion," 417.

60. Eidelberg, *Encyclopedia of Psychoanalysis*, 166; Buhle, *Feminism and Its Discontents*, 221. There existed, however, a small group who worked to maintain Freud's reputation against the feminist attack, and some women psychoanalysts, while sympathetic and even supportive of the women's rights movement, continued to champion the work of Karen Horney and her emphasis on the vagina. Buhle, *Feminism and Its Discontents*.

61. Pines, "Human Sexual Response," 48.

62. Buhle, *Feminism and Its Discontents*, 223, 220.

63. This division is largely one of historical convenience and did not seem to have played out consistently, especially perhaps at the local level. For example, see Ezekiel, *Feminism in the Heartland*.

64. Rosen, *The World Split Open*; Davis, *Moving the Mountain*; Houck, "What Do These Women Want?"; Stansell, *The Feminist Promise*. See also Evans, *Personal Politics*.

65. Buhle, *Feminism and Its Discontents*, 212.

66. Stansell, *Feminist Promise*, 244–45.

67. Morgen, *Into Our Own Hands*, 11, 71–72, 120–21.

68. Houck, "What Do These Women Want?," 107.

69. Boston Women's Health Book Collective, *Our Bodies, Ourselves* (1976), 10.

70. "Anatomy," *off our backs*.

71. Kline, *Bodies of Knowledge*, 4. Kline also argued, however, that this privileging of the individual experience assumed that such experience was universal among women, an assumption later challenged.

72. Murphy, "Immodest Witnessing"; Morgen, *Into Our Own Hands*; *Circle One: Self Help Handbook*.

73. Bailey, *Sex in the Heartland*, 10, 160.

74. Buhle, *Feminism and Its Discontents*, 214.

75. Davidson, *Loose Change*, 179–83.

76. Buhle, *Feminism and Its Discontents*, 209–10.

77. Person, "As the Wheel Turns," 1277. Person additionally noted the importance of the gay liberation movement in pushing for changes within psychoanalysis.

78. Buhle, *Feminism and Its Discontents*, 216.

79. Shulman, "Organs and Orgasms," 200.

80. Koedt, "Myth of the Vaginal Orgasm"; Jenny Knauss Collection, Chicago Liberation Union, Box 3, Folder 7, Deering Library Special Collections, Northwestern University, Evanston, Illinois.

81. Stansell, *Feminist Promise*, 253. Stansell here, however, mistakenly refers to Masters and Johnson's 1966 findings as coming from the Kinsey Institute during her discussion of the politics of the female orgasm.

82. Buhle, *Feminism and Its Discontents*, 217; emphasis in original.

83. Koedt, "Myth of the Vaginal Orgasm," 312, 320.

84. Some twenty years later, Jane Gerhard noted that Koedt's influential article "appeared when the concern with sexual freedom as a weapon in the battle against repression had yet to be challenged as having gendered implications." Gerhard, "Revisiting 'The Myth of the Vaginal Orgasm,'" 464, 468.

85. Lydon, "Understanding Orgasm," 59–63.

86. Atkinson, "Vaginal Orgasm," 5–7. Atkinson spends more time on the vaginal orgasm in her "The Institution of Sexual Intercourse," included in this same text.

87. Cathy, "Sex or Hey, I Thought This Was Supposed to Be Fun!"

88. Gerhard, *Desiring Revolution*, 5–7.

89. Gerhard, *Desiring Revolution*, 5–7. See also Buhle's discussion in *Feminism and Its Discontents*.

90. For Betty Dodson, masturbation was a route to autonomy, both sexually and psychologically. Dodson, *Liberating Masturbation*. Dodson's influence extended

beyond the feminist movement however; for example, Robyn Leary in a 1980 *Harper's Bazaar* article wrote that, "once a taboo topic, masturbation is now considered to be vital to our total awareness," enabling women to establish "loving contact with our own bodies" and "define and accept," even "heighten" individual as well as partner sex. Leary, "Masturbation and Orgasm," 200–201.

91. Stansell, *Feminist Promise*, 260.

92. Gerhard, *Desiring Revolution*, 2, 6. Not all women within the movement saw sexual empowerment as important, however. Betty Friedan and some older feminists were "bewildered by young women's obsessive discussions about sexuality" and thought such attention "distracted feminists from the more important subjects of employment and poverty." Rosen, *World Split Open*, 152.

93. Murphy, "Immodest Witnessing"; *Our Bodies, Ourselves*, various editions.

94. Murphy, "Immodest Witnessing," 122.

95. Frankfort, *Vaginal Politics*, 212. Examining one's own external and internal genitals was not just a practice within consciousness-raising sessions or within gynecology self-help meetings; such an examination also occurred within sex therapy such as in the practice of Philip and Lorna Sarrel, directors of the Sex Counseling Program at Yale University, who beginning in 1974 encouraged women and their partners to learn about the female genitalia. Sarrel and Sarrel, "Your Most Intimate You."

96. Boston Women's Health Book Collective, *Our Bodies, Ourselves* (1971), 16.

97. Horos, *Vaginal Health*, 16–18.

98. Cook and Dworkin, *Ms. Guide to a Woman's Health* (1979), 387; Cook and Dworkin, *The Ms. Guide to a Woman's Health* (1981), 423.

99. The Diagram Group, *Woman's Body*, 26.

100. National Women's Health Network, *Self Help*, 10–11.

101. Federation of Feminist Women's Health Centers, *New View of a Woman's Body*, 17, 33–35; emphasis in original.

102. Fugh-Berman, "Self-Help," 14.

103. The differences in *A New View* when compared to standard anatomy texts are a matter of semantics. While language and labeling matter greatly, the implication, as presented by *A New View*, was that this was not just a renaming of the female genitals but also a discovering of a hidden truth. I am not arguing whether *A New View*'s labels were more "truthful" about the female body, rather I am arguing that the information about the external and internal extensiveness of the clitoris, and its interconnectedness to the rest of the female genitalia, had existed in anatomy texts for decades prior to *A New View*.

104. The 1970s critique of the expansion of medicine had roots in the 1950s. Conrad, "Medicalization and Social Control."

105. Conrad, "The Shifting Engines of Medicalization." Though medicalization has often been seen as driven by physicians, patients were also active in medicalizing that which was previously not seen as under medical purview, including childbirth and premenstrual syndrome. Conrad, "Medicalization and Social Control."

106. Conrad and Schneider, *Deviance and Medicalization*.

107. On women actively seeking certain medical treatments, see Powderly, "Patient Consent and Negotiation"; Conrad, "Shifting Engines of Medicalization," 3–14; and Conrad, *Medicalization of Society*.

108. Haiken, *Venus Envy*, 10.

109. Stroman, *The Quick Knife*, 3.

110. Jacobson, *Cleavage*.

111. Isenberg and Elting, "A Guide to Sexual Surgery," 104.

112. Haldane, "Clitoral Circumcision," 46.

113. Kellison was writing in *Playgirl*, and though not necessarily regarded as a feminist magazine, it was advocating a feminism of a certain sort, especially regarding sexual empowerment.

114. Kellison, "Circumcision for Women," 124–25.

115. Ibid. The statement that Daniels had been practicing the surgery since 1961 again alludes to the use of this surgery when the vaginal orgasm dominated popular ideas about sex.

116. Kellison, "$100 Surgery," 55, 53.

117. Haldane, "Clitoral Circumcision," 45.

118. Schultz, "Female Circumcision," 53–54.

119. Haldane, "Clitoral Circumcision," 48. I do not know any more about her study than what Haldane reported.

120. Schultz, "Female Circumcision," 105.

121. Haldane, "Clitoral Circumcision," 46–47.

122. Isenberg and Elting, "Guide to Sexual Surgery," 104.

123. Kentsmith and Eaton, *Treating Sexual Problems in Medical Practice*, 159.

124. Schultz, "Female Circumcision," 104.

125. Ibid.

126. Haldane, "Clitoral Circumcision," 46–47.

127. Schultz, "Female Circumcision," 104.

128. Wolkoff, "Surgery of the Clitoris," 106.

129. Huffman, "Some Facts about the Clitoris," 245–47; emphasis in original.

130. Lauersen and Whitney, *It's Your Body*, 384–85.

131. Semmens, "Clitoral Surgery," 169, 220.

132. Kolodny, Masters, and Johnson, *Textbook of Sexual Medicine*, 192.

133. "Better Orgasms?," *Big Mama Rag*, 7.

134. Cook and Dworkin, *"Ms." Guide to a Woman's Health* (1979), 395; Cook and Dworkin, *"Ms." Guide to a Woman's Health* (1981), 431; emphasis in original.

135. For example, Reuben, *Everything You Always Wanted to Know about Sex*; Reuben, *Any Woman Can!*; and Comfort, *Joy of Sex*. *Everything* became the number one nonfiction book in the United States in 1971, spending six months on the *New York Times* bestsellers list with more than eight million paperback copies sold by 1975. Peterson, "Sex Texts," 88.

136. Gerhard, *Desiring Revolution*, 74.

137. Hite, *Hite Report*, 58–59, 134, 232, 251.

138. Kaplan, *New Sex Therapy*, 28, 341.

139. Barbach, "Five Myths about the Big O," 200.

140. For example, in his 1973 book, *The Female Orgasm*, Seymour Fisher argued for the vaginal over the clitoral orgasm. In a 1970 article, Richard Robertiello stated that for women who had both kinds of orgasms there was a clear distinction and that the "vaginal one is generally preferred." Robertiello, "Clitoral versus Vaginal Orgasm," 308. Rachel Copeland asserted in her 1971 sex manual that the sexually fulfilled

woman did not need clitoral stimulation and that the vaginal orgasm was the better, more mature orgasm. Copeland, *Sexually Fulfilled Woman.*

141. Oliven, *Clinical Sexuality*, 187.

142. Gray, "Women's Preferences regarding Clitoral Stimulation," 32, 39, 42.

143. Erickson with Steffen, *Kiss and Tell*, 6.

144. Hite, *Hite Report*, 58–59, 134, 232, 251.

145. Tavris and Sadd, *Redbook Report on Female Sexuality*, 20, 76, 79 (emphasis in original). Though one hundred thousand women responded to the survey, the study itself only used 2,278 of the replies, representational of the original sample.

146. Shulman, "Organs and Orgasms," 200.

147. Hite, *Women as Revolutionary Agents of Change*, 185–97.

148. Wolfe, *Cosmo Report*, 21, 101, 109, 104, 131.

149. Collier, "It *Is* Different for Women," 84–86.

150. Hartman and Fithian, *Treatment of Sexual Dysfunction*, 200.

151. Kline-Graber and Graber, *Woman's Orgasm*, 143.

152. Clark, *101 Intimate Sexual Problems Answered*, 59–60.

153. Kellison, "Circumcision for Women," 125; emphasis in original.

154. Nellis, "Hite Report," 121.

155. Crist, "Female Circumcision," 77.

Chapter Seven

1. Demick, "Love Surgery," 19.

2. Ibid.

3. Helgason and Davis, "Media Has Accepted"; Direct examination of Janet Phillips at 1278, *Phillips v. Burt*, 77 Ohio St. 3d 1229.

4. Search for James C. Burt, Ohio License Center, License and Registration, accessed January 11, 2007, https://license.ohio.gov/Lookup/SearchDetail.asp?ContactIdnt=2998932&DivisionIdnt=78.

5. Helgason and Davis, "Media Has Accepted."

6. Ibid.

7. Laskas, "Crime against Nature"; Holoweiko, "Why Was the Love Surgeon."

8. Brower, "James Burt's 'Love Surgery,'" 100.

9. Holoweiko, "Why Was the Love Surgeon," 126; Hennessee, "Love Surgeon," 207.

10. Williams, *Williams Obstetrics*, 450.

11. Demick, "Love Surgery," 18.

12. Holoweiko, "Why Was the Love Surgeon," 126; Demick, "Love Surgery." 18.

13. Burt was neither the first nor the last to consider the extent of the distance between the clitoris and the vaginal opening in relation to female orgasm during penetrative sex. See Wallen and Lloyd, "Female Genital Arousal."

14. Demick, "Love Surgery," 18.

15. Burt and Burt, *Surgery of Love*, 264–65.

16. Demick, "Love Surgery," 18–19.

17. Holoweiko, "Why Was the Love Surgeon," 132.

4

4

18. Helgason and Davis, "Media Has Accepted."
19. Demick, "Love Surgery," 18.
20. Brower, "James Burt's 'Love Surgery,'" 97, 98.
21. Helgason and Davis, "Media Has Accepted."
22. Brower, "James Burt's 'Love Surgery,'" 97.
23. Burt and Burt, *Surgery of Love*, 20, 27.
24. Ibid., 271.
25. Brower, "James Burt's 'Love Surgery,'" 98.
26. Burt and Burt, *Surgery of Love*, 266, 271.
27. Burt and Burt, *Surgery of Love*, 260.
28. Helgason and Davis, "Media Has Accepted."
29. Demick, "Love Surgery," 18.
30. Ibid. 20; Burt and Burt, *Surgery of Love*.
31. Holoweiko, "Why Was the Love Surgeon," 128.
32. Burt and Burt, *Surgery of Love*, n.p.
33. Ibid., 14–15, 67, 74–75.
34. Ibid., 83, 158–59, 57, 35, 40, 41, 262.
35. Ibid., 44, 11, 7, 17, 40.
36. Ibid., 40–41.
37. Bird, *How to Be a Happily Married Mistress*.
38. Burt and Burt, *Surgery of Love*, 8, 153, 66, 176, 57, 72.
39. Ibid., 153–54, 57, 200–201, 208.
40. Ibid., 70.
41. D'Emilio and Freedman, *Intimate Matters*, 280.
42. Heidenry, *What Wild Ecstasy*.
43. D'Emilio and Freedman, *Intimate Matters*, 328. The movie *Deep Throat* broke many social taboos concerning pornography. Released in 1972, the main female character discovers she has a clitoris in her throat and derives great pleasure from giving men oral sex. Holson, "Long View on *Deep Throat*." While this obviously reflected the popularity of the organ during this time, one does have to wonder whether some men confused the location of the organ, believing it to be down his lover's throat, not between her legs. But it also reflects the tension surrounding the clitoris—not just where it was but how men were to stimulate it while stimulating themselves. While challenging the cultural taboos regarding pornography, *Deep Throat* did little to challenge the taboos regarding women's sexual pleasure, for here a woman received pleasure with men by giving men pleasure, in keeping with the traditional scenario.
44. D'Emilio and Freedman, *Intimate Matters*, 300, 336, 340.
45. Weiss, *To Have and to Hold*, 157.
46. Demick, "Love Surgery," 21.
47. Burt and Burt, *Surgery of Love*, author's autobiographies, 195, 196; emphasis in original.
48. Ibid., 196, 15.
49. D'Emilio and Freedman, *Intimate Matters*, 330–33.
50. Knout, "Local Doctor Develops Corrective Surgery."
51. Demick, "Love Surgery,"18.

52. *Goldfarb v. Virginia State Bar*, Ameringer, "Organized Medicine on Trial." According to Ameringer, many of the ethical restrictions against advertising, solicitation, and contract practice (another core component of the Federal Trade Commission action), were enacted in the nineteenth century and were core components of the AMA's Principles of Medical Ethics as revised in 1957 (448). See also *AMA v. FTC.*

53. Demick, "Love Surgery"; Helgason and Davis, "Media Has Accepted"; Shah with Maier, "Heeere's . . . Donahue"; Holoweiko, "Why Was the Love Surgeon."

54. Laskas, "Crime against Nature," 64.

55. Demick, "Love Surgery," 20.

56. Helgason and Davis, "Media Has Accepted."

57. Demick, "Love Surgery," 20.

58. Burt and Burt, *Surgery of Love*, 265, 269.

59. "Furor over Vaginal Surgery for Anorgasmy," *Medical World News.*

60. Hite, *Hite Report*, 58–59, 134, 232.

61. Burt and Burt, *Surgery of Love*, 41.

62. Reiss and Reiss, *Solving America's Sexual Crises*, 174.

63. Ibid., 177. Reiss found Burt's response a "most revealing commentary on our culture"; women "will undergo major surgery but men will not wear a simple sex gadget." Reiss further found Burt's reason for love surgery—to cure women of what Masters and Johnson labeled a dysfunction—problematic. Because the term "sexual dysfunction" was lifted from the discipline of physiology (since many of the early sex therapists, like William Masters and Helen Singer Kaplan, were physicians) and referred to the disruptive operations of bodily organs, it implied that there was something wrong with the way women physically functioned sexually. Masters and Johnson, according to Reiss, defined sexual dysfunction as "conditions in which the ordinary physical responses of sexual function are impaired." But what exactly were ordinary sexual functions? wondered Reiss. Since the majority of women responded mostly to clitoral stimulation, Reiss considered that to be a woman's "ordinary physical response." Reiss and Reiss, *Solving America's Sexual Crises*, 176, 190.

64. Holoweiko, "Why Was the Love Surgeon," 131.

65. "Furor over Vaginal Surgery," *Medical World News*, 16.

66. Plaintiff's Witness List, in 1 Appellant's Supplement, at 480, *Phillips v. Burt*; Plaintiff's Exhibits, in 1 Appellant's Supplement at 492, *Philips v. Burt*; "Frederick P. Zuspan, M.D. 1922–2009," *UChicago News*, accessed March 18, 2014, http://news.uchicago.edu/article/2009/06/16/frederick-p-zuspan-md-1922-2009.

67. Demick, "Love Surgery," 18.

68. Holoweiko, "Why Was the Love Surgeon," 128.

69. Ashley, *Hospitals, Paternalism, and the Role of the Nurse*, 130.

70. Ibid., 131; Group and Roberts, *Nursing, Physician Control, and the Medical Monopoly.*

71. Law and Polan, *Pain and Profit*, 210.

72. Demick, "Love Surgery," 21.

73. Modic, "5-Week Burt Trial Down to Closing Arguments," 3A.

74. Modic, "St. Elizabeth Asks Judge for Immunity," 3A.

75. Laskas, "Crime against Nature," 66.

76. Modic and Beyerlein, "Judge Allows More Evidence in Burt Case," 3A.

77. "Looking Back," *Dayton Daily News*, 6A–7A.

78. Laskas, "Crime against Nature," 66.

79. Demick, "Love Surgery," 21.

80. Ibid. Emphasis in original.

81. American Cancer Society, "Laetrile," accessed October 24, 2012, http://www.cancer.org/treatment/treatmentsandsideeffects/complementaryandalternativemedicine/pharmacologicalandbiologicaltreatment/laetrile. According to the National Cancer Institute, Laetrile is a compound that has been used to treat cancer but has not been approved for cancer treatment or any other medical condition by the FDA. Cyanide is believed to be the active ingredient. "Questions and Answers about Laetrile/Amygdalin," National Cancer Institute, February 20. 2013, http://www.cancer.gov/cancertopics/pdq/cam/laetrile/patient/page2.

82. Holoweiko, "Why Was the Love Surgeon," 131.

83. Safran, "Gynecologist from Hell," 76.

84. Holoweiko, "Why Was the Love Surgeon," 131.

85. Modic and Hills, "Peers Criticized Burt in '78."

86. Holoweiko, "Why Was the Love Surgeon," 131, 132.

87. Modic and Hills, "Peers Criticized Burt in '78."

88. Hennessee, "Love Surgeon," 246.

89. Modic and Hills, "Peers Criticized Burt in '78"; Holoweiko, "Why Was the Love Surgeon," 132.

90. Demick, "Love Surgery," 21.

91. Holoweiko, "Why Was the Love Surgeon," 132.

92. Ibid.; Lander, *Defective Medicine*, 69–70.

93. Demick, "Love Surgery," 19.

94. "Furor over Vaginal Surgery," *Medical World News*, 15.

95. Ibid., 16.

96. Demick, "Love Surgery," 18–19.

97. Burt and Burt, *Surgery of Love*, 47–48.

98. Demick, "Love Surgery," 19.

99. Ibid.

100. Ibid., 19–20.

101. Ibid., 19.

102. Ibid., 20.

103. Ibid., 21.

104. Demick, "Love Surgery," 20.

105. Ibid., 21. The Women's Community Health Center's papers are archived at the Schlesinger Library at Harvard University, but the letter they sent out was not among the collection. E-mail to author, Amanda Strauss response to author e-mail query regarding letter, December 13, 2011.

106. Sommers, Bell, Wolhandler, and Stein, "Report from Women's Community."

107. "Regional Reports," *Health Right*, 11.

108. Downer, "Self-Help for Sex," 268.

109. Marieskind, *Women in the Health System*, 273.

110. Dejanikus, "Vaginal Mutilation American Style," 13.

111. "In Brief," *National NOW Times*. Though the latter does not note obtaining the information from the publication *Seven Days*, the *National NOW Times* brief contains the same quotations and information as several other stories that appeared regarding Burt in 1978 and that referenced *Seven Days* or *HerSay* as the source. I have been unable to find any reference to a *Seven Days* publication. The Reader's Guide Retrospective, for instance, does not record that name (searched on December 19, 2011).

In addition to these publications, others ran stories about Burt. The feminist publication *HerSay: A Woman's News Service* based in San Francisco report was subsequently picked up by a few other women's publications, such as *Big Mama Rag*. In their July/August 1978 issue, *Big Mama Rag* criticized Burt and his surgery in its briefs section. Under the title "More Genital Mutilation," the article quoted Burt saying the operation could benefit "millions of American women" by enabling them to have "more frequent and more intense orgasms" through the reconstruction of their vaginas "to make the clitoris more accessible to direct penile stimulation." The brief noted that Burt used his wife, Joan Burt, as "demonstrable proof that the operation works" (6). The Northwestern University library's collection of *HerSay* starts with the August 21, 1978, issue, so I did not have access to the original story in *HerSay*. The *New Women's Times*, a newspaper out of Rochester, New York, also published a brief about Burt. Under the headline "Doctor 'Fixes' Women's Vaginas," this article used the same information about the surgery that appeared in *Big Mama Rag*, again noting that it was taken from *HerSay*.

Interestingly, the women's publications that carried stories on Burt were not based in Ohio. For example, *off our backs* was out of Washington, DC, and *Big Mama Rag* was out of Denver. *What She Wants*, which billed itself as Cleveland's only women's paper, did not carry any story on Burt from January 1975 through January 1980. *What She Wants*, January 1975–January 1980, Northwestern University Deering Library's Special Collections. The other Cleveland feminist paper, the *Cleveland Feminist*, ceased publication in 1974, as did the Dayton *Women's Liberation Newsletter*, neither of which carried any stories about Burt before they folded, not unexpectedly since coverage of Burt in the feminist press did not appear until later in the 1970s. Both the *Cleveland Feminist* and the Dayton *Women's Liberation Newsletter* are at Northwestern University Deering Library's Special Collections, in Evanston, IL.

112. Sealander and Smith, "Rise and Fall of Feminist Organizations in the 1970s."

113. Ezekiel, *Feminism in the Heartland*. Unlike in other areas of the country, women's liberation predated liberal feminism in Dayton, Ezekiel notes.

114. Bronstein, *Battling Pornography*, 2.

115. Stansell, *Feminist Promise*, 288, 344–46. Lynne Segal noted in her introduction to an early 1990s volume on the feminist pornography debate that pornography divided feminists "like no other" issue in the late 1970s and 1980s. Feminists who were opposed to pornography, Segal argued, were concerned that it reduces women to passive bodies, something they considered inherently violent. Pornography became "*the* feminist issue of the 1980s" (emphasis in original), Segal wrote, based upon the dual ideas that sexuality is at the core of men's oppression of women and that pornography is the basis of male sexual practices. Pornography was regarded

as part of the spectrum of male violence. As Segal saw it a decade later, the focus on pornography by feminists was a sign of defeat: the religious right was gaining power, abortion rights were under attack, and the federal Equal Rights Amendment was being seriously undermined by those in the New Right. Feminists, according to Segal, were "retreating into defensive politics, isolating sexuality and men's violence from other issues of women's inequality." Segal, introduction to *Sex Exposed*, 1, 3, 5.

116. Gerhard, *Desiring Revolution*, 87.

117. Bronstein, *Battling Pornography*. Bronstein contended that though later depicted as such, most women in the antipornography movement were against violence, not sex.

118. LaBelle, "Snuff."

119. Lederer, introduction to *Take Back the Night*, 19–20.

120. Segal, introduction to *Sex Exposed*, 4.

121. Lederer, introduction to *Take Back the Night*, 19–20.

122. Bronstein, *Battling Pornography*.

123. Corea and de Wit, "Current Developments and Issues," 153.

124. "Robin Morgan," *Big Mama Rag*.

125. E. J. Leschansky to James C. Burt, July 1, 1979, at 320, *Philips v. Burt*, 77 Ohio St. 3d 1229.

126. Lander, *Defective Medicine*, 6. Hennessee, "The Love Surgeon."

127. Linda Cook asked the Ohio State University gynecologist who performed her corrective surgery to testify, but he refused. With no local expert witness willing to testify, she ended up settling for $1,500, with nearly half going to cover her legal fees. Safran, "Gynecologist from Hell." Anna Mitchell sued Burt in 1975 and settled two years later for $5,000 because no doctor would testify on her behalf. Holoweiko, "Why Was the Love Surgeon"; Brower, "James Burt's 'Love Surgery.'" And Judith Romer sued Burt and St. Elizabeth Medical Center in 1980, claiming love surgery left her unable to have sex and that the hospital was negligent in allowing the surgery to take place as it was not considered standard medical practice, but her case was dismissed in 1981 when she failed to appear at the trial. "Looking Back," *Dayton Daily News*; "Malpractice Suit Hits St. E.," *Journal Herald*.

128. Affidavit of Janet Phillips at 52, *Phillips v. Burt* 77 Ohio St. 3d 1229; Direct examination of Janet Phillips at 1261, *Phillips v. Burt*, 77 Ohio St. 3d 1229.

129. Direct examination of Janet Philips at 1261, *Phillips v. Burt* 77 Ohio St. 3d 1229.

130. James Burt's medical notes for Janet Phillips at 993, *Phillips v. Burt* 77 Ohio St. 3d 1229; James Burt's medical notes for Janet Phillips at 996, *Phillips v. Burt*, 77 Ohio St. 3d 1229.

131. Direct examination of Janet Phillips at 1265, *Phillips v. Burt* 77 Ohio St. 3d 1229; St. Elizabeth Medical Center consent form at 983, *Phillips v. Burt* 77 Ohio St. 3d 1229.

132. Direct examination of Janet Phillips at 1267, *Phillips v. Burt* 77 Ohio St. 3d 1229; Safran, "Gynecologist from Hell," 74.

133. Direct examination of Janet Phillips at 1269, *Phillips v. Burt* 77 Ohio St. 3d 1229.

134. Affidavit of Carol M. Loechinger at 46, *Phillips v. Burt* 77 Ohio St. 3d 1229.

135. Merit Brief of Plaintiff-Appellee at 12, *Phillips v. Burt* 77 Ohio St. 3d 1229 (1997).

136. Merit Brief of Plaintiff-Appellee (March 14, 1996) at 12, *Phillips v. Burt* 77 Ohio St. 3d 1229.

137. Affidavit of Michael Clark at 49, *Phillips v. Burt,* Case 77 Ohio St. 3d 1229.

138. Merit Brief of Plaintiff-Appellee at 12, *Phillips v. Burt* 77 Ohio St. 3d 1229.

139. Mcinnis, "Burt Seeks Protection from Debts."

140. Helgason, "We Had No Way to Stop Burt, Physicians Say."

141. Modic, "Doctor or Devil."

142. "Network Show to Examine Area Doctor's Surgery Claims," *Dayton Daily News.*

143. "Love Surgery," *CBS News—West 57th.*

144. Ibid., transcript, 1–2.

145. Ibid., 2.

146. Ibid., 4.

147. Letter for James C. Burt, December 8, 1988, State of Ohio, State Medical Board, Citation—Based on alleged performance of experimental and medically unnecessary surgical procedures, in some instances without proper patient consent—Notice of opportunity for hearing, Ohio License Center, accessed January 11, 2007, https://license.ohio.gov/Lookup/SearchDetail.asp?ContactIdnt=2998932&DivisionIdnt=78&Type=L.

148. "Doctor Loses Practice over Genital Surgery," *New York Times.*

149. Letter from James Burt, January 25, 1989: Voluntary surrender—Permanent revocation; ineligible to apply for licensure or practice medicine anywhere in the United States, Ohio License Center, accessed January 11, 2007, https://license.ohio.gov/Lookup/SearchDetail.asp?ContactIdnt=2998932&DivisionIdnt=78&Type=L.

150. Helgason, "'Love Surgery' Might Be Allowed in Future."

151. Theis, "Burt Quits Medicine"; "Dayton Gynecologist Gives Up His License," *Plain Dealer.*

152. Helgason, "'Love Surgery' Might Be Allowed in Future." Although as far as I can ascertain Burt never taught either at a medical school or individual practitioners, his idea of a correct alignment for better heterosexual response did not end with his quitting medicine. See, for example, Eichel and Noble, *Perfect Fit.*

153. Modic, "Most Burt Suits Settled."

Conclusion

1. Examples of early articles in medical journals: Beadnell, "Circumcision and Clitoridectomy as Practiced by the Natives of British East Africa"; Brassington, "Notes on Female Circumcision as Practiced by the Ameru"; Fox, "Female Circumcision in Savage Tribes"; "Circumcision of Women," *Sexology;* Arthur, "'Female Circumcision' among the Kikuyu." For an excellent discussion (though I disagree with some of her framing of medical knowledge regarding the clitoris) of British attempts to stop the practice of female circumcision in Kenya in the early twentieth century, see Susan Pedersen, "National Bodies, Unspeakable Acts." Fran Hosken published a good deal on this issue. See, for example, Hosken, "Female Circumcision and Fertility in

Africa"; Hosken, *Genital Mutilation of Women in Africa*; Hosken, *Hosken Report* (1979); Hosken, *Hosken Report* (1993).

2. Rosenthal, "Female Genital Torture: How Many Millions More?"; Rosenthal, "Female Genital Mutilation"; Rosenthal, "Torture Continues"; Ibid., "Female Genital Torture." For a review of this media coverage, and for a call for greater accuracy in coverage, see Public Policy Advisory Network, "Seven Things to Know."

3. For example: Klein, *Prisoners of Ritual*; and Crossette, "Female Genital Mutilation."

4. Walker, *Possessing the Secret of Joy*. My first exposure to the practice of female circumcision and clitoridectomy in the United States as medical therapy was through this book. In the book, a white North American woman's clitoris was removed when she was a child in the early twentieth century in an attempt to stop her from masturbating. I had never heard of it used in this context, and curiosity prompted me to go looking to see whether this indeed had ever occurred in the United States.

5. Walker and Parmar, *Warrior Marks*, 18; Parmar and Walker, *Warrior Marks*.

6. Dugger, "New Law Bans Genital Cutting in United States." For an overview of the debates regarding female genital cutting in the United States from the late 1970s through the 1990s, see chapter three, "The Evolution of Debates over Female Genital Cutting," in Boyle, *Female Genital Cutting*. See also Wade, "Learning from 'Female Genital Mutilation'"; and Johnsdotter, "Projected Cultural Histories of the Cutting of Female Genitalia."

7. James, review of *Warrior Marks*, 596. See also Grewal and Kaplan, "*Warrior Marks*."

8. Morgan and Steinem, "International Crime," 65–69. Others followed their example; in her 1994 book, *Cutting the Rose: Female Genital Mutilation; The Practice and its Prevention*, Efua Dorkenoo referred to the work of Morgan and Steinem to highlight "the way in which FGM manifested itself in North American and in Europe" (30).

9. See, for example, Herlund and Shell-Duncan, *Transcultural Bodies*; Bell, "Genital Cutting and Western Discourses on Sexuality"; Berer, "Labia Reduction for Non-therapeutic Reasons"; Essen and Johnsdotter, "Female Genital Mutilation in the West"; Johnsdotter and Essen, "Genitals and Ethnicity"; Gunning, "Female Genital Surgeries and Multicultural Feminism"; and Gunning, "Arrogant Perception, World-Travelling and Multicultural Feminism."

10. Center for Reproductive Rights, *Legislation on Female Genital Mutilation in the United States*, accessed April 24, 2012, http://reproductiverights.org/en/document/legislation-on-female-genital-mutilation-in-the-united-states.

11. Committee on Bioethics, American Academy of Pediatrics, "Female Genital Mutilation"; Committee on Bioethics, American Academy of Pediatrics, "Policy Statement," 1092.

12. Ostrom, "Harborview Debates Issues of Circumcision in Muslim Girls."

13. Aubey, "Are You Out of Your Mind?"

14. Committee on Bioethics, American Academy of Pediatrics "Policy Statement," 191.

15. Thank you to Joseph Pincus.

16. Horowitz, Jackson, and Teklemariam, "Female Circumcision," 188. They were commenting on Toubia, "Female Circumcision as a Public Health Issue."

Appendix

1. Curtis, *Textbook of Gynecology* (1931): 310.

2. Disease-specific texts—for example texts on gynecological cancers—rarely discussed the clitoris beyond recommending removal if cancerous. See, for example, Sherman, *Cancer of the Female Reproductive Organs.*

3. Speert, *Obstetrics and Gynecology in America.*

Bibliography

Archival Collections

Alfred C. Kinsey Collection. The Kinsey Institute for Research in Sex, Gender, and Reproduction, Inc. Indiana University, Bloomington, Indiana.

Clerks of Court. Supreme Court of Ohio. Columbus, Ohio.

Dayton Metro Library. Dayton, Ohio.

Deering Library Special Collections, especially the Jenny Knauss Collection. Chicago Liberation Union. Northwestern University, Evanston, Illinois.

Ebling Library for the Health Sciences. Historical Pamphlet Collection. University of Wisconsin–Madison, Madison, Wisconsin.

Court Cases and Legal Records

AMA v. FTC, 455 U.S. 676 (1982).

Goldfarb v. Virginia State Bar, 421 U.S. 773 (1975).

Affidavit of Michael Clark, February 1987, in 1 Appellant's Supplement at 49, *Phillips v. Burt*, 77 Ohio St. 3d 1229 (1997) (95-1522).

Affidavit of Carol M. Loechinger, February 16, 1987, in 1 Appellant's Supplement at 46–47, *Phillips v. Burt*, 77 Ohio St. 3d 1229 (1997) (95-1522).

Affidavit of Janet Phillips, February 1987, in 1 Appellant's Supplement at 52–57, *Phillips v. Burt*, 77 Ohio St. 3d 1229 (1997) (95-1522).

Direct examination of Janet Phillips, May 14, 1991, in 3 Appellant's Supplement at 1258–1309, *Phillips v. Burt*, 77 Ohio St. 3d 1229 (1997) (95-1522).

E. J. Leschansky, St. Elizabeth chief of staff, letter to James C. Burt, July 1, 1979, in 1 Appellant's Supplement at 320–21, *Phillips vs. Burt*, 77 Ohio St. 3d 1229 (1997) (95-1522).

James Burt's medical notes for Janet Phillips, March 25, 1981, in 2 Appellant's Supplement at 993–94, *Phillips v. Burt*, 77 Ohio St. 3d 1229 (1997) (95-1522).

James Burt's medical notes for Janet Phillips, July 5, 1981, in 2 Appellant's Supplement at 996, *Phillips v. Burt*, 77 Ohio St. 3d 1229 (1997) (95-1522).

Merit Brief of Plaintiff-Appellee, March 20, 1996, *Phillips v. Burt*, 77 Ohio St. 3d 1229 (1997) (95-1522).

Plaintiff's Exhibits, in 1 Appellant's Supplement, at 487–94, *Phillips vs. Burt*, 77 Ohio St. 3d 1229 (1997) (95-1522).

Plaintiff's Witness List, in 1 Appellant's Supplement, at 477–80, *Phillips vs. Burt,* 77 Ohio St. 3d 1229 (1997) (No. 95-1522).

St. Elizabeth Medical Center consent form for "female coital area reconstruction," signed by Janet Phillips, October 22, 1981, in 2 Appellant's Supplement at 983, *Phillips v. Burt,* 77 Ohio St. 3d 1229 (1997) (95-1522).

Published Materials

Abbott, Wallace C. "The Importance of Circumcision of the Female." *Medical Council* (December 1904): 437–42.

Abelson, Elaine S. "The Invention of Kleptomania." In *Women and Health in America,* edited by Judith Walzer Leavitt, 390–404. 2nd ed. Madison: University of Wisconsin Press, 1999.

Adair, Fred L. *Obstetrics and Gynecology.* Vol. 2. Philadelphia: Lea and Febiger, 1940.

Alcott, William. *Physiology of Marriage.* 1866. Reprint, New York: Arno Press, 1972.

American College of Obstetricians and Gynecologists. "Vaginal 'Rejuvenation' and Cosmetic Vaginal Procedures." ACOG Committee Opinion no. 378. *Obstetrics and Gynecology* 110 (2007): 737–38.

American Medical Directory. Chicago: American Medical Association, 1955.

American Medical Directory. Chicago: American Medical Association, 1961.

Ameringer, Carl F. "Organized Medicine on Trial: The Federal Trade Commission vs. the American Medical Association." *Journal of Policy History* 12 (2000): 445–72.

"Anatomy: Dig Yourself." *off our backs,* Summer 1971, 10–11.

Appignanesi, Lisa, and John Forrester. *Freud's Women.* New York: Basic Books, 1992.

Arden, Theodore Z. *A Handbook for Husbands and Wives.* New York: Association Press, 1939.

Arthur, John W. "'Female Circumcision' among the Kikuyu." *British Medical Journal* (October 24, 1942): 498.

Ashley, Jo Ann. *Hospitals, Paternalism, and the Role of the Nurse.* New York: Teachers College Press, 1976.

Ashton, William Easterly. *A Text-Book of the Practice of Gynecology.* Philadelphia: W. B. Saunders, 1910.

Ashwell, Samuel. *A Practical Treatise on the Diseases Peculiar to Women.* Philadelphia: Blanchard and Lea, 1855.

Atkinson, Ti-Grace. "Vaginal Orgasm as a Mass Hysterical Survival Response." In *Amazon Odyssey.* New York: Links Books, 1975.

Atkinson, William B. *The Therapeutics of Gynecology and Obstetrics.* Philadelphia: D. G. Brinton, 1880.

Aubey, Benjamin R. "Are You Out of Your Mind?" e-letter, *Pediatrics,* May 8, 2010, http://pediatrics.aappublications.org/content/125/5/1088.full/reply#pediatrics_el_50116.

Auchincloss, W. "Expiration of Enlarged Clitoris." *Glasgow Medical Journal* (1829): 165–67.

Bacon, C. S. "Adhesions of the Female Prepuce." *American Gynecological and Obstetrical Society Journal* 21 (1898): 278–79.

Bailey, Beth. *Sex in the Heartland.* Cambridge, MA: Harvard University Press, 1999.

Bainbridge, W. "Case of Enlarged Clitoris." *Medical Times and Gazette* (1860): 45–50.

Balint, Michael. "On the Termination of Analysis." *International Journal of Psycho-Analysis* 31 (1950): 196–99.

Ballantyne, J. William. "Malformations of the Genital Organs in Woman." In *A System of Gynecology*. Edited by Thomas Clifford Allbutt. New York: Macmillan, 1896.

Barbach, Lonnie. "Five Myths about the Big O." *Mademoiselle*, February 1981, 145, 200, 202.

Barkan, Elezar. *The Retreat of Scientific Racism: Changing Concepts of Race in Britain and the United States between the World Wars*. Cambridge: Cambridge University Press, 1992.

Barker-Benfield, G. J. "A Historical Perspective on Women's Health Care—Female Circumcision." *Women & Health* 1 (1976): 13–15, 18–20.

———. *The Horrors of the Half-Known Life*. New York: Harper, 1976.

Battan, Jesse F. "'The World Made Flesh': Language, Authority, and Sexual Desire in Late Nineteenth-Century America." *Journal of the History of Sexuality* 3 (1992): 223–44.

Beacham, Daniel Winston, and Woodard Davis Beacham. *Synopsis of Gynecology*. 9th ed. St. Louis, MO: C. V. Mosby, 1977.

Beadnell, C. Marsh. "Circumcision and Clitoridectomy as Practiced by the Natives of British East Africa." *British Medical Journal* (April 29, 1905): 964–65.

Beardsley, Edward H. "Race as a Factor in Health." In *Women, Health, and Medicine in America*. Edited by Rima D. Apple, 121–40. New Brunswick, NJ: Rutgers University Press, 1992.

Beasley, Deena. "Gynecologists Alarmed by Plastic Surgery Trend," *Reuters*, August 25, 2012, http://www.reuters.com/article/2012/08/25/us-usa-health-gynecology-idUSBRE87O05520120825.

Beccalossi, Chiara. "Female Same-Sex Desires: Conceptualizing a Disease in Competing Medical Fields in Nineteenth-Century Europe." *Journal of the History of Medicine and Allied Sciences* 67 (2012): 7–35.

———. *Female Sex Inversion: Same-Sex Desire in Italian and British Sexology, c. 1870–1920*. New York: Palgrave Macmillan, 2012.

Beebe, H. E. "The Clitoris." *Journal of Orificial Surgery* 6 (1897–98): 8–12.

Behrman, Samuel J., and John R. G. Gosling. *Fundamentals of Gynecology*. New York: Oxford University Press, 1966.

Bell, Kirsten. "Genital Cutting and Western Discourses on Sexuality." *Medical Anthropology Quarterly* 19 (2005): 125–48.

Bell, W. Blair. *The Principles of Gynecology: A Manual for Students and Practitioners*. 3rd ed. London: Bailliere, Tindall and Cox, 1919.

Bennett, Paula. "Critical Clitoridectomy: Female Sexual Imagery and Feminist Psychoanalytic Theory." *Signs* 18 (1993): 235–59.

Benson, Ralph C. *Handbook of Obstetrics and Gynecology*. 6th ed. Los Altos, CA: Lange Medical, 1977.

Berer, Marge. "Labia Reduction for Non-therapeutic Reasons vs. Female Genital Mutilation: Contradictions on Law and Practice in Britain." *Reproductive Health Matters* 18 (2010): 106–10.

Bergler, Edmund. "Newer Genetic Investigations on Impotence and Frigidity." *Menninger Clinic Bulletin* 11 (March 1947): 50–59.

———. "The Problem of Frigidity." In *Selected Papers of Edmund Bergler, MD, 1933–1961.* New York: Grune and Stratton, 1969.

———. "Some A-typical Forms of Impotence and Frigidity." *Psychoanalytic Review* 41 (1954): 29–47.

———. *Unhappy Marriage and Divorce.* New York: International Universities Press, 1946.

Bergler, Edmund, and William S. Kroger. "The Dynamic Significance of Vaginal Lubrication to Frigidity." *Western Journal of Surgery, Obstetrics, and Gynecology* 61 (1953): 711–16.

———. "Sexual Behavior," letter to the editor, *Journal of the American Medical Association* 154 (January 9, 1954): 167–68.

Berkeley, Comyns, and Victor Bonney. *A Guide to Gynecology in General Practice.* 2nd ed. London: Frowde, 1919.

Bermosk, Loretta S., and Sarah E. Porter. *Women's Health and Human Wholeness.* New York: Appleton-Century-Crofts, 1979.

Bernardy, Eugene P. "One of the Causes of Aneroticism in Women." *Proceedings, Philadelphia County Medical Society* 15 (1894): 426–32.

———. "Report of Cases of Aneroticism in Women." *Medical Council* (1896): 51–52.

"Better Orgasms?" *Big Mama Rag* (June 1977): 7.

Bigelow, H. R. "An Aggravated Instance of Masturbation in the Female." *American Journal of Obstetrics* 15 (1882): 436–41.

Bird, Lois. *How to Be a Happily Married Mistress.* Garden City, NY: Doubleday, 1970.

Birn, Anne-Emanuelle, Yogan Pillay, and Timothy H. Holtz. *Textbook of International Health: Global Health in a Dynamic World.* New York: Oxford University Press, 2009.

Black, John. "Female Genital Mutilation: A Contemporary Issue, and a Victorian Obsession." *Journal of the Royal Society of Medicine* 90 (1997): 402–5.

Bland, Lucy. "Trial by Sexology? Maud Allan, *Salome* and the 'Cult of the Clitoris' Case." In *Sexology in Culture: Labeling Bodies and Desires*, edited by Lucy Bland and Laura Doan, 183–98. Chicago: University of Chicago Press, 1998.

Bloch, A. J. "Sexual Perversion in the Female." *New Orleans Medical and Surgical Journal* 22 (1894): 1–7.

Bolling, Richard Walker. *Surgery of Childhood.* New York: D. Appleton, 1928.

Bonaparte, Marie. *Female Sexuality.* 1953. Reprint, New York: International Universities Press, 1956.

Boston Women's Health Book Collective. *Our Bodies, Ourselves: A Course by and for Women.* Boston: New England Free Press, 1971.

Boston Women's Health Book Collective. *Our Bodies, Ourselves: A Book by and for Women.* 2nd ed. New York: Simon and Schuster, 1976.

Bovee, J. Wesley. *The Practice of Gynecology.* Philadelphia: Lea Brothers, 1906.

Boyle, Elizabeth Heger. *Female Genital Cutting: Cultural Conflict in the Global Community.* Baltimore: Johns Hopkins University Press, 2002.

Brady, John Paul. "Brevital-Relaxation Treatment of Frigidity." *Behavior Research and Therapy* 4 (1966): 71–77.

Brassington, H. W. "Notes on Female Circumcision as Practiced by the Ameru." *British Medical and Churgical Journal* 49 (1932): 237.

Braun, Virginia. "Female Genital Cosmetic Surgery: A Critical Review of Current Knowledge and Contemporary Debates." *Journal of Women's Health* 19 (2010): 1393–407.

Brill, A. A. *Basic Principles of Psychoanalysis*. 1949. Reprint, Westport, CT: Greenwood Press, 1976.

———. "Masturbation: Its Causes and Sequellae." *Woman's Medical Journal* 25 (1915): 97–100.

Brody, Jane E. "Blue Shield Acts to Curb Payment on Procedures of Doubtful Value," *New York Times*, May 19, 1977.

Bronstein, Carolyn. *Battling Pornography: The American Feminist Anti-pornography Movement, 1976–1986*. New York: Cambridge University Press, 2011.

Brower, Montgomery. "James Burt's 'Love Surgery' Was Supposed to Boost Pleasure, but Some Patients Say It Brought Pain." *People*, March 27, 1989: 97–98, 100.

Brown, Isaac Baker. *On the Curability of Certain Forms of Insanity, Epilepsy, Catalepsy, and Hysteria in Females*. London: Robert Hardwicke, 1866.

Buck, W. Penn. "Hypertrophy of the Clitoris." *Photographic Review of Medicine and Surgery* 2 (1871–72): 22–23.

Buhle, Mary Jo. *Feminism and Its Discontents: A Century of Struggle with Psychoanalysis*. Cambridge, MA: Harvard University Press, 2000.

Bullough, Vern L. *Science in the Bedroom: A History of Sex Research*. New York: Basic Books, 1994.

Bullough, Vern L., and Martha Voght. "Homosexuality and Its Confusion with the 'Secret Sin' in Pre-Freudian America." *Journal of the History of Medicine* 25 (1973): 143–55.

Bumstead, F. J. "Hypertrophied Clitoris." *Photographic Review of Medicine and Surgery* (1870): 11–12.

Burnett, J. A. "The Clitoris." *Regular Medical Visitor* 4 (September 15, 1903): 201–3.

Burnham, John C. *Paths into American Culture: Psychology, Medicine, and Morals*. Philadelphia: Temple University Press, 1988.

———. "Psychoanalysis and American Medicine: 1894–1918." *Psychological Issues*, vol. 5, Monograph 20. New York: International Universities Press, 1967.

Burt, James C., and Joan Burt. *Surgery of Love*. New York: Carlton Press, 1975.

Butterfield, Oliver. *Sex Life in Marriage*. 1940. Reprint, New York: Emerson Books, 1962.

Byford, Henry T. *Manual of Gynecology*. 3rd rev. ed. Philadelphia: P. Blakiston, Son, 1902.

Byrd, W. Michael, and Linda A. Clayton. *African American Health Dilemma: Race, Medicine, and Health Care in the United States, 1900–2000*. New York: Routledge, 2002.

Caprio, Frank S. *Female Homosexuality: A Psychodynamic Study of Lesbianism*. New York: Citadel Press, 1954.

Carlston, Erin. "'A Finer Differentiation': Female Homosexuality and the American Medical Community, 1926–1940." In *Science and Homosexualities*, edited by Vernon A. Rosario, 177–96. New York: Routledge, 1997.

"Case of Excessive Masturbation." *Transactions of the Philadelphia Obstetrical Society* 2 (1872): 141–42.

"Case of Idiocy in a Female, Accompanied with Nymphomania, Cured by the Excision of the Clitoris." *Lancet* 1 (1825/1826): 420–21.

Cathy. "Sex or Hey, I Thought This Was Supposed to Be Fun!" *Womankind* (1972), Chicago Women's Liberation Union Herstory Project. Accessed July 27, 2011, http://www.cwluherstory.org/sex-or-hey-i-thought-this-was-supposed-to-be-fun. html.

Celello, Kristin. *Making Marriage Work: A History of Marriage and Divorce in the Twentieth-Century United States.* Chapel Hill: University of North Carolina Press, 2009.

Circle One: Self Help Handbook. Colorado Springs, CO: Circle One, 1973.

"Circumcision of Women." *Sexology* 1 (1933): 82–84.

Chauncey, George, Jr. "From Sexual Inversion to Homosexuality: Medicine and the Changing Conceptualization of Female Deviance." *Salmagundi* (Fall 1982–Winter 1983): 114–46.

Childs, Dan. "Intimate Operations: OB-GYN Organization Issues Warning," *ABC News,* August 31, 2007, http://abcnews.go.com/Health/WomensHealth/story?id=3547373.

Christensen, John B., and Ira Rockwood Telford. *Synopsis of Gross Anatomy.* New York: Harper and Row, 1966.

Clark, A. L. *A Treatise on the Medical and Surgical Diseases of Women.* Chicago: Jansen, McLurg, 1881.

Clark, LeMon. "Adhesions between the Clitoris and Prepuce." In *Advances in Sex Research: A Publication of the Society for the Scientific Study of Sex,* edited by Hugo Beigel, 233–35. New York: Harper and Row, 1963.

———. *Emotional Adjustment in Marriage.* St. Louis, MO: C. V. Mosby, 1937.

———. *101 Intimate Sexual Problems Answered.* New York: Signet Books, 1968.

Cleveland, Clement. "Amputation of the Clitoris." *American Journal of Obstetrics and Diseases of Women and Children* 43 (1901): 722–23.

"Clitoridectomy." *Southern Journal of the Medical Sciences* (February 1867): 794.

Colby, C. D. W. "Mechanical Restraint of Masturbation on a Young Girl." *Medical Record* 52 (1897): 206.

Cole, Simon A. "Fingerprint Identification and the Criminal Justice System: Historical Lessons for the DNA Debate." In *DNA and the Criminal Justice System: The Technology of Justice,* edited by David Lazer, 63–87. Cambridge, MA: MIT Press, 2004.

Collier, James Lincoln. "It *Is* Different for Women." *Reader's Digest,* January 1982, 84–86.

Collins, Joseph. *The Doctor Looks at Marriage and Medicine.* Garden City, NY: Doubleday, 1929.

Collins, Patricia Hill. *Black Sexual Politics: African Americans, Gender, and the New Racism.* New York: Routledge, 2004.

Comfort, Alex. *The Joy of Sex: A Gourmet Guide to Lovemaking.* New York: Simon and Schuster, 1972.

Committee on Bioethics, American Academy of Pediatrics. "Female Genital Mutilation." *Pediatrics* 102 (1998): 153–56.

Committee on Bioethics, American Academy of Pediatrics. "Policy Statement—Ritual Genital Cutting of Female Minors." *Pediatrics* 125 (2010): 1088–93.

Committee on Bioethics, American Academy of Pediatrics. "Policy Statement—Ritual Genital Cutting of Female Minors." *Pediatrics* 126 (2010): 191.

Conrad, Peter. "Medicalization and Social Control." *Annual Review of Sociology* 18 (1992): 209–32.

———. *The Medicalization of Society: On the Transformation of Human Conditions into Treatable Disorders.* Baltimore: Johns Hopkins University Press, 2007.

———. "The Shifting Engines of Medicalization." *Journal of Health and Social Behavior* 46 (2005): 3–14.

Conrad, Peter, and Joseph W. Schneider. *Deviance and Medicalization: From Badness to Sickness.* St. Louis, MO: C. V. Mosby, 1980.

Conrad, Robert. "Side Lights on the History of Circumcision." *Ohio State Medical Journal* 50 (1954): 770–73.

Cook, Cynthia W., and Susan Dworkin. *The Ms. Guide to a Woman's Health.* Garden City, NY: Doubleday, 1979.

———. *The Ms. Guide to a Woman's Health.* Rev. ed. New York: Berkley Books, 1981.

Cooke, Nicholas. *Satan in Society.* Chicago: J. S. Goodman, 1871.

Coontz, Stephanie. *Marriage, a History: From Obedience to Intimacy; or, How Love Conquered Marriage.* New York, Viking, 2005.

Cooper, E. S. "Removing the Clitoris in Cases of Masturbation, Accompanied with Threatening Insanity." *San Francisco Medical Press* 3 (January 1862): 17–21.

Copeland, Rachel. *The Sexually Fulfilled Woman.* New York: Weybright and Talley, 1971.

Corea, Gena, and Cynthia de Wit. "Current Developments and Issues: A Summary." *Reproductive and Genetic Engineering* 2 (1989): 153.

Costain, T. E. "Circumcision." *Journal of Orificial Surgery* 9 (1900): 158–69.

Costler, A., and A. Willy. *Encyclopedia of Sexual Knowledge.* New York: Eugenics, 1940.

Cotton, Alfred Cleveland. *The Medical Diseases of Infancy and Childhood.* Philadelphia: J. B. Lippincott, 1906.

Council on Scientific Affairs, American Medical Association. "Female Genital Mutilation." *Journal of the American Medical Association* 274 (December 6, 1995): 1714–16.

Coventry, Martha. "Making the Cut." *Ms.*, October/November 2000, www.msmagazine.com/oct00/makingthecut.html.

Creed, Barbara. "Lesbian Bodies: Tribades, Tomboys and Tarts." In *Feminist Theory and the Body: A Reader,* edited by Janet Price and Margrit Shildrick, 111–24. Edinburgh: Edinburgh University Press, 1999.

Crenner, Christopher. "Race and Medical Practice in Kansas City's Free Dispensary." *Bulletin of the History of Medicine* 82 (2008): 820–46.

Crist, Takey. "Female Circumcision." *Medical Aspects of Human Sexuality* (August 1977): 77.

Crossen, Harry Sturgeon, and Robert James Crossen. *Diseases of Women.* St. Louis, MO: C. V. Mosby, 1944.

Crossen, Robert James. *Diseases of Women.* St. Louis, C. V. Mosby, 1953.

Crossette, Barbara. "Female Genital Mutilation by Immigrants Is Becoming Cause for Concern in the U.S." *New York Times,* December 10, 1995.

Crouch, Robert A. "Betwixt and Between: The Past and Future of Intersexuality." In *Intersex in the Age of Ethics,* edited by Alice Dreger, 29–49. Hagerstown, MD: University Publishing Group, 1999.

Cunningham, D. J. *Cunningham's Text-Book of Anatomy*. Edited by J. C. Brash and E. B. Jamieson. 7th ed. New York: Oxford University Press, 1937.

Curtis, Arthur Hale. *A Textbook of Gynecology*. Philadelphia: W. B. Saunders, 1931.

———. *A Textbook of Gynecology*. 3rd ed. Philadelphia: W. B. Saunders, 1938.

———. *A Textbook of Gynecology*. 4th ed. Philadelphia: W. B. Saunders, 1942.

Curtis, Arthur Hale, and John William Huffman. *A Textbook of Gynecology*. 6th ed. Philadelphia: W. B. Saunders, 1950.

Dally, Ann. *Women under the Knife: A History of Surgery*. New York: Routledge, 1991.

Davidson, Sara. *Loose Change: Three Women of the Sixties*. Garden City, NY: Doubleday, 1977.

Davis, Flora. *Moving the Mountain: The Women's Movement in America since 1960*. New York: Simon and Schuster, 1991.

Davis, Katherine B. *Factors in the Sex Life of Twenty-Two Hundred Women*. 1929. Reprint, New York: Arno Press, 1972.

Davison, Wilburt C. *The Complete Pediatrician: Practical, Diagnostic, Therapeutic, and Preventive Pediatrics*. Durham, NC: Duke University Press, 1934.

Dawson, Benjamin E. "Circumcision in the Female: Its Necessity and How to Perform It." *American Journal of Clinical Medicine* 22 (1915): 520–23.

Dawson, Helen L. *Basic Human Anatomy*. New York: Appleton-Century-Crofts, 1966.

Dawson, W. W. "Hypertrophy of the Clitoris—Removal." *Cincinnati Lancet and Observer* 11 (1868): 95–97.

"Dayton Gynecologist Gives Up His License," *Plain Dealer*, January 26, 1989.

Degler, Carl. "What Ought to Be and What Was: Women's Sexuality in the Nineteenth Century." *American Historical Review* 79 (1974): 1467–90.

Dejanikus, Tacie. "Vaginal Mutilation American Style." *off our backs*, July 31, 1978, 13.

Demick, Barbara. "Love Surgery: Sexual Panacea or Mutilation for Profit?" *Real Paper*, August 26, 1978, 18–21.

D'Emilio, John, and Estelle B. Freedman. *Intimate Matters: A History of Sexuality in America*. New York: Harper and Row, 1988.

Dennett, Mary Ware. *The Sex Side of Life: An Explanation for Young People*. New York: Mary Ware Dennett, 1919.

Deutsch, Helene. *The Psychology of Women: A Psychoanalytic Interpretation*. Vol. 2, *Motherhood*. New York: Grune and Stratton, 1945.

Dewees, William P. *A Treatise on the Diseases of Females*. Philadelphia: Carey and Lea, 1831.

Diagram Group. *Woman's Body: An Owner's Manual*. New York: Simon and Schuster, 1981.

Dickinson, Robert Latou. "The Gynecology of Homosexuality." In *Sex Variants: A Study of Homosexual Patterns*, by George W. Henry. One-volume edition, 1069–130. New York: Paul B. Hoeber, 1948.

———. *Human Sex Anatomy: A Topographical Hand Atlas*. 2nd ed. Baltimore: Williams and Wilkins, 1949.

———. "Hypertrophies of the Labia Minora and Their Significance." *American Gynecology* 1 (1902): 225–54.

———. "Medical Analysis of *A Thousand Marriages*." *Journal of the American Medical Association* 97 (August 22, 1932): 529–35.

———. *A Thousand Marriages: A Medical Study of Sex Adjustment.* Baltimore: Williams and Wilkins, 1931.

Dickinson, Robert Latou, and Henry H. Pierson. "The Average Sex Life of American Women." *Journal of the American Medical Association* 85 (October 10, 1925): 1113–17.

"Dr. Baker Brown of London." *Chicago Medical Examiner* (July 1867): 442.

"Doctor 'Fixes' Women's Vaginas." *New Women's Times,* July 1978.

Dr. Groves' Reproductive Physiology and New Marriage Guide. New York: Cook, 1872.

"Doctor Loses Practice over Genital Surgery," *New York Times,* January 26, 1989.

Dodson, Betty. *Liberating Masturbation: A Mediation on Self-Love.* New York: Betty Dodson, 1976.

Dorkenoo, Efua. *Cutting the Rose: Female Genital Mutilation; The Practice and Its Prevention.* London: Minority Rights Group, 1994.

Dorland's Illustrated Medical Dictionary. 31st ed. Philadelphia: Saunders, 2007.

Downer, Carol. "Self-Help for Sex." In *Women's Sexual Development: Exploration of Inner Space,* edited by Martha Kirkpatrick, 255–71. New York: Plenum Press, 1980.

Dreger, Alice D. *Hermaphrodites and the Medical Invention of Sex.* Cambridge, MA: Harvard University Press, 1998.

———. "Hermaphrodites in Love: The Truth of the Gonads." In *Science and Homosexualities,* edited by Vernon A. Rosario, 46–66. New York: Routledge, 1997.

Drennan, M. R. "Pudenda of South African Bushwoman." *Medical Review of Reviews* 40 (1934): 36–44.

Drenth, Jelto. *The Origin of the World: Science and Fiction of the Vagina.* Translated by Arnold and Erica Pomerans. London: Reaktion Books, 2005.

Drever, James. *A Dictionary of Psychology.* Baltimore: Penguin Books, 1964.

DuBois, Ellen Carol, and Linda Gordon. "Seeking Ecstasy on the Battlefield: Danger and Pleasure in Nineteenth Century Feminist Sexual Thought." In *Pleasure and Danger: Exploring Female Sexuality,* edited by Carole S. Vance, 31–49. New York: Pandora, 1989.

Dudley, E. C. *Diseases of Women: A Treatise on the Principles and Practice of Gynecology for Students and Practitioners.* Philadelphia: Lea Brothers, 1898.

———. *The Principles and Practice of Gynecology.* 3rd ed. Philadelphia: Lea Brothers, 1902.

———. *The Principles and Practice of Gynecology.* 5th ed. Philadelphia: Lea Brothers, 1908.

Duffy, John. "Masturbation and Clitoridectomy: A Nineteenth-Century View." *Journal of the American Medical Association* 19 (October 19, 1963): 246–48.

Dugger, Celia W. "New Law Bans Genital Cutting in United States." *New York Times,* October 12, 1996.

Dunglison, Robley. *Medical Lexicon: A Dictionary of Medical Science.* 11th ed. Philadelphia: Blanchard and Lea, 1854.

———. *Medical Lexicon: A Dictionary of Medical Science.* 22nd ed. Philadelphia: Lea Brothers, 1900.

Duvall, Evelyn Millis, and Rueben Hill. *When You Marry.* Boston: D. C. Heath, 1945.

Eder, Sandra. "The Volatility of Sex: Intersexuality, Gender and Clinical Practice in the 1950s." *Gender & History* 22 (November 2010): 692–707.

Editor's note. "Mary Jane Sherfey: 'The Evolution and Nature of Female Sexuality in Relation to Psychoanalytic Theory.'" *Journal of the American Psychoanalytic Association* 26 (1968): 405.

Editorial note. *American Journal of Obstetrics* 10 (1877): 33.

Editorial note. *American Journal of Obstetrics* 10 (1877): 256–58.

Egan, R. Danielle, and Gail L. Hawkes. "Imperiled and Perilous: Exploring the History of Childhood Sexuality." *Journal of Historical Sociology* 21 (2008): 354–67.

Eichel, Edward W., and Philip Noble. *The Perfect Fit: How to Achieve Mutual Fulfillment and Monogamous Passion through the New Intercourse.* New York: D. I. Fine, 1992.

Eidelberg, Ludwig. *Encyclopedia of Psychoanalysis.* New York: Free Press, 1968.

Ellis, Albert. *The Albert Ellis Reader: A Guide to Well-Being Using Rational Emotive Behavior Therapy.* Edited by Albert Ellis and Shawn Blau. New York: Citadel Press, 1998.

———. *The American Sexual Tragedy.* New York: Lyle Stuart, 1962.

———. "Guilt, Shame, and Frigidity." *Quarterly Review of Surgery, Obstetrics and Gynecology* 16 (1959): 259–61.

———. "Is Vaginal Orgasm a Myth?" In *Sex, Society and the Individual,* edited by A. P. Pillay and Albert Ellis, 155–62. Bombay: International Journal of Sexology, 1953.

———. "Towards the Improvement of Psychoanalytic Research." *Psychoanalytic Review* 36 (1949): 123–43.

Ellis, Havelock. *Psychology of Sex: A Manual for Students.* New York: Emerson Books, 1936.

Elting, L. M., and Seymour Isenberg. *The Consumer's Guide to Successful Surgery.* New York: St. Martin's Press, 1976.

Engel, Jonathan. *American Therapy: The Rise of Psychotherapy in the United States.* New York: Gotham Books, 2008.

Engelhardt, H. Tristram, Jr. "The Disease of Masturbation: Values and the Concept of Disease." In *Sickness and Health in America: Readings in the History of Medicine and Public Health,* edited by Judith Walzer Leavitt and Ronald L. Numbers, 13–21. 2nd ed. Madison: University of Wisconsin Press, 1985.

Engelmann, George J. "Clitoridectomy." *American Practitioner: A Monthly Journal of Medicine and Surgery* (January 1882): 1–2.

English, Horace B., and Ava C. English. *A Comprehensive Dictionary of Psychological and Psychoanalytical Terms: A Guide to Usage.* New York: David McKay, 1958.

Epstein, Julia. "Either/Or—Neither/Both: Sexual Ambiguity and the Ideology of Gender." *Genders* 7 (1990): 99–142.

Erickson, Julia A., with Sally A. Steffen. *Kiss and Tell: Surveying Sex in the Twentieth Century.* Cambridge, MA: Harvard University Press, 1999.

Eskridge, Belle C. "Why Not Circumcise the Girl as Well as the Boy?" *Texas State Journal of Medicine* 14 (1918): 17–19.

Essen, Birgitta, and Sara Johnsdotter. "Female Genital Mutilation in the West: Traditional Circumcision versus Genital Cosmetic Surgery." *Acta Obstetrica et Gynecologica Scandinavica* 83 (2004): 611–13.

Evans, Sara M. *Born for Liberty: The Roots of the Women's Liberation Movement in America.* New York: Free Press, 1997.

———. *Personal Politics: The Roots of Women's Liberation in the Civil Rights Movement and the New Left.* New York: Vintage Books, 1980.

Everett, Millard. *The Hygiene of Marriage: A Detailed Consideration of Sex and Marriage.* Cleveland, OH: World, 1939.

Eyer, Alvin. "Clitoridectomy for the Cure of Certain Cases of Masturbation in Young Girls." *International Medical Magazine* 3 (1894–95): 259–60.

Exner, M. J. *The Sexual Side of Marriage.* New York: W. W. Norton, 1932.

Ezekiel, Judith. *Feminism in the Heartland.* Columbus: Ohio State University Press, 2002.

Faulkner, Howard J., and Virginia D. Pruitt, eds. *Dear Dr. Menninger: Women's Voices from the Thirties.* Columbia: University of Missouri Press, 1997.

Fausto-Sterling, Anne. *Sexing the Body: Gender Politics and the Construction of Sexuality.* New York: Basic Books, 2000.

Federation of Feminist Women's Health Centers. *A New View of a Woman's Body.* New York: Simon and Schuster, 1981.

Feibleman, Peter. "Natural Causes." *Doubletake Magazine*, Winter 1997, www.fiction-writer.com/double.htm.

Fellman, Anita Claire, and Michael Fellman. "The Rule of Moderation in Late Nine-teenth-Century American Sexual Ideology." *Journal of Sex Research* 17 (1981): 238–55.

Fields, Jill. "From Black Venus to Blonde Venus: The Meaning of Black Lingerie." *Women's History Review* 15 (2006): 611–23.

———. *An Intimate Affair: Women, Lingerie, and Sexuality.* Berkeley: University of California Press, 2007.

Fine, Reuben. *The History of Psychoanalysis.* Northvale, NJ: Jason Aronson, 1990.

Fischer, Louis. *The Baby and Growing Child: Feeding and Health Care for Physicians, Mothers, and Nurses.* New York: Funk and Wagnalls, 1936.

Fisher, Seymour. *The Female Orgasm.* New York: Basic Books, 1973.

Fleming, J. B. "Clitoridectomy—the Disastrous Downfall of Isaac Baker Brown." *Journal of Obstetrics and Gynecology of the British Empire* 67 (1960): 1017–18.

Fodor, Nandor, and Frank Gaynor, eds. *Freud: Dictionary of Psychoanalysis.* 1950. Reprint, New York: Greenwood Press, 1962.

Ford, Clellan S., and Frank A. Beach. *Patterns of Sexual Behavior.* New York: Harper and Brothers / Paul B. Hoeber Medical Books, 1951.

Fort, C. H. "Some Corroborative Facts in Regard to the Anatomical Difference between the Negro and White Races." *American Journal of Obstetrics* 10 (1877): 258–59.

Foucault, Michael. *The History of Sexuality.* Vol. 1. New York: Pantheon Books, 1978.

Fox, W. J. "Female Circumcision in Savage Tribes." *Sexology* 2 (1934–35): 522–24.

Francis, Carl C. *Introduction to Human Anatomy.* 3rd ed. St. Louis, MO: C. V. Mosby, 1959.

Frankfort, Ellen. *Vaginal Politics.* New York: Bantam, 1973.

Fraser, Alasdair. "Female Genital Mutilation and Baker Brown." *Journal of the Royal Society of Medicine* 90 (1997): 586–87.

Frederick, Carlton C. "Nymphomania as a Cause of Excessive Venery." *American Journal of Obstetrics and Diseases of Women and Children* 56 (1907): 743–44.

Freeman, Rowland Godfrey. *Elements of Pediatrics for Medical Students.* New York: Mac-Millan, 1917.

Freud, Sigmund. *New Introductory Lectures on Psycho-Analysis.* Translated by W. J. H. Sprott. New York: W. W. Norton, 1933.

———. "On the Sexual Theories of Children (1908)." In *The Standard Edition of the Complete Psychological Works of Sigmund Freud,* translated and edited by James Strachey in collaboration with Anna Freud. 9:209–26. 1959. Reprint. London: Hogarth Press, 1968.

———. "Three Essays on the Theory of Sexuality (1905)." In *The Standard Edition of the Complete Works of Sigmund Freud,* translated and edited by James Strachey in collaboration with Anna Freud. 7:135–243. 1962. Reprint. London: Hogarth Press, 1968.

"Frigidity in Women: A Symptom Not a Diagnosis." *Minnesota Medicine* 49 (1966): 1879–84.

Fritsch, Heinrich. *The Diseases of Women: A Manual for Physicians and Students.* New York: William Wood, 1883.

Fugh-Berman, Adrianne. "Self-Help: The Movement and a Book." *off our backs,* July 31, 1982, 14.

"Furor over Vaginal Surgery for Anorgasmy." *Medical World News* (April 17, 1978): 15–16.

Gallabin, Alfred Lewis. *A Handbook of the Diseases of Women.* Philadelphia: P. Blakiston, Son, 1882.

Gamwell, Lynn, and Nancy Tomes. *Madness in America: Cultural and Medical Perceptions of Mental Illness before 1914.* Ithaca, NY: Cornell University Press, 1995.

Gardetto, Darlaine. "Engendered Sensations: Social Construction of the Clitoris and Female Orgasm, 1650–1975." PhD diss., University of California, Davis, 1992.

Gardner, Ernest, and Donald J. Gray, and Ronan O'Rahilly. *Anatomy: A Regional Study of Human Structure.* Philadelphia: W. B. Saunders, 1960.

———. *Anatomy: A Regional Study of Human Structure.* 2nd ed. Philadelphia: W. B. Saunders, 1963.

———. *Anatomy: A Regional Study of Human Structure.* 3rd ed. Philadelphia: W. B. Saunders, 1969.

———. *Anatomy: A Regional Study of Human Structure.* 4th ed. Philadelphia: W. B. Saunders, 1975.

Gardner, Weston D., and William A. Osburn. *Structure of the Human Body.* Philadelphia: W. B. Saunders, 1967.

Gathorne-Hardy, Jonathan. *Sex the Measure of All Things: A Life of Alfred C. Kinsey.* Bloomington: Indiana University Press, 1998.

Gay, Peter. *Freud: A Life for Our Time.* New York: W. W. Norton, 1988.

"Genital Peculiarities of the Negro." *Atlanta Journal-Record of Medicine* 4 (1903): 842–44.

Gerhard, Jane. *Desiring Revolution: Second-Wave Feminism and the Writing of American Sexual Thought, 1920–1982.* New York: Columbia University, 2001.

———. "Revisiting 'The Myth of the Vaginal Orgasm': The Female Orgasm in American Sexual Thought and Second Wave Feminism." *Feminist Studies* 26 (2000): 449–76.

Gibbs, Philip A. "Self Control and Male Sexuality in the Advice Literature of Nineteenth Century America, 1830–1860." *Journal of American Culture* 9 (1986): 37–41.

Gibson, Margaret. "Clitoral Corruption: Body Metaphors and American Doctors' Constructions of Female Homosexuality, 1870–1900." In *Science and Homosexualities*, edited by Vernon A. Rosario, 108–32. New York: Routledge, 1997.

Giddings, Paula. "The Last Taboo." In *Words of Fire*, edited by Beverly Guy-Sheftall, 414–28. New York: New Press, 1995.

Giles, Arthur E. *Anatomy and Physiology of the Female Generative Organs and of Pregnancy.* London: Bailliere, Tindall and Cox, 1909.

Gillett, Myrtle Mann. "Normal Frigidity in Women: A Plea to the Family Physician." *Medical Woman's Journal* 57 (1950): 29–32.

Gillis, Jonathan. "The History of the Patient History since 1850." *Bulletin of the History of Medicine* 80 (2006): 490–512.

Gilman, Sander. *Difference and Pathology: Stereotypes of Sexuality, Race, and Madness.* Ithaca, NY: Cornell University Press, 1985.

Glenn, Jules, and Eugene H. Kaplan. "Types of Orgasm in Women: A Critical Review and Redefinition." *Journal of the American Psychoanalytic Association* 16 (1968): 549–64.

Gollaher, David L. *Circumcision: A History of the World's Most Controversial Surgery.* New York: Basic Books, 2000.

———. "From Ritual to Science: The Medical Transformation of Circumcision in America." *Journal of Social History* (1994): 5–36.

Goodell, William. "Masturbation in the Female." *Medical Bulletin* 6 (1884): 226.

Goodhart, James Frederic, and George Frederic Still. *The Diseases of Children.* Philadelphia: P. Blakiston's Son, 1910.

Goodman, Michael, Otto J. Placik, Royal H. Benson, John R. Miklos, Robert D. Moore, Robert A. Jason, David L. Malock, Alex F. Simopoulos, Bernard H. Stern, Ryan A. Stanton, Susan E. Kolb, and Federico Gonzalez. "A Large Multicenter Outcome Study of Female Genital Plastic Surgery." *Journal of Sexual Medicine* 7 (2010): 165–77.

Gordon, Linda. *The Moral Property of Women: A History of Birth Control Politics in America.* Urbana: University of Illinois Press, 2002.

Gordon, Michael. "From an Unfortunate Necessity to a Cult of Mutual Orgasm: Sex in American Marital Education Literature 1830–1940." In *Studies in the Sociology of Sex*, edited by James Henslin, 53–77. New York: Appleton-Century-Crofts, 1971.

Gould, George M., and Walter L. Pyle. *Anomalies and Curiosities of Medicine.* Philadelphia: W. B. Saunders, 1897.

Gould, Stephen Jay. "Freudian Slip." *Natural History* 96 (1987): 14–21.

———. "The Hottentot Venus." In *The Flamingo's Smile: Reflections on Natural History*, 291–301. New York: W. W. Norton, 1985.

———. "Of Wasps and WASPS." In *The Flamingo's Smile: Reflections on Natural History*, 155–66. New York: W. W. Norton, 1985.

Graber, Benjamin, and Georgia Miller Graber. "You and Your Sexuality." *Playgirl* (April 1974): 83.

Graetzer, E. *Practical Pediatrics: A Manual of the Medical and Surgical Diseases of Infancy and Childhood.* Translated with additions by Herman B. Sheffield. Philadelphia: F. A. Davis, 1905.

Graham, Edwin C. *Diseases of Children.* Philadelphia: Lea and Febiger, 1916.

Grandin, Egbert H. "The Role of the Clitoris in the Production of Neuroses." *Pediatrics* 3 (February 15, 1897): 145–48.

Grant, J. C. Boileau. *An Atlas of Anatomy by Regions.* Vol. 1. Baltimore: Williams and Wilkins, 1943.

———. *An Atlas of Anatomy by Regions.* 3rd ed. Baltimore: Williams and Wilkins, 1951.

———. *An Atlas of Anatomy by Regions.* 4th ed. Baltimore: Williams and Wilkins, 1956.

———. *An Atlas of Anatomy by Regions.* 5th ed. Baltimore: Williams and Wilkins, 1962.

———. *Method of Anatomy: Descriptive and Deductive.* 3rd ed. Baltimore: Williams and Wilkins, 1944.

———. *Method of Anatomy: Descriptive and Deductive.* 4th ed. Baltimore: Williams and Wilkins, 1948.

———. *Method of Anatomy: Descriptive and Deductive.* 6th ed. Baltimore: Williams and Wilkins, 1958.

Gray, Henry. *Anatomy: Descriptive and Surgical.* Philadelphia: Blanchard and Lea, 1859.

———. *Anatomy: Descriptive and Surgical.* 2nd American edition from the revised and enlarged London ed. Philadelphia: Blanchard and Lea, 1862.

———. *Anatomy: Descriptive and Surgical.* New American edition from the 5th English ed. Philadelphia: Henry C. Lea, 1870.

———. *Anatomy: Descriptive and Surgical.* New American edition from the 8th English ed. Philadelphia: Henry C. Lea, 1878.

———. *Anatomy: Descriptive and Surgical.* Edited by T. Pickering Pick. New American edition from the 10th English ed. Philadelphia: Lea and Sons, 1883.

———. *Anatomy: Descriptive and Surgical.* Edited by T. Pickering Pick and William W. Keen. New American edition from the 11th English ed. Philadelphia: Lea Brothers, 1887.

———. *Anatomy: Descriptive and Surgical.* Edited by T. Pickering Pick. New American edition from the 13th English ed. Philadelphia: Lea Brothers, 1893.

———. *Anatomy: Descriptive and Surgical.* Edited by T. Pickering Pick. New American edition from the 13th English ed. Philadelphia: Lea Brothers, 1897.

———. *Anatomy: Descriptive and Surgical.* Edited by T. Pickering Pick and Robert Howden. Revised American edition from the 15th English ed. Philadelphia: Lea and Febiger, 1901.

———. *Anatomy: Descriptive and Surgical.* Edited by Pick and Howden. 16th ed. New American ed. Revised and reedited by John Chalmers DaCosta. Philadelphia: Lea Brothers, 1905.

———. *Anatomy: Descriptive and Surgical.* Edited by John Chalmers DeCosta and Edward Anthony Spitzka. 17th ed. Philadelphia: Lea and Febiger, 1908.

———. *Anatomy: Descriptive and Applied.* Edited by Edward Anthony Spitzka. New American edition from the 18th English ed. Philadelphia: Lea and Febiger, 1913.

———. *Anatomy of the Human Body.* Edited by Warren H. Lewis. 20th ed. Philadelphia: Lea and Febiger, 1918.

———. *Anatomy of the Human Body.* Edited by Warren H. Lewis. 21st ed. Philadelphia: Lea and Febiger, 1924.

———. *Anatomy of the Human Body.* Edited by Warren H. Lewis. 22nd ed. Philadelphia: Lea and Febiger, 1930.

———. *Anatomy of the Human Body.* Edited by Warren H. Lewis. 23rd ed. Philadelphia: Lea and Febiger, 1936.

———. *Anatomy of the Human Body.* Edited by Warren H. Lewis. 24th ed. Philadelphia: Lea and Febiger, 1942.

———. *Anatomy of the Human Body.* Edited by Charles Mayo Goss. 25th ed. Philadelphia: Lea and Febiger, 1948.

———. *Anatomy of the Human Body.* Edited by Charles Mayo Goss. 26th ed. Philadelphia: Lea and Febiger, 1954.

———. *Anatomy of the Human Body.* Edited by Charles Mayo Goss. 27th ed. Philadelphia: Lea and Febiger, 1959.

Gray, Mary Jane. "Women's Preferences regarding Clitoral Stimulation." *Medical Aspects of Human Sexuality* 12 (1978): 32–42.

Green, Charles M. *Case Histories in Diseases of Women.* Boston: W. M. Leonard, 1915.

Greene, Ryland W., ed. *Lippincott's Medical Dictionary.* Philadelphia: J. L. Lippincott, 1897.

Greenhalgh, Robert. Letter to the editor. *British Medical Journal* (December 29, 1866): 730.

Greenhill, J. P. "Frigidity in Women." *Postgraduate Medicine* 12 (August 1952): 145–51.

———. *Obstetrics.* 13th ed. Philadelphia: W. B. Saunders, 1965.

Greenlee-Donnell, Cynthia. "'A White Man Has Got Hattie': Black Families, Child Rape, and Law in South Carolina, 1885–1905." Paper presented at the Organization of American Historians, Milwaukee, WI, April 19, 2012.

Grewal, Inderpal, and Caren Kaplan. "*Warrior Marks*: Global Womanism's Neo-colonial Discourse in a Multi-cultural Context." *Camera Obscura* 13 (1996): 4–33.

Griffith, J. P. Crozer, and A. Graeme Mitchell. *The Diseases of Infants and Children.* 2nd ed. Vol. 2. Philadelphia: W. B. Saunders, 1927.

———. *The Diseases of Infants and Children,* 3rd ed. Philadelphia: W. B. Saunders, 1933.

Griswold, Rufus. "Some Observations on the Physiology of Coitus from the Female Side of the Matter." *Clinical News* (1880): 445–49.

Groneman, Carol. *Nymphomania: A History.* New York: W. W. Norton, 2000.

Grossman, Elliott A., and Norman Ames Posner. "The Circumcision Controversy: An Update." *Obstetrics and Gynecological Annual* 13 (1984): 181–95.

Group, Thetis M., and Joan I. Roberts. *Nursing, Physician Control, and the Medical Monopoly: Historical Perspectives on Gendered Inequality in Roles, Rights, and Range of Practice.* Bloomington: Indian University Press, 2001.

Groves, Ernest. *The Marriage Crisis.* New York: Longmans, Green, 1928.

Guernsey, Henry. *Plain Talk on Avoided Subjects.* Philadelphia: F. A. Davis, 1907.

Gunning, Isabelle R. "Arrogant Perception, World-Travelling and Multicultural Feminism: The Case of Female Genital Surgeries." *Columbia Human Rights Legal Review* 23 (1991–92): 189–248.

———. "Female Genital Surgeries and Multicultural Feminism: The Ties That Bind; The Differences That Distance." *Third World Legal Studies* 13 (1995): 17–47.

Guy, Nichol. "The Clitoris Martyr." *World Medicine* 4 (May 6, 1969): 59, 63, 65.

Guy-Sheftall, Beverly. "The Body Politic: Sexuality, Violence, and Reproduction." In *Words of Fire: An Anthology of African-American Feminist Thought,* edited by Beverly Guy-Sheftall, 1–22. New York: New Press, 1995.

Gwillim, C. M. "President's Address: A Meeting of the Royal Medical and Chirurgical Society in the Session 1861–62." *Proceedings of the Royal Society of Medicine* 55 (1862): 89–90.

Haiken, Elizabeth. *Venus Envy: A History of Cosmetic Surgery.* Baltimore: Johns Hopkins University Press, 1997.

Haldane, David. "Clitoral Circumcision: Will It or Won't It Help a Woman Obtain Orgasm?" *Penthouse Forum* (October 1978): 45–49.

Hale, Edwin M. "Two Cases of Imprisoned Clitoris." *Homeopathic Journal of Obstetrics, Gynecology and Pediatrics* 18 (1896): 446.

Hale, Nathan G, Jr. *The Beginnings of Psychoanalysis in the United States, 1876–1917.* New York: Oxford University Press, 1971.

———. *Rise and Crisis of Psychoanalysis in the United States: Freud and the Americans.* New York: Oxford University Press, 1995.

Hall, G. Stanley. *Adolescence: Its Psychology and Its Relations to Physiology, Anthropology, Sociology, Sex, Crime, Religion, and Education.* Vol. 1. New York: D. Appleton, 1905.

Haller, John S., Jr. *Outcasts from Evolution: Scientific Attitudes of Racial Inferiority, 1859–1900.* Urbana: University of Illinois Press, 1971.

———. "The Physician versus the Negro: Medical and Anthropological Concepts of Race in the Late Nineteenth Century." *Bulletin of the History of Medicine* 44 (1970): 154–67.

Haller, John S., Jr., and Robin M. Haller. *The Physician and Sexuality in Victorian America.* Urbana: University of Illinois Press, 1974.

Hamilton, Eugene G. "Frigidity in the Female." *Missouri Medicine* 58 (1961): 1040–51.

Hamilton, G. V. *A Research in Marriage.* New York: Albert and Charles Boni, 1929.

Hansen, Bert. "American Physicians' 'Discovery' of Homosexuals, 1880–1900: A New Diagnosis in a Changing Society." In *Sickness and Health in America,* edited by Judith Waltzer Leavitt and Ronald L. Numbers, 13–31. 3rd rev. ed. Madison: University of Wisconsin Press, 1997.

Hardenbergh, E. W. "The Psychology of Female Sex Experience." *International Journal of Sexology* 2 (1949): 224–28.

Harding, Celia. "Introduction: Making Sense of Sexuality." In *Sexuality: Psychoanalytic Perspectives,* edited by Celia Harding, 1–17. Philadelphia: Brunner-Routledge, 2001.

Harris, Frederick M. *Essays on Marriage.* New York: Association Press, 1931.

Hartman, William E., and Marilyn A. Fithian. *Treatment of Sexual Dysfunction.* New York: Jason Aronson, 1974.

Hassler, M. Margaret. "Preputial Adhesions in Little Girls." *Hahnemannian Monthly* (March 1897): 182–85.

Hausman, Bernice. *Changing Sex: Transsexualism, Technology, and the Idea of Gender.* Durham, NC: Duke University Press, 1995.

Hawkes, W. J. "Rational Treatment of Prepuce and Clitoris in Children." *Medical and Surgical Reporter* 17 (1909): 352–56.

Heidenry, John. *What Wild Ecstasy: The Rise and Fall of the Sexual Revolution.* New York: Simon and Schuster, 1997.

Heiman, Marcel. "Discussion," *Journal of the American Psychoanalytic Association* 26 (July 1968): 406–16.

Helgason, Julia. "'Love Surgery' Might Be Allowed in Future, St. E President Says." *Dayton Daily News*, January 27, 1989.

———. "We Had No Way to Stop Burt, Physicians Say; Strict Rules Govern Complaints, Privileges." *Dayton Daily News*, November 13, 1988.

Helgason, Julia, and Dave Davis. "'Media Has Accepted Lies as Truth,' Says Burt." *Dayton Daily News*, November 20, 1988.

Helmuth, William Tod. *A Dozen Cases of Clinical Surgery*. Albany: Weed, Parsons, 1876.

Henry, George W. *Sex Variants: A Study of Homosexual Patterns*. One-volume edition. New York: Paul B. Hoeber, 1948.

Hennessee, Judith Adler. "The Love Surgeon." *Mademoiselle*. August 1989: 206–7, 245–47.

Herlund, Ylva, and Bettina Shell-Duncan, eds. *Transcultural Bodies: Female Genital Cutting in Global Context*. New Brunswick, NJ: Rutgers University Press, 2007.

Hite, Shere. *The Hite Report: A Nationwide Study on Female Sexuality*. New York: Macmillan, 1976.

———. *Women as Revolutionary Agents of Change: The Hite Reports and Beyond*. Madison: University of Wisconsin Press, 1994.

Hitschmann, Edward. "Frigidity in Women—Restatement and Renewed Experiences." *Psychoanalytic Review* 36 (1949): 45–53.

Hitschmann, Edward, and Edmund Bergler. *Frigidity in Women: Its Characteristics and Treatment*. Washington: Nervous and Mental Disease, 1936.

Hobson, Janell. *Venus in the Dark: Blackness and Beauty in Popular Culture*. New York: Routledge, 2005.

Hoffman, Frederick L. "The Race Traits and Tendencies of the American Negro." *Publications of the American Economic Association* 11 (1896): 1–329.

———. "Vital Statistics of the Negro." *Arena* 29 (April 1892): 529–41.

Hollander, Marc H. "The 51st Landmark Article." *Journal of the American Medical Association* 250 (July 8, 1983): 228–29.

Holoweiko, Mark. "Why Was the Love Surgeon Allowed to Keep Cutting?" *Medical Economics*, July 17, 1989, 125–28, 131–33, 136–38.

Holson, Laura M. "The Long View on *Deep Throat*." *New York Times*, September 5, 2004.

Holt, L. Emmett. *The Care and Feeding of Children: A Catechism for the Use of Mothers and Children's Nurses*. New York: D. Appleton, 1915.

———. *Diseases of Infancy and Childhood*. 4th ed. New York: D. Appleton, 1908.

Holt, L. Emmett, and John Howland. *Diseases of Infancy and Childhood*. 7th rev. ed. New York: D. Appleton, 1916.

———. *Diseases of Infancy and Childhood*. Revised by L. Emmett Holt Jr. and Rustin McIntosh. 10th ed. New York: D. Appleton, 1933.

———. *Holt's Diseases of Infancy and Childhood*. Revised by L. Emmett Holt Jr. and Rustin McIntosh. 11th ed. New York: D. Appleton, 1940.

Hor and Sprague. "Case of Nymphomania." *Boston Medical and Surgical Journal* 25 (1841–42): 62.

Horn, David G. "This Norm Which Is Not One: Reading the Female Body in Lombroso's Anthropology." In *Deviant Bodies: Critical Perspectives on Difference in Science and Popular Culture*, edited by Jennifer Terry and Jacqueline Urla, 109–28. Bloomington: Indiana University Press, 1995.

Horos, Carol V. *Vaginal Health*. New Canaan, CT: Tobey, 1975.

Horowitz, Carol, J. Carey Jackson, and Mamae Teklemariam. "Female Circumcision." *New England Journal of Medicine* 332 (January 19, 1995): 188.

Hosken, Fran. "Female Circumcision and Fertility in Africa." *Women and Health* 1 (1976): 3–11.

———. *Genital Mutilation of Women in Africa*. Pasadena, CA: Munger Africana Library, California Institute of Technology, 1976.

———. *The Hosken Report: Genital and Sexual Mutilation of Females*. 2nd ed. Lexington, MA: Women's Institute Network News, 1979.

———. *The Hosken Report: Genital and Sexual Mutilation of Females*. 4th rev. ed. Lexington, MA: Women's International Network News, 1993.

Houck, Judith A. *Hot and Bothered: Women, Medicine, and Menopause in Modern America*. Cambridge, MA: Harvard University Press, 2006.

———. "'What Do These Women Want?' Feminist Responses to *Feminine Forever*, 1963–1980." *Bulletin of the History of Medicine* 77 (2003): 103–32.

Howe, Joseph. *Excessive Venery, Masturbation, and Continence. The Etiology, Pathology, and Treatment of the Diseases Resulting from Venereal Excess, Masturbation, and Continence*. New York: Bermingham, 1883.

Howell, A. Brazier. *Gross Anatomy: A Brief Systematic Presentation of the Macroscopic Structure of the Human Body*. New York: D. Appleton-Century, 1939.

Hsu, Chi-yuan. "Orificial Surgery: A History." MD thesis, Harvard University, 1993.

Hudgins, Archibald Perrin. "The Doctor as Marital Counselor." *International Record of Medicine and General Practice Clinics* 164 (1951): 472–81.

Huffman, John W. "Some Facts about the Clitoris." *Postgraduate Medicine* 60 (1976): 245–47.

Hyatt, H. Otis. "A Note on the Normal Anatomy of the Vulvo-Vaginal Orifice." *American Journal of Obstetrics* 10 (April 1877): 253–56.

Hyde, Frank E. "Frigidity and the Clitoris." Letter to Queries and Minor Notes. *Journal of the American Medical Association* 130 (February 23, 1946): 546.

Iiams, Frank J. "Female Circumcision." *Medical Record and Annals* 31 (April 1937): 171–73.

"In Brief." *National NOW Times*, October 1978.

Irvine, Janice M. *Disorders of Desire: Sex and Gender in Modern American Sexology*. Philadelphia: Temple University Press, 1990.

Isenberg, Seymour, and L. Melvin Elting. "A Guide to Sexual Surgery." *Cosmopolitan*, November 1976, 104, 108, 110, 164.

Jackson, Margaret. "Sex Research and the Construction of Sexuality: A Tool of Male Supremacy?" *Women's Studies International Forum* 7 (1984): 43–51.

Jacobs, Maurice S. "Circumcision." *Annals of Medical History* 1 (1939): 68–73.

Jacobson, Nora. *Cleavage: Technology, Controversy, and the Ironies of the Man-Made Breast*. New Brunswick, NJ: Rutgers University Press, 2000.

James, Stanlie. Review of *Warrior Marks*, by Alice Walker and Pratibha Parmar. *American Historical Review* 102 (1997): 595–96.

Jeffcoate, T. N. A. *Principles of Gynaecology*. 3rd ed. New York: Appleton-Century-Crofts, 1967.

Johnsdotter, Sara. "Projected Cultural Histories of the Cutting of Female Genitalia: A Poor Reflection in the Mirror." *History and Anthropology* 23 (2012): 91–114.

Johnsdotter, Sara, and Birgitta Essen. "Genitals and Ethnicity: The Politics of Genital Modifications." *Reproductive Health Matters* 18 (2010): 29–37.

Jones, James H. *Alfred C. Kinsey: A Public/Private Life.* W. W. Norton, 1997.

Jordan, William George. *Little Problems of Married Life: The Baedeker to Matrimony.* New York: Fleming H. Revell, 1910.

Jung, Frederic Theodore, Anna Ruth Benjamin, and Elizabeth Carpenters Earle. *Anatomy and Physiology.* Philadelphia: F. A. Davis, 1939.

Jung, Moses. "The Course in Modern Marriage at the State University of Iowa." *Living: The Journal of Marriage and the Family* 1 (1939): 43, 50.

Kaplan, Helen Singer. *The New Sex Therapy: Active Treatment of Sexual Dysfunctions.* New York: Brunner/Mazel, 1974.

Katz, Jonathan Ned. *The Invention of Heterosexuality.* New York: Dutton, 1995.

Keating, John M., ed. *Clinical Gynecology, Medical and Surgical.* Philadelphia: J. B. Lippincott, 1896.

Kellison, Catherine. "Circumcision for Women." *Playgirl,* October 1973, 76, 124–25.

———. "$100 Surgery for a Million-Dollar Sex Life." *Playgirl,* May 1975, 52–55.

Kellogg, J. H. *Plain Facts for Old and Young.* Burlington, IA: I. F. Segner, 1886.

Kelly, G. Lombard. "Operations on Clitoris for Frigidity." Letter to Queries and Minor Notes. *Journal of the American Medical Association* 130 (March 30, 1946): 908.

———. *Sexual Feeling in Women.* Augusta, GA: Elkay, 1930.

Kelly, Howard A. "Elephantiasis of the Clitoris." *Report of the Director of the Johns Hopkins Hospital* 2 (1891): 227–30.

———. *Medical Gynecology.* New York: D. Appleton, 1908.

Kelly, Howard A., and Charles P. Nobel. *Gynecology and Abdominal Surgery.* Vol. 1. Philadelphia: W. B. Saunders, 1907.

Kenen, Stephanie Hope. "Scientific Studies of Human Sexual Difference in Interwar America." PhD diss., University of California, Berkeley, 1998.

Kent, James. *Sexual Neuroses.* St. Louis, MO: Maynard & Tedford, 1879.

Kentsmith, David K., and Merrill T. Eaton Jr. *Treating Sexual Problems in Medical Practice.* New York: Arco, 1979.

Kerley, Charles Gilmore. *Treatment of the Diseases of Children.* Philadelphia: W. B. Saunders, 1907.

Kerr, Le Grand. *The Care and Training of Children.* New York: Funk and Wagnalls, 1910.

Kessler, Suzanne J. *Lessons from the Intersexed.* New Brunswick, NJ: Rutgers University Press, 1998.

———. "The Medical Construction of Gender: Case Management of Intersexed Infants." *Signs* 16 (1990): 3–26.

Kestenberg, Judith S. "Discussion." *Journal of the American Psychoanalytic Association* 16 (July 1968): 417–23.

Kinsey, Alfred, Wardell B. Pomeroy, Clyde E. Martin, and Paul H. Gebhard. *Sexual Behavior in the Human Female.* Philadelphia: Saunders, 1953.

Kisch, E. Heinrich. *The Sexual Life of Woman.* New York: Rebman, 1910.

Kistler, S. L. "Rapid Bloodless Circumcision of Male and Female and its Technic." *Journal of the American Medical Association* 54 (May 28, 1910): 1782–83.

Kistner, Robert W. *Gynecology: Principles and Practice.* 2nd ed. Chicago: Year Book Medical, 1973.

————. *Gynecology: Principals and Practice.* 3rd ed. Chicago: Year Book Medical Publications, 1979.

Kleegman, Sophia J. "Frigidity in Women." *Quarterly Review of Surgery, Obstetrics and Gynecology* 16 (October–December 1959): 243–48.

Klein, Hanny Lightfoot. *Prisoners of Ritual: An Odyssey into Female Genital Mutilation in Africa.* New York: Haworth Press, 1989.

Kline, Wendy. *Bodies of Knowledge: Sexuality, Reproduction, and Women's Health in the Second Wave.* Chicago: University of Chicago Press, 2010.

Kline-Graber, Georgia, and Benjamin Graber. *Woman's Orgasm: A Guide to Sexual Satisfaction.* Indianapolis: Bobbs-Merrill, 1975.

Knott, John. "Normal Ovariotomy, Circumcision, Clitoridectomy and Infibulation." *Medical Press and Circular* (1890): 33–39.

Knout, Jo Ann. "Local Doctor Develops Corrective Surgery." *Dayton Daily News,* September 3, 1975.

Koedt, Anne. "The Myth of the Vaginal Orgasm." In *Liberation Now! Writings from the Women's Liberation Movement,* compiled by Deborah Babcox and Madeline Belkin, 311–20. New York: Dell, 1971.

Kolischer, G. "Sexual Frigidity in Women." *American Journal of Obstetrics and Diseases of Women and Children* 32 (1905): 416.

Kolodny, Robert C., William H. Masters, and Virginia E. Johnson. *Textbook of Sexual Medicine.* Boston: Little, Brown, 1979.

Koplik, Henry. *The Diseases of Infancy and Childhood Designed for Students and Practitioners of Medicine.* 3rd ed. New York: Lea and Febiger, 1910.

Kroger, William S. "Psychosomatic Aspects of Frigidity and Impotence." In *Psychosomatic Obstetrics, Gynecology and Endocrinology,* edited by William S. Kroger, 383–85. Springfield, IL: Charles C. Thomas, 1962.

Kroger, William S., and S. Charles Freed. *Psychosomatic Gynecology, Including Problems in Obstetrical Care.* Philadelphia: W. B. Saunders, 1951.

————. "Psychosomatic Aspects of Frigidity and Impotence." *Journal of the American Medical Association* 143 (June 10, 1950): 526–32.

Kuhn, Thomas. *The Structure of Scientific Revolutions.* 2nd ed. Chicago: University of Chicago Press, 1970.

Kupperman, Herbert S. "Hormonal Aspects of Frigidity." *Quarterly Review of Surgery, Obstetrics, and Gynecology* 16 (October–December 1959): 254–57.

LaBelle, Beverly. "Snuff—the Ultimate in Woman-Hating." In *Take Back the Night: Women on Pornography,* edited by Laura Lederer, 272–78. New York: William Morrow, 1980.

Laipson, Peter. "'Kiss without Shame, for She Desires It': Sexual Foreplay in American Marital Advice Literature, 1900–1925." *Journal of Social History* (Spring 1996): 507–25.

Lander, Louise. *Defective Medicine: Risk, Anger, and the Malpractice Crisis.* New York: Farrar, Straus and Giroux, 1978.

Lane, Charles E. "Remarkable Results following Female Circumcision." *Journal of the American Institute of Homeopathy* 33 (March 1940): 155–56.

Laqueur, Thomas. "Amor Veneris, vel Dulcedo Appeletur." In *Fragments for a History of the Human Body,* edited by Michel Feher, 91–131. Part 3. Cambridge, MA: MIT Press, 1989.

————. *Making Sex: Body and Gender from the Greeks to Freud.* Cambridge, MA: Harvard University Press, 1990.

————. *Solitary Sex: A Cultural History of Masturbation.* New York: Zone Books, 2003.

Laskas, Jeanne Marie. "Crime against Nature." *Savvy Woman,* June 1989, 63–66.

Laumann, Edward O., Christopher M. Masi, and Ezra W. Zuckerman. "Circumcision in the United States: Prevalence, Prophylactic Effects, and Sexual Practice." *Journal of the American Medical Association* 277 (April 2, 1997): 1052–57.

Lauersen, Niels, and Steven Whitney. *It's Your Body: A Woman's Guide to Gynecology.* New York: Grosset and Dunlap, 1977.

La Vake, Rae Thornton. *A Handbook of Clinical Gynecology and Obstetrics.* St. Louis, MO: C. V. Mosby, 1928.

Law, Sylvia, and Steven Polan. *Pain and Profit: The Politics of Malpractice.* New York: Harper and Row, 1978.

Lawrence, Susan, and Kae Bendixen. "His and Hers: Female Anatomy in Anatomy Texts for U.S. Medical Students, 1890–1989." *Social Science and Medicine* 35 (1992): 925–34.

Layman, William A., Gerald H. Rozan, and Morton L. Kurland. "Frigidity in the Female." *General Practitioner* (October 1966): 103–6.

Leary, Robyn. "Masturbation and Orgasm." *Harper's Bazaar,* April 1980, 200–201.

Leavitt, Judith Walzer. *Brought to Bed: Childbearing in America, 1750–1950.* New York: Oxford University Press, 1986.

Lederer, Laura. Introduction to *Take Back the Night: Women on Pornography,* edited by Laura Lederer, 15–20. New York: William Morrow, 1980.

Levinson, Abraham. *Pediatric Nursing.* Philadelphia: Lea and Febiger, 1945.

Lewis, Carolyn Herbst. *Prescriptions for Heterosexuality: Sexual Citizenship in the Cold War.* Chapel Hill: University of North Carolina Press, 2010.

————. "Waking Sleeping Beauty: The Premarital Pelvic Exam and Heterosexuality during the Cold War." *Journal of Women's History* 17 (2005): 86–110.

Lewis, Denslow. "The Gynecologic Consideration of the Sexual Act." *Journal of the American Medical Association* 250 (July 8, 1983): 222–27.

Lichtenstein, Perry M. "The 'Fairy' and the Lady Lover." *Medical Review of Reviews* 27 (1921): 369–74.

Lindsey, Ben B., and Wainwright Evans. *The Companionate Marriage.* New York: Boni and Liveright, 1927.

Lief, Harold I. "Sex Education of Medical Students and Doctors." In *Human Sexuality in Medical Education and Practice,* edited by Clark E. Vincent, 19–33. Springfield, IL: Charles C. Thomas, 1968.

Liswood, Rebecca. *A Marriage Doctor Speaks Her Mind about Sex.* New York: Dutton, 1961.

Litchfield, Harry R., and Leon H. Dembo. *Therapeutics of Infancy and Childhood.* Vol. 2. 3rd ed. Philadelphia: F. A. Davis, 1947.

————. *Therapeutics of Infancy and Childhood.* Vol. 3, 3rd ed. Philadelphia: F. A. Davis, 1947.

Lloyd, Elisabeth. *The Case of the Female Orgasm: Bias in the Science of Evolution.* Cambridge, MA: Harvard University Press, 2005.

Long, H. W. *Sane Sex Life and Sane Sex Living.* Boston: R. G. Badger, 1922.

"Looking Back: 18 Years of Controversy." *Dayton Daily News,* August 4, 1991.

"The Love Surgery: A Sex Scandal," *CBS News—West 57th,* October 29, 1988, recording and transcript, possession of author.

Lowen, Alexander. "Frigidity: A Bioenergetic Study." *Quarterly Review of Surgery, Obstetrics and Gynecology* 16 (October–December 1959): 258.

Lucas, William Palmer. *The Modern Practice of Pediatrics.* New York: Macmillan, 1927.

Lumley, J. S. P., J. L. Craven, and J. T. Aitken. *Essential Anatomy and Some Clinical Applications.* Edinburgh: Churchill Livingstone, 1975.

Lundberg, Ferdinand, and Marynia F. Farnham. *Modern Woman: The Lost Sex.* New York: Harper and Brothers, 1947.

Lydon, Susan. "Understanding Orgasm." *Ramparts,* December 1969, 59–63.

M.D., New York. "Masturbation in Women." Letter to Queries and Minor Notes. *Journal of the American Medical Association* 109 (November 6, 1937): 1564.

Madden, Thomas More. *Clinical Gynecology.* Philadelphia: J. B. Lippincott, 1893.

Magubane, Zine. "Which Bodies Matter? Feminism, Post-structuralism, Race, and the Curious Theoretical Odyssey of the 'Hottentot Venus.'" In *Black Venus 2010: They Called Her 'Hottentot,'* edited by Deborah Willis, 47–60. Philadelphia: Temple University Press, 2010.

Maier, Thomas. *Masters of Sex: The Life and Times of William Masters and Virginia Johnson, the Couple Who Taught American How to Love.* New York: Basic Books, 2009.

Maines, Rachel. *The Technology of Orgasm: "Hysteria," The Vibrator, and Women's Sexual Satisfaction.* Baltimore: Johns Hopkins University Press, 1999.

Malchow, C. W. *The Sexual Life.* St. Louis, MO: C. V. Mosby, 1923.

"Malpractice Suit Hits St. E.," *Journal Herald* (Dayton, OH), May 31, 1980.

Marieskind, Helen I. *Women in the Health System: Patients, Providers, and Programs.* St. Louis, MO: C. V. Mosby, 1980.

Marmor, Judd. "Some Considerations concerning Orgasm in the Female." *Psychosomatic Medicine* 16 (1954): 240–45.

Marsh, Margaret, and Wanda Ronner. *The Fertility Doctor: John Rock and the Reproductive Revolution.* Baltimore: Johns Hopkins University Press, 2008.

Martensen, Robert L. "Physiology as Destiny: Medicine and Motherhood in the Progressive Era." *Journal of the American Medical Association* 275 (April 17, 1996): 1213.

Mason, Lyman W. "Hypertrophy of the Clitoris: Report of Two Cases." *American Journal of Obstetrics and Gynecology* 25 (January 1933): 144–46.

Masters, William H., and Virginia E. Johnson. *Human Sexual Response.* Boston: Little, Brown, 1966.

———. "Orgasm, Anatomy of the Female." In *The Encyclopedia of Sexual Behavior,* edited by Albert Ellis and Albert Abarbanel, 788–93. New York: Hawthorne Books, 1961.

———. "The Sexual Response Cycle of the Human Female: The Clitoris; Anatomic and Clinical Considerations." *Western Journal of Surgery, Obstetrics, and Gynecology* (September-October 1962): 248–57.

———. "The Sexual Response Cycles of the Human Male and Female: Comparative Anatomy and Physiology." In *Sex and Behavior,* edited by Frank A. Beach, 512–34. New York: John Wiley and Sons, 1965.

"Masturbation." *Boston Medical and Surgical Journal* (September 14, 1842): 102.

Matas, Rudolph. "The Surgical Peculiarities of the Negro: A Statistical Inquiry Based upon the Records of the Charity Hospital of New Orleans." *Transactions of the American Surgical Association* 14 (1896): 483–610.

May, Charles Henry. *May's Diseases of Women.* Edited by Leonard S. Rau. 2nd ed. Philadelphia: Lea Brothers, 1890.

May, Elaine Tyler. *Great Expectations: Marriage and Divorce in Post-Victorian America.* Chicago: University of Chicago Press, 1980.

———. *Homeward Bound: American Families in the Cold War Era.* New York: Basic Books, 1988.

McDonald, C. F. "Circumcision of the Female." *General Practitioner* 18 (1958): 98–99.

McGuire, Terence F., and Richard M. Steinhilber. "Sexual Frigidity." *Mayo Clinic Proceedings* 39 (1964): 416–26.

Mcinnis, Doug. "Burt Seeks Protection from Debts, Court Records Say." *Dayton Daily News,* November 8, 1988.

Meagher, John F. W. "Quackery de Luxe: A Form of Medical Charlatanism Known as Orificial or Constructive Surgery." *New York Medical Journal and Medical Record* (February 21, 1923): 224–30.

———. *A Study of Masturbation and the Psychosocial Life.* 2nd ed. New York: William Wood, 1929.

Melendy, Mary R. *Perfect Womanhood for Maidens-Wives-Mothers.* K. T. Boland, 1901.

Meyerowitz, Joanne. "Introduction: Women and Gender in Postwar America, 1945–1960." In *Not June Cleaver: Women and Gender in Postwar America, 1945–1960,* edited by Joanne Meyerowitz, 1–36. Philadelphia: Temple University Press, 1994.

Miller, C. Jeff. *An Introduction to Gynecology.* 2nd ed. St. Louis, MO: C. V. Mosby, 1934.

Miller, Heather Lee. "Sexologists Examine Lesbians and Prostitutes in the United States, 1840–1940." *Feminist Formations* 12 (Fall 2000): 67–91.

Mills, Charles K. "A Case of Nymphomania, with Hystero-Epilepsy Conditions and Peculiar Mental Perversions—the Results of Clitoridectomy and Oophorectomy—the Patient History as Told by Herself." *Medical Times* 15 (April 18, 1885): 534–40.

Mitchell, G. A. G. and E. L. Patterson. *Basic Anatomy.* Baltimore: Williams and Wilkins, 1954.

Mitchell, Graeme. *Mitchell-Nelson Textbook of Pediatrics.* Edited by Waldo E. Nelson. 4th ed. Philadelphia: W. B. Saunders, 1945.

———. *Mitchell-Nelson Textbook of Pediatrics.* Edited by Walden E. Nelson. 7th ed. Philadelphia: W. B. Saunders, 1959.

Mitchinson, Wendy. "Gynecological Operations on Insane Women: London, Ontario, 1895–1901." *Journal of Social History* 15 (1982): 467–84.

Modic, Rob. "'Doctor or Devil': Jurors to Deliberate." *Dayton Daily News,* June 20, 1991.

———. "5-Week Burt Trial Down to Closing Arguments." *Dayton Daily News,* June 19, 1991.

———. "Most Burt Suits Settled." *Dayton Daily News,* September 7, 1997.

———. "St. Elizabeth Asks Judge for Immunity." *Dayton Daily News,* June 18, 1991.

———. "Woman Testifies of Trust for Gynecologist Burt." *Dayton Daily News,* June 1, 1991.

Modic, Rob, and Tom Beyerlein. "Judge Allows More Evidence in Burt Case." *Dayton Daily News*, May 16, 1991.

Modic, Rob, and Wes Hills. "Peers Criticized Burt in '78." *Dayton Daily News*, June 13, 1991.

Moore, Burness E. "Frigidity in Women." *Journal of the Psychoanalytic Association* 9 (1961): 571–84.

Moore, Lisa Jean, and Adele E. Clarke. "Clitoral Conventions and Transgressions: Graphic Representations in Anatomy Texts, c. 1900–1991." *Feminist Studies* 21 (1995): 255–301.

Morantz-Sanchez, Regina. *Conduct Unbecoming a Woman: Medicine on Trial in Turn-of-the-Century Brooklyn.* New York: Oxford University Press, 1999.

———. "Negotiating Power at the Bedside: Nineteenth Century Patients and Their Gynecologists." *Feminist Studies* (Summer 2000): 287–309.

"More Genital Mutilation." *Big Mama Rag*, July/August 1978, 6.

Morgan, Robin, and Gloria Steinem. "The International Crime of Female Genital Mutilation." *Ms.*, September 1980, 65–69.

Morgen, Sandra. *Into Our Own Hands: The Women's Health Movement in the United States, 1969–1990.* New Brunswick, NJ: Rutgers University Press, 2002.

Morrill, C. *The Physiology of Woman and Her Disease from Infancy to Old Age.* 8th ed. Boston: James Campbell, 1870.

Morris, Desmond. *The Naked Woman: A Study of the Female Body.* New York: St. Martin's Press, 2004.

Morris, Henry. *Morris's Human Anatomy: A Complete Systematic Treatise.* 2nd ed. Philadelphia: P. Blakiston's Sons, 1898.

Morris, Robert T. "Circumcision in Girls." *International Journal of Surgery* (May 1912): 135–36.

———. "Is Evolution Trying to Do Away with the Clitoris?" In *Lectures on Appendicitis and Notes on Other Subjects.* New York: G. P. Putnam's Sons, 1895. 2nd ed. 1897.

Morse, John Lovett. *Case Histories in Pediatrics.* 2nd ed. Boston: W. M. Leonard, 1913.

Moseley, William E., and Robert B. Morison. "Elephantiasis Arabum of the External Genitals of a Negress." *Medical News* 50 (April 23, 1887): 462–63.

Muchembled, Robert. *Orgasm and the West: A History of Pleasure from the Sixteenth Century to the Present.* Translated by Jean Birrell. Cambridge: Polity, 2008.

Mudd, Emily Harthshorne, and Elizabeth Kirk Rose. "Development of Marriage Counsel of Philadelphia as a Community Service, 1932–1940." *Living: The Journal of Marriage and the Family* 2 (1940): 40–41.

Munde, Paul F. "Mental Disturbances in the Female Produced and Cured by Gynecological Operations." *American Gynecological and Obstetrical Record* 12 (1898): 53–55.

Murphy, Michelle. "Immodest Witnessing: The Epistemology of Vaginal Self-Help Examination in the U.S. Feminist Self-Help Movement." *Feminist Studies* 30 (Spring 2004): 115–47.

National Women's Health Network. *Self Help: Resource Guide 7.* Washington, DC: National Women's Health Network, 1980.

Nellis, Barbara. "The Hite Report: What Do Women Really Want?" *Playboy* 1977. Reprinted in *Readings in Human Sexuality 79/80*, edited by James R. Barnour, 120–22. Guilford, CT: Dushkin, 1979.

"Network Show to Examine Area Doctor's Surgery Claims." *Dayton Daily News*, October 29, 1988.

Neuhaus, Jessamyn. "The Importance of Being Orgasmic: Sexuality, Gender, and Marital Sex Manuals in the United States, 1920–1963." *Journal of the History of Sexuality* 9 (2000): 447–73.

Neuman, R. P. "Masturbation, Madness, and the Modern Concepts of Childhood and Adolescence." *Journal of Social History* (1975): 1–27.

Novak, Edmund R., and J. Donald Woodruff. *Novak's Gynecologic and Obstetric Pathology with Clinical and Endocrine Relations.* 5th ed. Philadelphia: W. B. Saunders, 1962.

Novak, Josef. *Gynecological Therapy.* New York: McGraw-Hill, 1960.

Numbers, Ronald L. "The Fall and Rise of America's Medical Profession." In *Sickness and Health in America: Readings in the History of Medicine and Public Health,* edited by Judith Walzer Leavitt and Ronald L. Numbers, 185–96. Madison: University of Wisconsin Press, 1985.

Odlum, Doris M. "Revision Corner: Treatment of Frigidity in Women." *Practitioner* (1955): 737–39.

Oliven, Joseph F. *Clinical Sexuality: A Manual for the Physician and the Professions.* 3rd ed. Philadelphia: J. B. Lippincott, 1974.

Omolade, Barbara. "Hearts of Darkness." In *Words of Fire: An Anthology of African-American Feminist Thought,* edited by Beverly Guy-Sheftall, 362–78. New York: New Press, 1995.

Ostrom, Carol. "Harborview Debates Issues of Circumcision in Muslim Girls." *Seattle Times,* September 13, 1996.

Pancoast, Seth. *The Ladies' New Medical Guide.* Chicago: Thompson and Thomas, 1890.

Parke, J. Richardson. *Human Sexuality: A Medico-Literary Treatise on the History and Pathology of the Sex Instinct.* Philadelphia: Professional, 1909.

Parmar, Pratibha and Alice Walker (writers and producers). *Warrior Marks.* directed by Pratibha Parmar. 1993; color; 54 minutes. Distributor: Women Make Movies, New York.

Parrish, J. "Tumors of Left Labium, Resembling Elephantiasis, Removed from a Negress." *Medical Examiner* 3 (1840): 229–32.

Parsons, Leonard, and Seymour Barling. *Diseases of Infancy and Childhood.* London: Oxford University Press, 1954.

"Participants." In *Sex and Behavior,* edited by Frank A. Beach, xi–xiii. New York: John Wiley and Sons, 1965.

Parvin, Theophilus. "Nymphomania and Masturbation." *Medical Age* 4 (February 10, 1886): 51.

Pedersen, Susan. "National Bodies, Unspeakable Acts: The Sexual Politics of Colonial Policy-making." *Journal of Modern History* 63 (1991): 647–80.

Perry, A. W. *Straight Talk about Cosmetic Surgery.* New Haven, CT: Yale University Press, 2007.

Perry, Ralph. "Sexual Hunger as a Factor in Diseases of Women." *American Journal of Dermatology and Genito-urinary Diseases* 3 (January 1899): 5–8.

Person, Ethel Spector. "As the Wheel Turns: A Centennial Reflection on Freud's 'Three Essays on the Theory of Sexuality.'" *Journal of the American Psychoanalytic Association* 53 (2005): 1257–82.

Petersen, Alan. "Sexing the Body: Representations of Sex Differences in *Gray's Anatomy*, 1858 to the Present." *Body and Society* 4 (1998): 1–17.

Peterson, Valerie Victoria. "Sex Texts: The Social Construction of Sex in Popular Manuals, 1962–1995." PhD diss., University of Iowa, 1999.

Philipp, Elliot E. *Obstetrics and Gynaecology: Combined for Students.* London: H. K. Lewis, 1962.

Philipp, Elliot E., Josephine Barnes, and Michael Newton, eds. *Scientific Foundations of Obstetrics and Gynaecology,* 2nd ed. London: William Heinemann Medical Books, 1977.

Pines, M. "'Human Sexual Response': A Discussion of the Work of Masters and Johnson." *Journal of Psychosomatic Research* 12 (1968): 39–49.

Pitzman, Marsh. *The Fundamentals of Human Anatomy: Including Its Borderland Districts, from the Viewpoint of a Practitioner.* St. Louis, MO: C. V. Mosby, 1920.

Platt, W. B. "Hypertrophy of the Clitoris." *Transactions of the Medical Chirurgical Facility of the State of Maryland* (1885): 104.

Podolsky, Edward. "The Causes and the Management of What Is Termed Frigidity." *Medical World* 64 (June 1946): 265–66.

———. "Sexual Frigidity in Women." *East African Medical Journal* 30 (1953): 459–65.

Polak, John O. "A Case of Nymphomania." *Medical News* (September 4, 1897): 301–2.

Potter, La Forest. "Case of Enormous Hypertrophy of Clitoris." *Medical Press* (1885): 120.

———. *Strange Loves: A Study in Sexual Abnormalities.* New York: Robert Dodsley, 1933.

Powderly, Kathleen. "Patient Consent and Negotiation in the Brooklyn Gynecological Practice of Alexander J. C. Skene: 1863–1900." *Journal of Medicine and Philosophy* 25 (2000): 12–27.

Pratt, Edwin H. "Circumcision of Girls." *Journal of Orificial Surgery* 6 (1898): 385–92.

Preves, Sharon. *Intersex and Identity: The Contested Self.* New Brunswick, NJ; Rutgers University Press, 2003.

———. "Sexing the Intersexed: An Analysis of Sociocultural Responses to Intersexuality." *Signs* 27 (2001): 523–56.

A Provincial F. R. C. P. "Mr. Baker Brown's Operation." *British Medical Journal* (May 5, 1866): 478.

Pryor, William R. *Gynaecology: A Textbook for Students and a Guide for Practitioners.* New York: D. Appleton, 1903.

Public Policy Advisory Network on Female Genital Surgeries in Africa. "Seven Things to Know about Female Genital Surgeries in Africa." *Hastings Center Report* (November–December 2012): 19–27.

Rado, Sandor. "Sexual Anesthesia in the Female." *Quarterly Review of Surgery, Obstetrics and Gynecology* 16 (1959): 249–53.

Rapaport, Lisa. "Designer Vagina Surgery is a $5,500 Risk, Doctors Say (Update 2)," *Bloomberg.com,* August 31, 2007, http://www.bloomberg.com/apps/news?pid=newsarchive&sid=a4XVbk.FZd4A.

Rathmann, W. G. "Female Circumcision: Indications and a New Technique." *GP: General Practitioner* 20 (1959): 115–17.

Reed, Charles A. *Diseases of Women: Medical and Surgical Gynecology.* New York: D. Appleton, 1913.

Reed, James. "Doctors, Birth Control, and Social Values, 1830–1970." In *The Therapeutic Revolution: Essays in the Social History of American Medicine*, edited by Morris J. Vogel and Charles E. Rosenberg, 109–33. Philadelphia: University of Pennsylvania Press, 1979.

"Regional Reports." *Health Right* 4 (1978): 11.

Reich, Wilhelm. "Function of Orgasm." *Archives of Psychoanalysis* 1 (1927): 1148.

Reis, Elizabeth. *Bodies in Doubt: An American History of Intersex.* Baltimore: Johns Hopkins University Press, 2009.

———. "Impossible Hermaphrodites: Intersex in America, 1620–1960." *Journal of American History* 92 (2005): 411–41.

Reiss, Ira. *An Insider's View of Sexual Science since Kinsey.* Lanham, MD: Rowman & Littlefield, 2006.

Reiss, Ira, and Harriet M. Reiss. *Solving America's Sexual Crises.* Amherst, NY: Prometheus Books, 1997.

"Removal of Hypertrophied Clitoris by Excision." *Medical Press* (December 23, 1891): 654.

Reuben, David R. *Any Woman Can! Love and Sexual Fulfillment for the Single, Widowed, Divorced . . . and Married.* New York: David McKay, 1971.

———. *Everything You Always Wanted to Know about Sex but Were Afraid to Ask.* New York: David McKay, 1969.

Reverby, Susan. *Examining Tuskegee: The Infamous Syphilis Study and Its Legacy.* Chapel Hill: University of North Carolina Press, 2009.

Review of *Kinsey's Myth of Female Sexuality,* by Edmund Bergler and William S. Kroger. "The Medical Facts." *Journal of the American Medical Association* 154 (April 17, 1954): 1390.

Review of *Sexual Behavior in the Human Female,* by Alfred Kinsey et al. *Journal of the American Medical Association* 154 (March 20, 1954): 1045–46.

Ritmiller, LeRoy F., and Roy E. Nicodemus. "Frigidity in the Female." *Pennsylvania Medical Journal* (August 1946): 1214–16.

Rivers, W. C. "A New Theory of Kissing, Cunnilingus, and Fellatio." *Alienist and Neurologist* 36 (1915): 253–68.

Robertiello, Richard. "The 'Clitoral versus Vaginal Orgasm' Controversy and Some of Its Ramifications." *Journal of Sex Research* 6 (1970): 307–11.

Roberts, Dorothy. "The Paradox of Silence and Display: Sexual Violation of Enslaved Women and Contemporary Contradictions in Black Female Sexuality." In *Beyond Slavery: Overcoming Its Religious and Sexual Legacies,* edited by Bernadette J. Brooten, 41–60. New York: Palgrave Macmillan, 2010.

Robie, W. F. *The Art of Love.* Boston: Richard G. Badger, 1921.

"Robin Morgan: Love Surgery." *Big Mama Rag,* November 1979, 20.

Robinett, Patricia. *The Rape of Innocence: Female Genital Mutilation and Circumcision in the USA.* Eugene, OR: Nunzio Press, 2010.

Robinson, Byron. "The Clitoris." *Interstate Medical Journal* 7 (1900): 18–23.

———. *Landmarks in Gynecology.* Vol. 1. Detroit: George S. Davis, 1894.

Robinson, Marie N. *The Power of Sexual Surrender.* Garden City, NY: Doubleday, 1959.

Robinson, Paul. *The Modernization of Sex: Havelock Ellis, Alfred Kinsey, William Masters and Virginia Johnson.* New York: Harper and Row, 1978.

Robinson, William J. *Woman: Her Sex and Love Life,* 19th ed. New York: Eugenics, 1929.

Roques, Frederick W., John Beattie, and Joseph Wrigley, eds. *Diseases of Women by Ten Teachers.* 10th ed. London: Edward Arnold, 1959.

Rosen, Ismond. "The Male Response to Frigidity." *Journal of Psychosomatic Research* 10 (1966): 135–41.

Rosen, Ruth. *The World Split Open: How the Modern Women's Movement Changed America.* New York: Viking Press, 2000.

Rosenberg, Charles E. *The Care of Strangers: The Rise of America's Hospital System.* Baltimore: Johns Hopkins University Press, 1987.

Rosenthal, A. M. "Female Genital Mutilation." *New York Times,* December 24, 1993.

———. "Female Genital Torture: How Many Millions More?" *New York Times,* December 29, 1992.

———. "Female Genital Torture." *New York Times,* November 12, 1993.

———. "The Torture Continues." *New York Times,* July 27, 1993.

Rosse, Cornelius. "Anatomical Atlases." *Clinical Anatomy* 12 (1999): 293–99.

Rothman, Ellen K. *Hands and Hearts: A History of Courtship in America.* New York: Basic Books, 1984.

Roy, Judith M. "Surgical Gynecology." In *Women, Health, and Medicine in America: A Historical Handbook,* edited by Rima D. Apple, 173–95. New Brunswick, NJ: Rutgers University Press, 1992.

Royal College of Obstetricians and Gynaecologists. "Ethical Considerations in Relation to Female Genital Cosmetic Surgery." RCOG Ethics Committee, Ethical Opinion Paper. October 2013. http://www.rcog.org.uk/files/rcog-corp/RCOG%20FGCS%20Ethical%20opinion%20paper.pdf.

Rudofsky, Bernard. *The Unfashionable Human Body.* Garden City, NY: Doubleday, 1971.

Russett, Cynthia Eagle. *Sexual Science: The Victorian Construction of Womanhood.* Cambridge, MA: Harvard University Press, 1989.

Rutgers, J. *How to Attain and Practice the Ideal Sex Life.* New York: Cadillac, 1940.

Rutherford, Robert N. "The Problem of Pelvic Dis-ease." *Journal of the Medical Women's Association* 20 (1965): 155–60.

Rutherford, Robert N., A. L. Banks, S. H. Davidson, W. A. Coburn, and J. Williams. "Frigidity in Women, with Special Reference to Postpartum Frigidity." *Postgraduate Medicine* 26 (1959): 76–84.

Rutherford, Robert N., A. L. Banks, S. H. Davidson, W. A. Coburn, J. Williams, and F. H. Zaffiro. "Psychosomatic Testings in Frigidity and Infertility." *Psychosomatics* (March–April 1960): 72–74.

Rutkow, Ira M. "Edwin Harley Pratt and Orificial Surgery: Unorthodox Surgical Practice in Nineteenth Century United States." *Surgery* 114 (1993): 558–63.

Ryan, James J. "Surgical Intervention in the Treatment of Sexual Disorders." In *Clinical Management of Sexual Disorders,* edited by Jon K. Meyer, 226–64. Baltimore: Williams and Wilkins, 1976.

Safran, Claire. "The Gynecologist from Hell." *Woman's Day,* August 15, 1989, 70, 74, 76, 87.

Sahli, Nancy. "Sexuality and Woman's Sexual Nature." In *Women, Health, and Medicine in America,* edited by Rima D. Apple, 81–99. New York: Garland, 1990.

Sarrel, Philip, and Lorna Sarrel. "Your Most Intimate You: What Every Woman Will Be Delighted to Know." *Redbook,* March 1978, 82, 86, 88, 90.

Sauer, Louis W. *From Infancy through Childhood.* New York: Harper Brothers, 1942.

———. *Nursery Guide for Mothers and Nurses.* St. Louis, MO: C. V. Mosby, 1923.

Savitt, Todd L. *Race and Medicine in Nineteenth- and Early-Twentieth-Century America.* Kent, OH: Kent State University Press, 2007.

Schauffler, Goodrich C. *Pediatric Gynecology.* Chicago: Year Book, 1942.

———. "Persistent Vaginal Discharge in Infants and in Little Girls." *American Journal of Diseases of Children* 34 (1927): 644–56.

Schiebinger, Londa. *Nature's Body: Gender in the Making of Modern Science.* New Brunswick, NJ: Rutgers University Press, 2004.

Scholes, Robert. *Semiotics and Interpretation.* New Haven, CT: Yale University Press, 1982.

Schroeder, Clarence W. "Background Factors in Divorce." *Living: The Journal of Marriage and the Family* 1 (1939): 71–72.

Schultz, Teri. "Female Circumcision: Operation Orgasm." *Viva,* 1975, 53–54, 104–5.

Schumann, Edward A. "Observations on the Comparative Anatomy of the Female Genitalia." *American Journal of Obstetrics* 64 (1911): 626–36.

Scull, Andrew, and Diane Favreau. "'A Chance to Cut Is a Chance to Cure': Sexual Surgery for Psychosis in Three Nineteenth Century Societies." In *Research in Law, Deviance and Social Control,* edited by Steven Spitzer and Andrew Scull, 3–39. Greenwich, CT: JAI Press, 1986.

———. "The Clitoridectomy Craze." *Social Research* 53 (1986): 243–60.

Sealander, Judith, and Dorothy Smith. "The Rise and Fall of Feminist Organizations in the 1970s: Dayton as a Case Study." *Feminist Studies* (Summer 1986): 320–41.

Segal, Lynne. Introduction to *Sex Exposed: Sexuality and the Pornography Debate,* edited by Lynne Segal and Mary McIntosh, 1–11. New Brunswick, NJ: Rutgers University Press, 1992.

Semmens, James P. "Clitoral Surgery." *Medical Aspects of Human Sexuality* 7 (1973): 169, 220.

Simmons, Christina. *Making Marriage Modern: Women's Sexuality from the Progressive Era to World War II.* New York: Oxford University Press, 2009.

Singer, Natasha. "'Recontouring' and Its Critics." *New York Times,* October 4, 2007.

Shah, Diane K., and Frank Maier. "Heeere's . . . Donahue!" *Newsweek,* March 13, 1978, 85.

Sharpley-Whiting, T. Denean. *Black Venus: Sexualized Savages, Primal Fears, and Primitive Narratives in French.* Raleigh, NC: Duke University Press, 1999.

Sheehan, Elizabeth. "Victorian Clitoridectomy: Isaac Baker Brown and His Harmless Procedure." *Feminist Issues* (Spring 1985): 39–53.

Sherfey, Mary Jane. "The Evolution and Nature of Female Sexuality in Relation to Psychoanalytic Theory." *Journal of the American Psychoanalytic Association* 14 (1966): 28–128.

———. *The Nature and Evolution of Female Sexuality.* New York: Random House, 1972.

Sherman, Alfred I. *Cancer of the Female Reproductive Organs.* St. Louis: C. V. Mosby Co., 1963.

Shoemaker, George E. "Malformations of Female Genitalia." *American Journal of Obstetrics* 32 (August 1895): 215–18.

Shorter, Edward. *From Paralysis to Fatigue: A History of Psychosomatic Illness in the Modern Era.* New York: Free Press, 1992.

Shulman, Alix. "Organs and Orgasms." In *Woman in Sexist Society: Studies in Power and Powerlessness*, edited by Vivian Gornick and Barbara Moran, 198–206. New York: Basic Books, 1971.

Sligh, J. M. "Adherent Prepuce in the Female." *Medical Sentinel* (1894): 215–17.

Small, M. F. "Frigidity and the Clitoris." Letter to Queries and Minor Notes. *Journal of the American Medical Association* 114 (February 24, 1940): 680.

Smith, Daniel Scott. "The Dating of the American Sexual Revolution: Evidence and Interpretation." In *The American Family in Social-Historical Importance*, edited by Michael Gordon, 312–35. New York: St. Martin's Press, 1973.

Smith, E. H. "Masturbation in the Female." *Pacific Medical Journal* (February 1903): 76–83.

Smith, Henry H. *Anatomical Atlas, Illustrative of the Structure of the Human Body*. Philadelphia: Lea and Blanchard, 1845.

Smith, Richard M. *The Baby's First Two Years*. 10th ed. Boston: Houghton Mifflin, 1921.

Smith-Rosenberg, Carol. *Disorderly Conduct: Visions of Gender in Victorian America*. New York: Oxford University Press, 1986.

Smith-Rosenberg, Carol, and Charles E. Rosenberg. "The Female Animal: Medical and Biological Views of Woman and Her Role in Nineteenth-Century America." In *Women and Health in America*, edited by Judith Walzer Leavitt, 111–30. 2nd ed. Madison: University of Wisconsin Press, 1999.

Smout, C. F. V. *Basic Anatomy and Physiology*. London: Edward Arnold, 1962.

Sommers, Elizabeth, Susan Bell, Jill Wolhandler, and Jodi Stein. "A Report from Women's Community Health Center." *Quest: A Feminist Quarterly* 4 (Summer 1977): 13–21.

Somerville, Siobhan. "Scientific Racism and the Emergence of the Homosexual Body." *Journal of the History of Sexuality* 5 (October 1994): 243–66.

Sorrells, Morris L. "The History of Circumcision in the United States: A Physician's Perspective." In *Male and Female Circumcision: Medical, Legal, and Ethical Considerations in Pediatric Practice*, edited by George C. Denniston, Frederick M. Hodges, and Marilyn F. Milos, 331–38. New York: Kluwer Academic / Plenum, 1999.

Southwick, G. R. *A Practical Manual of Gynecology*. Boston: Otis Clapp and Son, 1891.

Spaltheholz, Werner. *Hand-Atlas of Human Anatomy*. Translated by Lewellys F. Barker. Vol. 3. 4th ed. Philadelphia: J. B. Lippincott, 1923.

Speert, Harold. *Obstetrics and Gynecology in America: A History*. Chicago: American College of Obstetricians and Gynecologists, 1980.

Spitz, Rene A. "Authority and Masturbation: Some Remarks on a Bibliographical Investigation." In *Masturbation: From Infancy to Senescence*, edited by Irwin M. Marcus and John J. Francis, 381–409. New York: International Universities Press, 1975.

Spock, Benjamin. *The Common Sense Book of Baby and Childcare*. New York: Duell, Sloan and Pearce, 1945.

Spongberg, Mary. "Are Small Penises Necessary for Civilization? The Male Body and the Body Politic." *Australian Feminist Studies* 12 (1997): 19–28.

Stansell, Christine. *The Feminist Promise: 1792 to the Present*. New York: Modern Library, 2010.

Starr, Paul. *The Social Transformation of American Medicine.* New York: Basic Books, 1982.

Stearns, Carol, and Peter Stearns. "Victorian Sexuality: Can Historians Do It Better?" *Journal of Social History* (Summer 1985): 624–34.

Stengers, Jean, and Anne Van Neck. *Masturbation: The History of a Great Terror.* New York: Palgrave, 2001.

Stewart, Douglas H. "Circumcision of the Preputium Clitoridis." *American Practitioner and News* 10 (1912): 216–17.

Stewart, Felicia Hance, Gary K. Stewart, Felicia Jane Guest, and Robert A. Hatcher. *My Body, My Health: The Concerned Woman's Guide to Gynecology.* Clinician's Edition. New York: John Wiley and Sons, 1979.

Stoddard, F. Jackson. *Case Studies in Obstetrics and Gynecology.* Philadelphia: W. B. Saunders, 1964.

Stone, Abraham. "Marriage Education and Marriage Counseling in the United States." *Marriage and Family Living* 11 (May 1949): 38–39, 50.

Stone, Hannah M., and Abraham Stone. *A Marriage Manual: A Practical Guide-Book to Sex and Marriage.* New York: Simon and Schuster, 1935.

Storer, Horatio R. "On Self Abuse in Woman, Its Causation and Rational Treatment." *Western Journal of Medicine* (August 1867): 456.

Stroman, Duane F. *The Quick Knife: Unnecessary Surgery USA.* Port Washington, NY: National University Publications, 1979.

Sutcliffe, J. A. "Excision of the Clitoris in a Child for Nymphomania." *Indiana Medical Journal* 8 (1889): 64–65.

Tait, Lawson. *Diseases of Women.* New York: William Wood, 1879.

Tanner, Thomas Hawkes. "On Excision of the Clitoris as a Cure for Hysteria, Etc." *Transactions of the Obstetrical Society of London* 8 (1866): 369–70.

Task Force on Circumcision, American Academy of Pediatrics. "Circumcision Policy Statement." *Pediatrics* 103 (March 1, 1999): 686–93.

Task Force on Circumcision, American Academy of Pediatrics. "Circumcision Policy Statement." *Pediatrics* 130 (September 1, 2012): 585–86.

Tavris, Carol, and Susan Sadd. *The Redbook Report on Female Sexuality: 100,000 Married Women Disclose the Good News about Sex.* New York: Delacorte Press, 1975.

Taylor, Robert W. *A Practical Treatise on Sexual Disorders of the Male and Female.* 3rd ed. New York: Lea Brothers, 1905.

Terry, Jennifer. *An American Obsession: Science, Medicine, and Homosexuality in Modern Society.* Chicago: University of Chicago Press, 1999.

———. "Anxious Slippages between 'Us' and 'Them': A Brief History of the Scientific Search for Homosexual Bodies." In *Deviant Bodies: Critical Perspectives on Difference in Science and Popular Culture,* edited by Jennifer Terry and Jacqueline Urla, 129–69. Bloomington: Indiana University Press, 1995.

———. "Lesbians under the Medical Gaze: Scientists Search for Remarkable Differences." *Journal of Sex Research* 27 (1990): 317–39.

Terry, Jennifer, and Jacqueline Urla. "Introduction: Mapping Embodied Deviance." In *Deviant Bodies: Critical Perspectives on Difference in Science and Popular Culture,* edited by Jennifer Terry and Jacqueline Urla, 1–10. Bloomington: Indiana University Press, 1995.

Theis, Sandy. "Burt Quits Medicine; No Hearing." *Dayton Daily News*, January 26, 1989.

Theriot, Nancy. "Negotiating Illness: Doctors, Patients, and Families in the Nineteenth Century." *Journal of the History of Behavioral Sciences* 37 (2001): 349–68.

———. "Women's Voices in Nineteenth-Century Medical Discourse: A Step toward Deconstructing Science." *Signs* 19 (1993): 1–31.

Thompson, Clara. "Penis Envy in Women." *Psychiatry* 6 (1943): 123–25.

———. "Some Effects of the Derogatory Attitude towards Female Sexuality." *Psychiatry* 13 (1950): 349–54.

Tiefer, Leonore. "Activism on the Medicalization of Sex and Female Genital Cosmetic Surgery by the New View Campaign in the United States." *Reproductive Health Matters* 18 (2010): 56–63.

Tomes, Nancy. *The Gospel of Germs: Men, Women, and the Microbe in American Life.* Cambridge, MA: Harvard University Press, 1998.

Toubia, Nahid. "Female Circumcision as a Public Health Issue." *New England Journal of Medicine* 331 (September 14, 1994): 712–16.

Traub, Valerie. "The Psychomorphology of the Clitoris." In *Feminist Approaches to Theory and Methodology*, edited by Sharlene Hesse-Biber, Christina Gilmartin, and Robin Lydenberg, 301–29. New York: Oxford University Press, 1999.

Tuana, Nancy. "Coming to Understand: Orgasm and the Epistemology of Ignorance." *Hypatia* 19 (2004): 194–232.

———. "The Speculum of Ignorance: The Women's Health Movement and Epistemologies of Ignorance." *Hypatia* 21 (2006): 1–19.

Turnispeed, Edward B. "Some Facts in Regard to the Anatomical Difference between the Negro and White Races." *American Journal of Obstetrics* 10 (1877): 32–33.

Tuttle, George M. *Diseases of Children.* Philadelphia: Lea Brothers, 1899.

Tyrer, Alfred Henry. *Sex Satisfaction and Happy Marriage.* New York: Emerson Books, 1940.

Ullman, Sharon R. *Sex Seen: The Emergence of Modern Sexuality in America.* Berkeley: University of California Press, 1997.

Ussher, Jane M. "Biology as Destiny: The Legacy of Victorian Gynaecology in the 21st Century." *Feminism & Psychology* 13 (2003): 17–22.

Van de Velde, Theodore. *Ideal Marriage: Its Physiology and Technique.* New York: Random House, 1930.

Wade, Lisa. "Learning from 'Female Genital Mutilation': Lessons from 30 Years of Academic Discourse." *Ethnicities* 12 (2012): 26–49.

Waiss, A. S. "Reflex Neuroses from Adherent Prepuce in the Female." *Chicago Clinical School* (1900): 279–83.

Walden, William D. "MD Feedback." *Playgirl*, October 1975, 6.

Walker, Alice. *Possessing the Secret of Joy.* New York: Harcourt Brace Jovanovich, 1992.

Walker, Alice, and Pratibha Parmar. *Warrior Marks: Female Genital Mutilation and the Sexual Blinding of Women.* New York: Harcourt Brace, 1993.

Walkowitz, Judith R. "Dangerous Sexualities." In *A History of Women: Emerging Feminism from Revolution to World War*, edited by Genevieve Fraisse and Michelle Perrot, 369–98. Vol. 4 Cambridge, MA: Harvard University Press, 1993.

Wallen, Kim, and Elisabeth Lloyd. "Female Genital Arousal: Genital Anatomy and Orgasm in Intercourse." *Hormones and Behavior* 59 (2011): 780–92.

Wallerstein, Edward. *Circumcision: An American Health Fallacy.* New York: Springer, 1980.

——. "Circumcision: The Uniquely American Medical Enigma." *Urologic Clinics of North America* 12 (1985): 123–32.

Walls, C. B. "Circumcision—Is It a Fad?" *Journal of Orificial Surgery* 5 (1896): 504–12.

Walters, Ronald. *Primers for Prudery.* Englewood Cliffs, NJ: Prentice Hall, 1973.

Warner, John Harley. "From Specificity to Universalism in Medical Therapeutics: Transformation in the 19th Century United States." In *Sickness and Health in America: Readings in the History of Medicine and Public Health,* edited by Judith Walzer Leavitt and Ronald L. Numbers, 87–101. 3rd rev. ed. Madison: University of Wisconsin Press, 1997.

——. "The Uses of Patient Records by Historians—Patterns, Possibilities and Perplexities." *Health & History* 1 (1999): 101–11.

Weiner, Marli F., and Mazie Hough. *Sex, Sickness, and Slavery: Defining Illness in the Antebellum South.* Urbana: University of Illinois Press, 2012.

Weiss, Jessica. *To Have and to Hold: Marriage, the Baby Boom, and Social Change.* Chicago: University of Chicago Press, 2000.

Wiener, Daniel N. *Albert Ellis: Passionate Skeptic.* New York: Praeger Press, 1988.

Wilcox, Sidney F. "Phimosis and Adherent Hood of the Clitoris—Their Effects on Children and Methods of Treatment." *Hahnemannian Monthly* (May 1906): 336–40.

Wilde, Sally. "Truth, Trust, and Confidence in Surgery: Patient Autonomy, Communications, and Consent." *Bulletin of the History of Medicine* 83 (2009): 302–30.

Willard, De Forest. *The Surgery of Childhood, including Orthopedic Surgery.* Philadelphia: J. B. Lippincott, 1910.

Williams, J. Whitridge. *Williams Obstetrics.* Edited by Nicholas J. Eastman. 11th ed. New York: Appleton-Century-Crofts. 1956.

Willis, Deborah. "Introduction: The Notion of Venus." In *Black Venus 2010: They Called Her "Hottentot,"* edited by Deborah Willis, 3–11. Philadelphia: Temple University Press, 2010.

Willman, Reinhold. *Married Life: A Family Handbook.* Chicago, J. S. Hyland, 1917.

Wilson, Doris Burda, and Wilfred J. Wilson. *Human Anatomy.* New York: Oxford University Press, 1978.

Winckel, Franz. *Diseases of Women: A Handbook for Physicians and Students.* Translated by Joseph H. Williamson. Philadelphia: P. Blakiston Son, 1887.

Winslow, Forbes. Letter to editor. *British Medical Journal* (December 22, 1866): 706.

Wise, P. M. "Case of Sexual Perversion." *Alienist and Neurologist* 1 (1883): 87–91.

Wolfe, Linda. *The Cosmo Report.* New York: Arbor House, 1981.

Wolkoff, A. Stark. "Surgery of the Clitoris." In *The Clitoris,* edited by Thomas P. Lowry, 104–10. St. Louis, MO: Warren H. Green, 1976.

Wollman, Leo. "Hooded Clitoris." *Journal of the American Society of Psychosomatic Dentistry and Medicine* 20 (1973): 3–4.

Wood, Ann Douglas. "'The Fashionable Diseases': Women's Complaints and Their Treatment in Nineteenth-Century America." In *Women and Health in America: Historical Readings,* edited by Judith Walzer Leavitt, 222–38. Madison: University of Wisconsin Press, 1984.

Wortis, S. Bernard. "Counseling in the Premarital Interview." *Marriage and Family Living* 7 (November 1945): 86.

Wylie, W. Gill. "Amputation of the Clitoris." *American Journal of Obstetrics and Diseases of Women and Children* 43 (1901): 722.

Young, James. *A Text-Book of Gynecology for Students and Practitioners.* 6th rev. ed. London: Adam and Charles Black, 1944.

Young-Bruehl, Elizabeth, ed. *Freud on Women: A Reader.* New York: W. W. Norton, 1990.

Zaretsky, Eli. *Secrets of the Soul: A Social and Cultural History of Psychoanalysis.* New York: Knopf, 2004.

Zimmerman, Ernest L. "A Comparative Study of Syphilis in Whites and in Negroes." *Archives of Dermatology and Syphilogy* (1921): 75–88.

Index

Printed in the United States
by Baker & Taylor Publisher Services